Nursing: Beyond the Basics

Nursing: Beyond the Basics

Editor: Helen Hayden

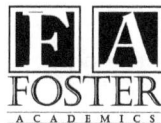

FA
FOSTER
A C A D E M I C S

www.fosteracademics.com

www.fosteracademics.com

FA
FOSTER
ACADEMICS

Cataloging-in-Publication Data

Nursing : beyond the basics / edited by Helen Hayden.
    p. cm.
Includes bibliographical references and index.
ISBN 978-1-63242-851-6
1. Nursing. 2. Nursing--Practice. 3. Care of the sick. 4. Clinical medicine. I. Hayden, Helen.
RT41 .N87 2019
610.73--dc23

Foster Academics,
118-35 Queens Blvd., Suite 400,
Forest Hills, NY 11375, USA

ISBN 978-1-63242-851-6 (Hardback)

Contents

Preface

Nursing is a primary division of healthcare. It can be referred to as the use of clinical judgement in order to provide autonomous or collaborative care to patients. It involves the achievement of optimal health and quality of life for individuals, families or communities. Nurses help in developing a plan of care to treat illnesses by working in coordination with physicians and therapists. Clinical nurse specialists may also diagnose health problems and prescribe medications accordingly. Nursing care can be provided in diverse settings such as hospitals, homes, schools, occupation health settings, etc. This book unfolds the innovative aspects of nursing which will be crucial for the progress of this field in the future. While understanding the long-term perspectives of the topics, this book makes an effort in highlighting their impact as a modern tool for the growth of the discipline. It is appropriate for students seeking detailed information in this area as well as for experts.

This book is a result of research of several months to collate the most relevant data in the field.

When I was approached with the idea of this book and the proposal to edit it, I was overwhelmed. It gave me an opportunity to reach out to all those who share a common interest with me in this field. I had 3 main parameters for editing this text:

1. Accuracy – The data and information provided in this book should be up-to-date and valuable to the readers.

2. Structure – The data must be presented in a structured format for easy understanding and better grasping of the readers.

3. Universal Approach – This book not only targets students but also experts and innovators in the field, thus my aim was to present topics which are of use to all.

Thus, it took me a couple of months to finish the editing of this book.

I would like to make a special mention of my publisher who considered me worthy of this opportunity and also supported me throughout the editing process. I would also like to thank the editing team at the back-end who extended their help whenever required.

Editor

"We'll check vital signs only till we finish the school": experiences of student nurses regarding intra-semester clinical placement in Ghana

Charles Ampong Adjei[1*] , Collins Sarpong[2], Priscilla Adumoah Attafuah[2], Ninon P. Amertil[2] and Yaw Abayie Akosah[2]

Abstract

Background: Clinical practicum is an integral part of nursing education because it provides students with opportunities to perform nursing care and practice specific nursing tasks. In Ghana, little is known about the experiences of baccalaureate student nurses with regard to intra-semester clinical practicum. This study therefore, explored perceptions, challenges, and how the intra-semester clinical practicum affects the learning process of student nurses in a private university in Ghana.

Methods: Exploratory descriptive phenomenological design was used. Nine in-depth interviews and three focus group discussions were conducted for baccalaureate student nurses in their second, third and fourth years of study. Only those who have attended intra-semester clinical practicum for at least two semesters in the course of their study were recruited. Purposive sampling technique was used to select the participants. The sample size was based on data saturation, however, a total of 33 participants were recruited. Data was analysed using content analysis technique.

Results: The findings show that baccalaureate student nurses perceive the intra-semester clinical practicum as beneficial. It affords the opportunity to translate theoretical knowledge into practice concurrently. However, students recounted their stressful experiences during the clinical period which negatively affected their academic work. Additionally, staff nurses assigned the students to do menial jobs instead of appropriate nursing tasks.

Conclusions: A review of the "block" method in which students will go to clinicals for a stipulated number of consecutive days in a month and then resume lectures, is worth considering.

Keywords: Experience, Baccalaureate, Student nurses, Intra-semester, Clinical practicum

Background

Nursing is a practice-based profession and therefore the clinical setting is an essential part of the training [1–3].The preparation of student nurses involves rigorous theoretical and practical instruction [4]. However, effective training is dependent on appropriate supervision and mentorship particularly in the clinical environment [5–7].

It is well established that student nurses perceive clinical placement as rewarding [8] since it has the tendency to improve their clinical skills, connect theory with practice and support their professional growth [8–12]. Notwithstanding, the clinical environment presents numerous challenges to students [3, 13–15]. For instance, in South Africa, nursing students complained of lack of support by staff nurses [15]. Some incidents of bullying of student nurses were documented in other countries [14, 16]. These incidents created anxiety and depression among the students and consequently affected the care they offered to their clients. Despite all

* Correspondence: chadjei@ug.edu.gh
[1]Department of Community Health Nursing, School of Nursing, College of health Sciences, University of Ghana, Accra, Ghana
Full list of author information is available at the end of the article

these occurrences, the overall positive effect of clinical placement of nursing students cannot be underestimated.

Furthermore, different nursing practical methodologies are used by various nursing schools all over the world. For example, in the United Kingdom (UK), student nurses are placed in the clinical learning environment for 6 weeks continuously which enables them in gaining self-confidence and improves their communication with clients and nursing staff [17]. What is unique about this approach is that registered nurses who participate in the Nursing and Midwifery Council's (NMC) approved mentorship programme, support the students professionally [17]. On the contrary, South African student nurses are in the clinical environment for only 14 days, a time period which they perceive as too short for acquisition of nursing skills [18].

In Ghana, a recent curriculum designed by the NMC requires each student nurse to obtain clinical contact of 432 h, 624 h, and 576 h during the first, second and third year of training respectively [19].This curriculum allows nursing schools in the country to adopt either of the acceptable clinical placement schedules; intra-semester and inter-semester clinical placement [19].

For the past 3 years, Valley View University has implemented these two methodologies prescribed by the council. During vacation, students are assigned to hospitals for clinical attachment for a maximum of 8 weeks (inter-semester practicum). Then when classes are in session, the students attend lectures 3 days in a week and spend the remaining 2 days in the clinical setting to ensure that they satisfy the NMC's intra-semester practicum requirement. This means that teaching and practical attachment are done concurrently during the course of the semester. This study therefore was aimed at documenting the perception and challenges that students face during intra-semester clinical placement since the limited literature in Ghana focuses primarily on student's attitude toward clinical work [2].

Methods
Study design
This study used exploratory descriptive phenomenological design. Considering the fact that intra-semester clinical practicum is a new practical methodology used by the University, this design was best suited to explore the experiences of the students.

Study setting
The study was conducted in the Greater Accra region of Ghana. The region is the capital town of the country and shares borders with the Eastern region to the north, Central region to the west, Volta region to the east and the Gulf of Guinea to the south [20]. About 4,010,050 people reside in the region [20].The study was conducted

at Valley View University which was established in 1979 by the West Africa Union Mission of the Seventh-Day Adventist Church. The baccalaureate nursing programme of the institution commenced in September, 2007. Currently, it has a student population of 462.

Participant's eligibility
Inclusion criteria
Participants were included in the study if they were baccalaureate student nurses who have completed at least two semesters of their 4 year programme and have attended intra-semester clinical practicum at least twice in the course of their study and consented to participate.

Exclusion criteria
First year baccalaureate student nurses were excluded.

Sample and sampling methods
Participants were selected purposively. In all, 33 participants took part in the study. The study objectives were shared with the students in class. Those who were interested to participate and met the inclusion criteria were recruited. Nine in-depth interviews made up of three students each from year two, three and four were conducted. In addition, three focus group discussions, which consisted of eight students from each of the three levels, were done.

Data collection tool
A semi-structured interview guide was used to conduct the in-depth interviews and the focus group discussions. The guide had both open and closed ended questions such as: "How do you perceive intra-semester clinical practicum?"; "Did the clinical practicum have any effect (positive or negative) on your learning?"; "Did you face any challenges with intra-semester clinical practicum?" The guide was designed based on literature and experts' contributions (refer to Additional file 1).

Data procedure
Data collection started between June and August, 2016 following ethical clearance and permission from University authorities. On the day of the scheduled interview/ discussion, the researchers met the participants at the agreed venues which included classrooms and conference rooms in the school. The study aims were explained to the participants and their written consents were obtained. In addition, their consent to audio record the interviews/discussions were sought. The in-depth interviews lasted between 45 min and 1 h. However, the focus group discussions lasted between 60 min and 90 min. None of the participants experienced any psychological disturbances in the course of narrating their experience.

Data analysis

Data were analysed using content analysis technique. The recorded interviews were played and listened to by the researchers. Each researcher coded the data, which was followed by a series of group discussions by the research team. Finally, major themes and sub-themes were generated and presented as findings of the study.

Methodological rigour

Rigour refers to trustworthiness. Rigour in qualitative study must satisfy the following criteria: credibility, transferability, dependability, and confirmability [21]. In this study, credibility was achieved by piloting the interview guide using baccalaureate student nurses who shared similar characteristics but were not part of the study participants. Transferability was ensured by the use of direct quotes from participants and a thick description of the study setting. An audit trail with the voice records, transcripts, field notes and diaries was kept to ensure dependability and confirmability.

Ethic approval

The study was ethically approved by the Dodowa Health Research Center of the Ghana Health Service (protocol Number-DHRCIRB/07/06/16). Permission was also sought from the Head of the Nursing Department of the University. In addition, participants' written consents were obtained after the rationale of the study was explained. Pseudonyms are used to ensure anonymity of the participants.

Results

Socio-demographic characteristics

The study involved thirty three (33) baccalaureate student nurses in their second, third and final year of the nursing programme. They ranged in age from 19 to 24 years. Each participant had attended intra-semester clinical practicum at least twice in the course of their study. In all, three themes and seven sub-themes emerged from the data and are presented below.

Perception about intra-semester clinical practicum

This theme describes how the students perceived intra-semester clinical practicum. A number of the participants indicated that the practicum was very beneficial. However, some added that it was associated with stress, which consequently affected their academic work.

Benefits of intra-semester clinical practicum

The study revealed how clinical practicum presents an opportunity for student nurses to appreciate what they are taught in the classroom, particularly courses that are practically oriented. Some shared their thoughts:

"Intra-semester clinical is very helpful because aside the lectures and the skills lab, you need a real patient to try your hands on. It is only on the ward that you get such cases and time to practice." **[Kofi – 300]**

"Intra-semester clinical is important. For example, you can only appreciate a course like community health nursing when you see it being practiced and not that you learn and wait till a certain period of time before you go and practice." **[Akua – 300]**

Notwithstanding, some students indicated that they only derived the full benefit of the clinical practicum when they were assigned to wards that offered care to patients with conditions that were in line with the topics being discussed in class.

"When you are placed on a ward that is related to what you are studying in class, it helps you better understand the theoretical aspects of the nursing course" **[Afia – 400]**

Stress

Almost all the participants during the interview expressed their concerns about the stressful nature of the intra-semester clinical practicum. According to the participants, long distance to the hospitals and the fact that they must attend lecture the next day compounds the situation.

They lamented:

"Going for the clinical is stressful, I mean very stressful. The long distance from the school to the hospital makes it very stressful." **[Adwoa-300]**

"Going for afternoon shift especially is very tiring. We come back from clinical very late in the evening meanwhile, we have lectures early in the morning on the next day. So I think it's too stressful." **[Akosua-400]**

Effects on academic performance

Some participants echoed the effect of the intra-semester clinical on their academic performance. According to them, they were unable to prepare adequately for class the next day especially when they returned to campus very late. The carry over effect of the stress also influenced most students to sleep in class during lecture periods.

"...when you go for afternoon shift and come around 9pm, you will be tired, and learning your books before the next lectures becomes very difficult. You are unable to revise your lecture notes and so you get confused when you're taught new things in class" [**Kwaku-400**]

"We mostly sleep in class because of the tiredness we experience. Also, we don't have time to read on our previous lessons" [**Akua – 300**]

Learning environment

The study revealed that there is a huge gap between what students learn in class and what is being practiced in the hospitals. In addition, some participants reported that they were not supported by the staff nurses.

Theory and practice gap

The majority of the participants indicated that a gap existed between theory and practice. According to them, the nurses in the hospitals did not follow standard protocols in providing nursing care. This contradicts the systematic way in which they are taught in the school's skill laboratory. Some shared their frustrations:

"The procedures that they use at the wards mostly don't follow protocol like how we're taught in the school's skills laboratory. The way they (nurses) do things on the ward is different. They (the nurses) want to be able to serve everybody quickly and therefore do not follow the exact protocol that we've been taught" [**Nii-200**]

One participant argued why it may be better to learn the practical component of nursing from the literature rather than going to the hospital. He said:

"Sometimes I think it seems better reading the literature and getting things right about practical aspect of nursing than going to the ward where improvisation is the theme of the day. You can imagine if you pick the wrong things there by doing them, it'll be very difficult to conform to standards" [**Kojo-400**]

Student-nurse relationship

Some participants mentioned that the learning environment was not friendly due to a lack of bonding between the students and the staff nurses. This was attributed to the fact that students were placed in the hospital twice a week and therefore were unable to acquaint themselves very well with the staff nurses.

"...because the practicum is not continuous, there is absence of that kind of close relationship and cordial relationship with the nurses." [**Akweley-300**]

Furthermore, some participants expressed that the poor relationship had a negative impact on their skill acquisition on the ward. A student said:

"Because we go twice a week, we're always new on the ward so the ward in-charges do not have confidence in us to let us do much of the procedures. They think we still don't know..., we're still novice on the ward because they don't see us every day." [**Kwabena – 400**]

One participant was afraid that continuing with just the 2 day contacts in a week at the hospital will not give him the chance to practice advanced nursing procedures but only the checking of vital signs.

"When we continue to go twice a week, we'll always check vital signs only till we finish the school." [**Kofi-200**]

Challenges of intra-semester clinical practicum

This theme describes the challenges that confronted the students during the intra-semester clinical practicum. Some participants indicated that they were only used for menial jobs in the hospitals. Others also mentioned that the twice a week contact at the hospital did not afford them opportunity to know the outcome of their patients' conditions.

Break in continuity of care

The study revealed that most participants were unable to follow their patient's progress to the end and therefore were not able to measure their success.

"When we go twice a week and we care for patients, it takes another week before we meet them again. Sometimes, it is very difficult to follow up... you have to pick a new patient again." [**Kwesi-300**]

"when you're on the ward and you nurse a patient for a particular week, by the time you go for the following week you'll realize that the patient has been discharged and you can't get access to the folder so it seems you've done nothing for the patient." [**Adwoa-400**]

Messenger role

A number of the participants expressed how the staff nurses used them for menial jobs on the ward instead of allowing them to spend productive hours with their patients.

Yaw had this to say:

"They (nurses) *kept on sending me everywhere, I went to the orthopedic unit, and many places. Anytime I return they will say that I have the long legs so I have to be transporting patients to other units. Sometimes, I don't even get time with the patients. I sometimes spent a maximum of five minutes with my patients the whole day."* [**Yaw-200**]

Discussion

This study explored the experiences of baccalaureate student nurses regarding intra-semester clinical practicum. The findings showed that students perceived intra-semester clinical practicum as beneficial since it afforded the opportunity to translate theory into practice concurrently as previously reported in other studies [8, 10, 22]. For instance, in Saudi Arabia, about 75.6% (*n* = 205) of nursing students were satisfied with their clinical practicum [10]. The similarities may have resulted from the fact that student nurses recognised nursing as both an art and science and therefore understood the importance of the practical component.

The study also found that clinical placement was associated with stress. The long distance (35.5 km) to the hospitals and early morning class schedules for the next day, compounded the participants' stressful experiences. Previous studies have also documented stress as one challenge that negatively affected the learning processes and the general health of nursing students [12, 23, 24]. According to Jamshidi et al. [23], student nurses in Iran were stressed by the new experience of being in the hospital and also by the complexities of devices they observed on patients. Other related studies supported the experiences of stress in the clinical environment for students [24, 25]. It is worth considering repackaging the clinical placement schedule such that students spend sometime in the classsroom and subsequently halt for practicum during the course of the semester.

Many studies have reported on the existence of a gap between theory and practice in relation to nursing education [8, 18]. Some participants in this study mentioned that the systematic way of carrying out nursing procedures was missing in the hospitals. Students were therefore in a state of dilemma as to whether or not they should copy the practices of staff nurses, which were not evidence supported. The non-compliance to standard procedures by the staff nurses is not surprising since it appears there is an imbalance in the nurse-to-patient ratio which increases the workload of nurses. Also, we can speculate that some nurses are not confident enough to demonstrate nursing procedures to students. Clinical supervisors need to be guided by clinical objectives before assigning students to the hospital wards. In addition, preceptors must be trained and assigned to students for supervision and assessment. This will bridge the extensively reported gap between theory and practice.

The study also found that the learning environment was unsupportive and this was evidenced by the poor relationship that existed between students and staff nurses. This corroborated a study by Mabuda, Potgieter & Alberts [15] which found that nurses failed to support students during clinical attachment. Perhaps the behaviour of students, including lateness to work, the use of mobile phones on duty, lack of commitment to clinical work and absenteeism without permission as documented in a similar study in Ghana [2], might have influenced the reaction of the staff nurses toward the students. It is therefore important to orient students on their clinical objectives before commencing their clinical schedules. It is also important to have the students followed by experienced clinical instructors to ensure the best learning results [2]. Faculty support in the clinical environment has significant impact, particurlarly in facilitating, evaluating and monitoring the students during the clinical period [13], and therefore it is worth strengthening. Moreover, staff nurses need to recognise themselves as mentors and important stakeholders in the training of student nurses.

The findings further showed that some staff nurses treated the students as messengers instead of learners. It was widely reported that student nurses were used for errands and were further tasked to do menial jobs instead of providing nursing care. This finding is not peculiar to Ghana but is also present in other countries [3, 18]. This obviously has an implication for nursing skill acquisition since the students are not encouraged to take on challenging tasks to develop their professional skills. It is important to assign students to specific tasks as soon as they report to the hospital and these tasks should be evaluated at the end of the shift by a preceptor or clinical instructor.

Conclusions

The findings of this study provide insight to nursing students' experiences in the clinical environment. It reveals that student nurses perceive intra-semester clinical practicum as a good approach for acquisition of skills. However, there are some challenges that require an immediate review of the methodology so as to help students derive the full benefit of the intra-semester clinical practicum. One suggestion may be an adoption of the "block" method where students will go for clinical attachment for a stipulated number of consecutive days in a month and then resume lectures.

Abbreviation
NMC: Nursing and Midwifery Council of Ghana

Acknowledgements
The authors acknowledge the contribution of the students who participated in the study.

Authors' contributions
CAA and CS conceptualised the study. CAA, CS and PAA collected the data. CAA, NPA, YAA drafted the manuscript. Critical review of manuscript was done by CAA, PAA, YAA and NPA. All authors read and approved the final manuscript.

Competing interests
The authors declare that they have no competing interests.

Author details
[1]Department of Community Health Nursing, School of Nursing, College of health Sciences, University of Ghana, Accra, Ghana. [2]Department of Nursing, Valley View University, Box AF 595, Adenta, Accra, Ghana.

References
1. Jonsén E, Melender HL, Hilli Y. Finnish and Swedish nursing students' experiences of their first clinical practice placement - a qualitative study. Nurse Educ Today. 2013;33(3):297–302.
2. Awuah-Peasah D, Sarfo LA, Asamoah F. The attitudes of student nurses toward clinical work. Int J Nurs Midwifery. 2013;5(2):22–7. Retrieved from http://doi.org/10.5897/IJNM12.017
3. Shoqirat N. Clinical placement in Jordan : qualitative views of final year nursing students. Aust J Adv Nurs. 2010;30(4):49–58.
4. Rajeswaran L. Clinical experiences of nursing students at a selected Institute of Health Sciences in Botswana. Health Sci J. 2017;10(6):1–6.
5. International Confederation of Midwives. Global standards for midwifery education. 2010 http://www.internationalmidwives.org. Accessed 3 Oct 2017.
6. World Health Organization. Global standards for the initial education of professional nurses and midwives. (2009). http://apps.who.int/iris/handle/10665/44100. Accessed 4 Oct 2017.
7. Rooke N. An evaluation of nursing and midwifery sign off mentors, new mentors and nurse lecturers understanding of the sign off mentor role. Nurse Educ Pract. 2014;14:43–8.
8. Tiwaken SU, Caranto LC, David JJT. The real world: lived experiences of student nurses during clinical practice. Int J Nurs Sci. 2015;5(2):66–75.
9. Lamont S, Brunero S, Woods KP. Satisfaction with clinical placement-the perspectives of nursing students from multiple universities. Collegian. 2015; 22:125–33.
10. Abouelfettoh A, Mumtin SA. Nursing Students' Satisfaction with their Clinical Practicum. J Sci Res Rep. 2015;4(6):490–500.
11. Wang H, Li X, Chen H. Perceptions of nursing profession and learning experiences of male students in baccalaureate nursing program in Changsha, Chian. Nurse Educ Today. 2010;31(1):36–42.
12. Sharif F, Masoumi SA. Qualitative study of nursing student experiences of clinical practice. BMC Nurs. 2005;4(1):1–7.
13. Killam LA, Carter IM. Challenges to the student nurse on clinical placement in the rural setting: a review of the literature. Rural Remote Health. 2010; 10(3) https://www.rrh.org.au/journal/article/1523. Accessed 7 Oct 2017
14. Mabrouk A, Rahman R. Perception of student nurses' bullying behaviors and coping strategies used in clinical settings [paper presented at the sigma Theta tau international, nursing education research conference, Indianapolis]. 2014. http://www.nursinglibrary.org/vhl/handle/10755/316820. Accessed October 2017.
15. Mabuda BT, Potgieter E, Alberts UU. Student nurses' experiences during clinical practice in the Limpopo province. Curationis. 2008;31(1):19–27.
16. Budden LM, Birks M, Cant R, Bagley T, Park T. Australian nursing students' experience of bullying and/or harassment during clinical placement. Collegian. 2017;24(2):125–33.
17. Bembridge E, Jeong S. Student Nurse Confidence - A Reflection. 2013. http://journals.sfu.ca/hneh/index.php/hneh/article/view/25. Accessed 20 Oct 2017.
18. Botman Y, Ria L. Preparation of clinical preceptors. Trends in Nursing. 2012;1(1): 1–12.
19. Nursing and Midwifery Council of Ghana. Curriculum for the Registered General Nursing (RGN) Programme. 2015. Unpublished. http://www.nmcgh.org.
20. Ghana Statistical Service. 2010 Population and Housing Census Regional analytical report-Greater Accra Region. 2013. http://www.statsghana.gov.gh/docfiles/2010phc/2010_PHC_Regional_Analytical_Reports_Greater_Accra_Region.pdf. Accessed 12 Aug 2016.
21. Lincoln Y, Guba E. Naturalistic Inquiry. Beverly Hills: Sage publication inc; 1985. p. 290.
22. Cameron-jones M, Hara PO. Practicum as part of higher education. Kluwer Academic Publisher. 2015;19(3):341–9.
23. Jamshidi N, Molazem Z, Sharif F, Torabizadeh C, Kalyani MN. The challenges of nursing students in the clinical learning environment: a qualitative study. Sci World J. 2016;2016:1–7. https://www.hindawi.com/journals/tswj/2016/1846178/.
24. Zupiria X, Huitzi X, Jose M, Erice A, Jose M, Iturriotz U. Stress sources in nursing practice. Evolution during nursing training. Nurse Educ Today. 2007; 27:777–87.
25. Berntsen K. Nursing students' perceptions of the clinical learning environment in nursing homes. J Nurs Educ. 2010;49(1):17–22.

2

Nurses' attitude and perceived barriers to pressure ulcer prevention

Werku Etafa[1*], Zeleke Argaw[2], Endalew Gemechu[2] and Belachew Melese[3]

Abstract

Background: The presence or absence of pressure ulcers has been generally regarded as a performance measure of quality nursing care and overall patient health. The aim of this study- wasto explorenurses' attitude about pressure ulcer prevention'and to identify staff nurses' perceived barriers to pressure ulcer prevention public hospitals in Addis Ababa, Ethiopia.

Methods: A self-reported multi-center institutional based cross sectional study design was employed to collect data from staff nurses ($N = 222$) working in six (6) selected public hospitals in Addis Ababa, from April 01–28/2015.

Results: Majority of the nurses had ($n = 116$, 52.2%) negative attitude towards pressure ulcer prevention. The mean scores of the test for all participants was 3.09out of 11(SD =0.92, range = 1–5). Similarly, the study revealed several barriers need to be resolved to put in to practice the strategies of pressure ulcer prevention; Heavy workload and inadequate staff (lack of tie) (83.1%), shortage of resources/equipment (67.7%) and inadequate training (63.2%) were among the major barriers identified in the study.

Conclusions: The study finding suggests that Addis Ababa nurses have negative attitude to pressure ulcer prevention. Also several barriers exist for implementing pressure ulcer prevention protocols in public hospitals in Addis Ababa, Ethiopia. Suggestion for improving this situation is attractive.

Keywords: Wound, Pressure ulcer prevention, Nurses attitude, Perceived barrier

Background

Pressure ulcers are defined as localized injury to the skin and/or underlying tissue usually over a bony prominence, as a result of pressure, or pressure in combination with shear [1]. PUs significantly limits many aspects of an individual's well-being, including general health and physical, social, financial, and psychological quality of life [2]. In United States nearly 1 million people develop pressure ulcers annually, while approximately 60,000 acute care patients die from related complications [3]. The estimated cost of managing stage III/IV pressure injury per patient is $70–150 thousand, and the total cost for treatment of pressure ulcers in the United States is estimated at $9–11 billion per year [4].

Research evidences displayed that Pressure ulcer prevalence is varying from country to country For example, prevalence of pressure ulcer in Jordan (12%),

Nigeria (3.22%), (Norway, 17%, Irish, 16%, Denmark, 15%, Sweden, 25%), Irish (9%), (Norwegian, 54% & Irish, 12%), Wales (8.9%) [5–10].

One study [11] identified risks for the development of pressure ulcers/injuries included advanced age, immobility, incontinence, inadequate nutrition and hydration, neurosensory deficiency, device-related skin pressure, multiple comorbidities and circulatory abnormalities.

A systematic review reported that pressure ulcer incidence rates vary considerably by clinical setting; ranging from 0.4 to 38% in acute care, from 2.2 to 23.9% in long term care, and from 0 to 17% in home care [12]. A retrospective secondary analysis of database studies have shown that an estimated 3.5–4.5% of all hospitalized patients are developing potentially preventable, hospital-acquired pressure ulcers, despite heightened awareness [3]. Hospital-acquired pressure ulcers/injuries (HAPU/I) result in significant patient harm, including pain, expensive treatments, increased length of institutional stay and, in some patients, premature mortality [13].

* Correspondence: witafay@gmail.com
[1]Department of Nursing, College of Health Science, Wollega Unversity, Samara, Ethiopia
Full list of author information is available at the end of the article

A single published study by Haileyesus & Mignote [14] conducted in Ethiopia in Felegehiwot referral hospital, among 422 found the overall prevalence rate of 16.8%. Of this, 62%, 26.8% and 2.8% developed stage I, II and stage IV pressure ulcer, respectively, based on European Pressure Ulcer Advisory Panel (EPUAP). This research also reported that the significant variables with the presence of PU such as stay in hospital for a long, slight limit of sensory perception, and friction and shearing forces.

Fishbein & Ajzen [15] explicated that attitude is learned and is affected by knowledge, behavioral intent and the amount of affection for or against an object. Aperson who holds a positive attitude toward an issue will have a greater possibility of performing a supportive behavior related to that issue [15]. For example, the more positive attitude of nurses to PU prevention, the better practice of PU prevention care demonstrated [16].

Evidence-based clinical guideline has a significant correlation with positive feeling to pressure ulcer prevention [17]. Grimshaw et al. [18] stated that lack of knowledge, negative attitudes, or underdeveloped skills are the principal barriers to evidence-based practice at the level of the individual health care professional. Ayello & Meaney [19] also explicated negative attitude of nurses to PU prevention increase the prevalence rate of pressure ulcers. Similarly, Hill [20] expressed that nurses' negative attitude could be affected by shortage of staff, lack of time, lack of knowledge and insufficient equipment.

Among the researched and published documents on the same topic, six studies concluded that most nurses hold a positive attitude to PU prevention (Moore & Price 2004, Kallman & Suserud 2009, Islam 2010, Demarré et al. 2011, Tubaishat et al. 2013, and Uba et al. 2014) [21–26]. In addition to attitude of nurses explored, three papers identified the major barriers for nurses' to demonstrate PU prevention practice such as lack of time, staff and uncooperative patient [21, 22, 25].

However, a study conducted among 145 Belgian nursing homes by Beeckman et al. [17] using convenience sampling found that poor attitude to PU prevention. Similarly, another data collected from 105 health care professionals (nurses, physical therapist, occupational therapist and physician medicine) in the rehabilitation at Fahad Medical College city, Riyadh found unsatisfactory attitude of health care professionals to PU prevention [27]. A cross sectional study among Jordanian nurses also found a positive relationship between positive attitude of nurses and longer year of experience [25].

Pressure ulcer prevention is a priority for nurses, healthcare professionals and healthcare organizations throughout the world, and a key factor in pressure ulcer prevention and management is individual nurse decision making [28]. Nurses hold the most responsibility for prevention and management of pressure ulcers though it is a multidisciplinary team approach [29].

Padula et al. [3] described that hospitals adhering to PU updates had significant pressure injury reductions by average hospital 7.5 pressure injury case reductions and $500,000 + savings per year. Moore & Price [21] suggested that pressure ulcer prevention and management involves both emphasizing on educational strategies and promoting a positive attitude of nurses towards PU care.

To date, no similar studies have been conducted in Ethiopia to examine nurses' attitude and perceived barriers to PU prevention. Therefore, this study was undertaken to assess attitude of nurses in Public Hospitals in Addis Ababa to PU prevention.

Objectives

The objective of this study was to explore nurses' attitudes toward the prevention of pressure ulcers, and to identify staff nurses' perceived barriers to pressure ulcers prevention in Public hospitals in Addis Ababa, Ethiopia.

Methods
Study design

Institutional based cross sectional multi-center study using quantitative method was employed from April 01–28, 2015.

Study setting and sample

The study was in Addis Ababa, the capital city of Ethiopia which contains 13 public referral hospitals (each contains from 120 to 400 beds for admission). There are 34 private hospitals, 86 health centers and various NGOs and health institutions. The data in this study included nurses working from patient admission units in six randomly selected public referral hospitals (46%). The units included were medical, surgical, orthopedics, intensive care unit, gynecology, pediatrics, dermatology, burn and oncology.

Sample size and sampling procedure

The sample size was determined using a formula of estimating a single population proportion for cross sectional study. Since the population size is less than 10, 000 ($N = 534$), the final sample size was estimated using correction formula. The final sample size obtained including 10% non-response rate was 252. Then, the number of participants in each selected hospitals to obtain similar proportion of participants were determined using the population proportionate sampling (PPS). It is estimated using the formula: n = (nf * N in a health facilities)/N $_{total}$, where, n = Proportion of nurses participate in the study in a given public hospital, nf = Final sample size obtained using correction formula (252), N = is the total number of nurses in the selected public hospitals (534).

Study instrument

A questionnaire used for gathering data contained three parts. For the purpose of the current study, demographic information which may or may not have an impact on the nurses' attitude towards pressure ulcer prevention (age, sex, clinical working experience, educational level, and the nurses received training on PU prevention and read research articles about it) were added.

Part two of the data collection tool was Pressure Ulcer Attitude Test tool contained 11 statements developed and validated by Moore & Price [21]. In this section, the response option utilized a 5 point Likert scale from strongly disagree to strongly agree. It was chosen since it allows scaling of an individual's attitude and is more sensitive to the full range of attitude than a simple dichotomous agree/disagree option. The validity of instrument were assessed by nursing instructors holding MSc (Assistant professors) and had research experience (n = 3) before and after pilot study.

Piloted test was conducted at St. Peters hospital Research after Review Ethical Committee granted us a letter of permission. After pilot test, marginal corrections such as order and wording of questions were assessed. Similarly, the questionnaire was pilot tested (n = 25). The internal consistency reliability (Cronbach's α) was 0.76.

Part three of the data collection tool in the questionnaire was comprised a closed-ended questions ('Yes' or 'No' response) to identify nurses' barriers to implement pressure ulcer prevention protocol adapted by reviewing different literatures [21, 22, 25].

The hospital which agreed for participation was asked to give the list of their participants through matron. The head nurses at study site were asked for their assistance to distribute questionnaires and were cooperative. The participants were selected using random sampling table (Fig. 1).

Data analysis

The data cleaning was done, entered in to computer using EPI data version 3.1 statistical packages, and 10% of the response was randomly selected and checked for the consistency of data entry. SPSS version 20 was used for data analysis. Frequencies and percentages were calculated to all variables which were related to the objectives of the study. The mean score attained from the scale was used to measure nurses' attitude. A numeric value was assigned for each attitude test items: 5 = strongly agree, 4 = Agree, 3 = neither agree nor

disagree, 2 = disagree, and 1 = strongly disagree. The questions include both positive and negative statements. But for negatively stated questions the score is reversed. The attitude mean was obtained by collapsing the Likert scales strongly disagree, disagree and neither agree nor disagree to the negative attitude, and strongly agree and agree to the positive attitude. Appropriate inferential test like ANOVA (analyses of variance) were used to test the effect of demographics on attitude. Results for p- value < 0.05 were considered significant.

Results

Demographic characteristics of the nurses

A total of 252 professional nurses were invited to participate in the study, 222 fully participated in the study, for a response rate of 78.7%. Among 369 nurses 128 (36%) were males. The mean ages of participants were 29 with minimum 20 and 61 years maximum. Most participants had a bachelor's degree in (n = 140, 63%), while 11% (n = 24) were enrolled in masters of Science degree in nursing. Nurses who are counted for their experiences in more than 10 years were 20.2% while majority of them 54% have 1–4 years of experience in nursing profession. Sixteen nurses (n = 16, 7.2%) reported that they had received and the largest proportion of them (n = 148, 66.7%) never received any training in PU prevention, while majority of them (n = 191, 86%) had not previously read research articles about PU compared to 31 (14%) who had read it. A limited number of nurses had attended PU training on conference. The majority of the participants were from medical ward (30.0%) as shown in Table 1.

Nurses' attitude towards pressure ulcer prevention

The study result indicated that more than half (n = 116, 52.2%) of nurses' attitude towards pressure ulcer prevention were negative (mean = 3.09, SD = 0.92, range = 1–5). The lowest possible score (negative attitude) was 11 whilst the highest possible score (positive attitude) was 55.

Data analysis of the nurses' attitudes showed some interesting points in relation to certain statements (Table 2). More than half of staff nurses (n = 126, 56.6%) felt that all patients are at risk of developing PUs, and around three quarter of the participants (n = 162, 72.9%) thought PU treatment was seen as lesser priority than its prevention. Nurses also believed that PU could be voided (n = 153, 68.8%), PU prevention care was not time consuming (n = 129, 58%), and 69% was considered continuous assessment of patient would give an accurate process of identifying patient at risk for PU.

The only statistically significant association in this study was gender of staff nurses (P = 0.032). It found that

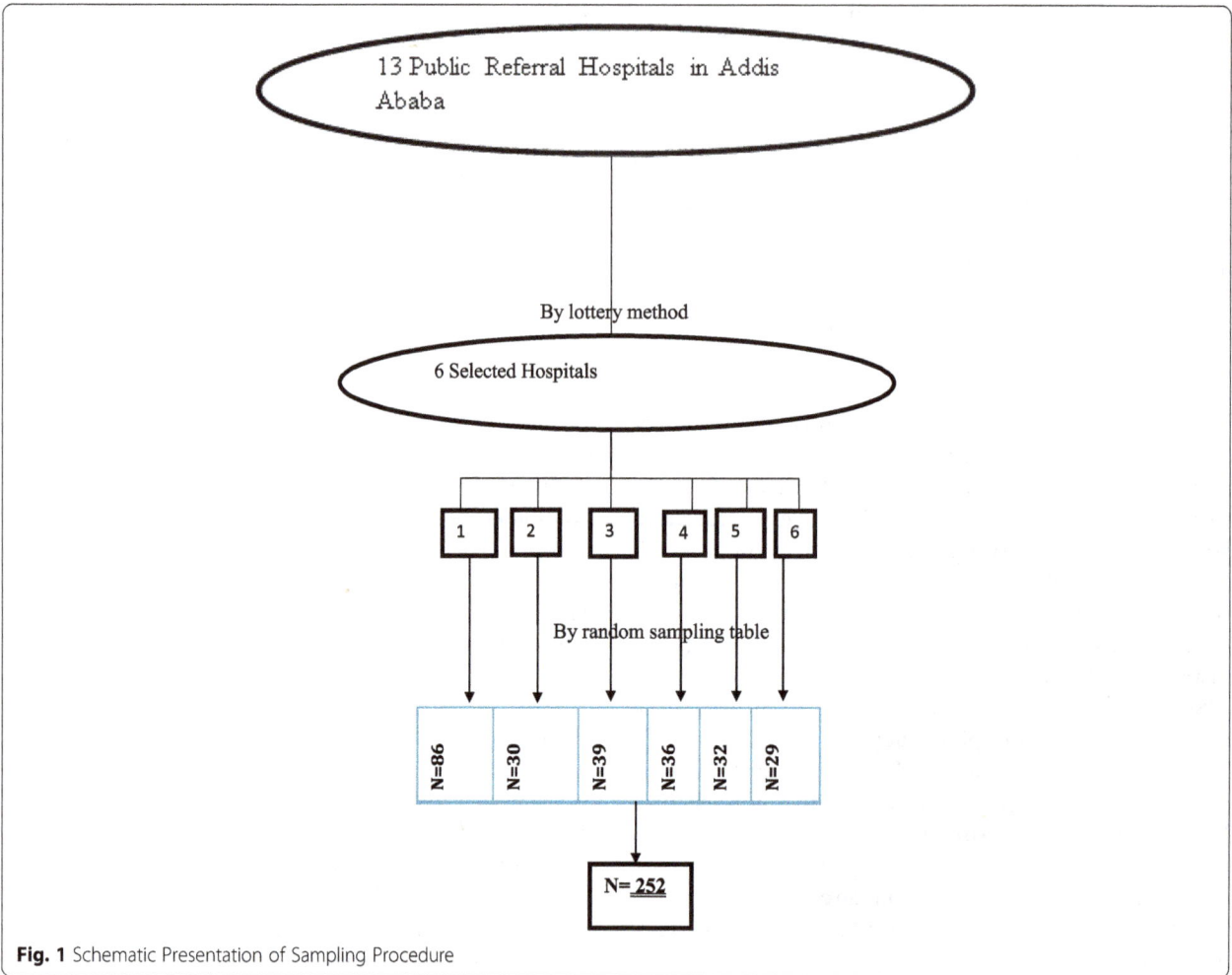

Fig. 1 Schematic Presentation of Sampling Procedure

male staff nurses showed that more positive attitude to PU prevention than female staff nurses. Other variables like age group, educational level, whether PU training received and reading research articles about PU had no effect on the nurses' attitude to pressure ulcer prevention.

Nurses' perceived barriers for practicing PU prevention care

Among thestaff nurses participated in the study (n = 222), only 2% of them had not reported any challenge for preventing pressure ulcer while majority (98%) of them had reported different challenges. The most frequently cited barriers were heavy work load and inadequate staff (n = 185, 83.1%), shortage of pressure relieving devices (inadequate equipment and devices), (n = 150, 67.7%), inadequate training about PUprevention (n = 140, 63.22%), lack of job satisfaction (n = 125, 56.2%), presence of other priorities than PU (n = 130, 58.7%) and lack of universal guide lines (n = 133, 59.3%) as illustrated in (Table 3).

Discussion

The results of this cross-sectional study explored that Addis Ababa nurses' hold a negative attitude to PU prevention. Similarly, major staff nurses' barriers to practice PU prevention such as heavy workload/inadequate staff, shortage of resources and inadequate training about PU prevention were identified. The present research result contradicted with several other previous study results [21–26]. This may be due to this study participants' included were from inpatient units. However, the present study result is in agreement with study conducted by Beeckman et al. [17] and Kaddourah et al. [27].

According to Moore and Price [21], the presence of barriers and obstacles (lack of time and staff, training, resources, and guideline) could prevent positive attitudes of nurses' from being reflected in practice. So, for the current study, it can be interpreted that the major barriers identified by staff nurses to practice PU prevention such as heavy workload and inadequate staff, and shortage of resources and inadequate training about PU prevention could be the possible reasons for most nurses' negative attitude.

Table 1 Frequency distribution of nurses' socio-demographic variables (N = 222)

Variables	N (%)
Sex	
• Male	77 (34.7)
• Female	145 (65.3)
Age (M = 29, SD = 6.65,max = 61,min = 20)	
• 20–29 years	148 (66.7)
• 30–39 years	49 (22)
• > = 40 years	25 (11.3)
Level of education	
• Diploma in nursing	58 (26)
• Degree in nursing	140 (63)
• Masters in nursing	24 (11)
Working experience (max = 41, min = 1)	
• 1–4 years	115 (51.8)
• 5–10 years	55 (24.8)
• Above 10 years	52 (23.4)
Where you received training on PU prevention?	
• In-service	16 (7.2)
• Course	37 (16.7)
• Conference	2 (0.9)
• Workshop	19 (8.5)
• Never	148 (66.7)
Have you read researchs about pressure ulcers?	
• Yes	31 (14)
• No	191 (86)

The Knowledge, Attitude and Practice (KAP) model [29] explained that individual's ability to perform actions can be influenced by certain knowledge, and attitude affects individual towards practice. Beeckman, et al. [17] suggested the more positive attitude towards prevention of PU, the more adequate preventive care patients will receive. This is supported by two other studies [18, 20]. In addition to identified barriers, for this study poor knowledge of nurses could be another possible reason for staff nurses' negative attitude towards PU prevention.

This paper showed that male nurses hold more positive attitude than female nurses ($p = 0.032$) to PU prevention though no similar researched topic agree with this point. The current study is in line with Moore and Price (2004) [22], who found that nurses' level of education and year of clinical working experience had no significant effect on nurses' attitude. Although Tubaishat et al. [25] found that nurses who had more year of experience, showed more positive attitude, our study did not support it. In addition, the respondents who had received PU care training and read research articles about PU did not scored higher attitudes than their counter parts. This supported by other research results [21, 22].

However, Kallman and Suserud [22] identified perceived barriers such as lack of time and un-cooperative patients, and lack of pressure relieving devices as the possible barriers, whereas as, Tubaishat et al. [25] identified as lack of policies and guidelines about PU prevention (50%), lack of cooperation with other health professionals (51%) and lack of job satisfaction (57%) as the major barriers to prevent PU cited by most of the nurses. Similarly, this study displayed heavy workload and inadequate staff (lack of time) as the major barrier

Table 2 Nurses' attitude towards pressure ulcer prevention, 2015 (N = 222)

Variables	Nurses' attitude rate				
	Strongly agree N (%)	Agree N (%)	Neither agree nor disagree N (%)	Disagree N (%)	Strongly disagree N (%)
All patients are at risk of developing PUs	64 (28.8)	62 (28)	46 (20.7)	28 (12.6)	22 (9.9)
PU prevention is time consuming for me	34 (15.3)	59 (26.6)	39 (17.6)	34 (15.3)	56 (25.2)
In my opinion, patients tend not to get as many PUs now days.	24 (10.8)	56 (25.2)	56 (25.2)	49 (22.1)	37 (16.7)
I do not need to concern myself with PU prevention in my job.	25 (11.3)	32 (14.4)	36 (16.2)	47 (21.2)	82 (36.9)
PU treatment is greater priority than its prevention.	37 (16.7)	23 (10.4)	17 (7.7)	27 (12.1)	118 (53.1)
Most pressure ulcers can be avoided	107 (48.1)	46 (20.7)	36 (16.2)	14 (6.3)	19 (8.7)
Continuous assessment of patient will give an accurate account of their PU risk	90 (40.6)	63 (28.4)	27 (12.1)	23 (10.3)	19 (8.6)
I am less interested in PU prevention than other aspects of care	22 (9.9)	34 (15.3)	2 6 (11.8)	46 (20.7)	94 (42.3)
My clinical judgment is better than any PU risk assessment tool available to me	34 (15.3)	31 (14)	32 (14.5)	36 (16.2)	89 (40)
In comparison with other areas of care, PU prevention is a low priority for me.	48 (21.5)	51 (22.9)	70 (31.4)	33 (14.8)	21 (9.4)
PU risk assessment should be regularly carried out on all patients during their stay in hospital	94 (42.3)	46 (20.7)	34 (15.3)	26 (11.7)	22 (10)

Table 3 Nurses' perceived barriers practice to prevent pressure ulcer prevention (N = 222)

Nurses' perceived barriers for preventing PU	Frequency (%)
Poor access to literature and reading facilities	110 (49.7)
Heavy workload and inadequate staff	185 (83.1)
Lack of universal guide line on prevention of pressure ulcer	133 (59.8)
Inadequate training coverage of pressure ulcer prevention	140 (63.2)
Uncooperative patients	87 (39.3)
Lack of job satisfaction in nursing profession	125 (56.2)
Presence of other priorities than pressure ulcer	130 (58.7)
Shortage of resources (equipment/resource)	150 (67.7)
Inadequate knowledge about pressure ulcer among nurses	60 (27)
Lack of multidisciplinary among staff nurses	64 (28.9)
I don't have any challenge	4 (2)

for being practicing PUP care, whilst, uncooperative patients as not cited as a major barrier to PU prevention. But, majority (58%) of them believed that PU is not consuming. This could be they had not sufficient time and adequate man powerto provide PU prevention.

This study described that 70.7% of nurses believed that their clinical judgment is better than risk assessment tool. This indicated they can assess PU clinically better than using risk assessment tool. Bergstrom et al. [30] found that risk assessment tool is more accurate and reliable than clinical judgment to who are at risk for PU development. However, Samuriwo, & Dowding [28] indicated that assessment tools were not routinely used to identify pressure ulcer risk, and that nurses rely on their own knowledge and experience rather than research evidence to decide what skin care to deliver.

Almost three quarter (74.8%) of the respondents also more interested in PU prevention than other aspects of nursing care. This is in line with Moore and Price study result [21] and Kaddourah et al. [27]. This suggested nurses had high interest in PU care; but, priority was given to other illnesses. This is why most of the staff nurses (n = 130, 58.7%) complained priority for other illnesses rather than PU as a barrier.

A significant number of the staff nurses (66.7%) surveyed had received no training to PU prevention, 191 (86%) have not ever read research about PU while 133 (59.8%) identified lack of universal guide line among the major barriers to practice prevent PU care. This idea is strengthened by the participants' response for which majority of them had disagreed that patients are tends not to get as many PUs now days. Further, poor access to literatures and journals due to lack of electronic libraries near the nurse' working units/wardswas another cited barrier to practice PU prevention. Hunt [31] stated that

if nurses did not read scientific journals, they will not be able to integrate research into their practice.

From researchers' experience in developing countries it is obvious that nursing care provided for patients are not adequate. This is highly due to shortage of resources. According to this study, one of the most commonly cited barriers was shortage of equipment/resource or facilities (67.7%) which is in agreement with the study finding among (Irish, Belgian and Jordanian nurses [21, 24, 25]. The shortage of resources in developed countries (among Belgian [24] and Irish [21] nurses) may be due to the participants were nurses who give caring at home. Lack of job satisfaction (56.2%) may be another reason behind for not practicing PU prevention care. According to Tubaishat et al. [25] lack of job dissatisfaction (25%) was also among the most commonly cited barrier. In Ethiopia,there is scarcity of pressure ulcer relieving devices which help nurses lifting patient or changing the patient position paying off the minimum energy particularly for severely ill patients in addition to time it saves.

Majority (66.7%) of the nurses that participated in this study reported that they never attended any training concerning pressure ulcersand about 133 (59.8) of participants reported lack of universal guideline for PUP. This indicates how much attention is paid to prevent PU in Addis Ababa. Padula et al. [4] stated hospitals adhering to PU updates had significant pressure injury reductions and $500,000+ savings per year. Currently evidences exhibited that prevalence of pressure ulcer is vary from country to country. This is supported by study results [5–10].

As observed from the participants' characters only 26 (11%) were second degree holders and 58 58 (26%) were diploma holders in nursing. It is reported that educational program will improve the knowledge of PU prevention. Similarly, updating nurses' education is the cardinal to increase nurses' competency to help them better clinical decision maker [32]. Generally, authors noted that lack of knowledge, negative attitudes, or underdeveloped skills are the principal barriers to PU prevention [18, 19].

Limitations

The data are from self-report questionnaires and qualitative method was not employed. But, since there is similar educational setting and resources fairly distributed to all hospitals, the result of the study can be generalizableto all nurses working from Addis Ababa region.

Conclusions

In the current study, the attitude of most nurses towards PUP was negative. The study also identified the major barriers to carry out PUP practice: Heavy work load/

inadequate staff or lack of time 185 (83.3%), Shortage of resources (equipment/resources) 150 (67.6%), Inadequate training coverage of pressure ulcer prevention140 (63%) and lack of universal guide line on prevention of pressure ulcer 133 (59.9%) are the most commonly cited barriers. Further research into nurses' attitude to pressure ulcer is needed using structured interview questionnaire.

Abbreviation
NGO: Non-Governmental organization; SD: Standard Deviation; SPSS: Statistical Package for Social Sciences

Acknowledgements
We would like to extend our sincere gratitude to thedata collectors, participants, hospitals directors, matrons and head nurses for their great assistance and cooperation.

Funding
The cost of data collection for this research was funded by Addis Ababa University.

Authors' contributions
WE contributed to the drafting of proposal, design, analysis and interpretation of the data, and manuscript preparation. ZA and BM were also involved in data analysis as well as drafting and revising this research paper. EG and BM were involved in the interpretation of the data and contributed to manuscript preparation. All authors were informed and gave the go ahead to publish the work. WE agrees to be held accountable for all aspects of the work hence any questions related to the accuracy or integrity of the work should be directed to WE. The authors declare that this manuscript has not been presented to any other journal for publication. All authors read and approved the final manuscript.

Ethics approval and consent to participate
Initially ethical clearance was obtained from Addis Ababa University, College of Health Sciences, Department of Nursing and Midwifery Research Review Ethical Committee(Protocol number was 18/Nurse and approved on 27/03/150), and Addis Ababa Regional Health Bureau Ethical Clearance Committee for four hospitals includedin the study (Yekatit 12 Medical College, ZewdituMemoriall Hospital, Tirunesh Beijing Hospital, Menilik II Hospital and RasDesta Memorial Hospital)(reference number: A.A.H/5973/227 and approved on 24/04/2015) to obtain participants in each hospitals. The sixth hospital is teaching hospital (Black Lion Hospital) administered by Addis Ababa University. These findings were part of a research titled "An assessment Nurses' knowledge, attitude and practice towards pressure ulcer prevention in admitted patients in Public referral hospitals in Addis Ababa. Permissions to obtain participants secured from each hospital medical directors, matrons and head nurses for the research to be undertaken at each hospital. The anonymity of the participants was respected. The names of the participants were not mentioned to keep the confidentiality. A signed written consent was obtained from participants before participation.

Competing interests
This manuscript maintains no competing financial interest declaration from any person or organization, or non-financial competing interests such as political, personal, religious, ideological, academic, intellectual, commercial or any other.

Author details
[1]Department of Nursing, College of Health Science, Wollega Unversity, Samara, Ethiopia. [2]School of Nursing, College of Health Science, Addis Ababa University, Addis Ababa, Ethiopia. [3]Department of Statistics, College of Natural and Computational Sciences, Arsi University, Asella, Ethiopia.

References
1. NPUAP, EPUAP and PPPIA. In: Haesler E, editor. Prevention and treatment of pressure ulcers: quick reference guide. Osborne Park: Western Australia, Cambridge Media; 2014. p. 2014.
2. Baranoski S, & Ayello, EA. Wound care essentials: practice principles. (3rd edition) Springhouse PA: Lippincott Williams & Wilkins. 2012, (4).
3. LyderCH WY, MeterskyM CM, KlimanR VNR, Hunt DR. Hospital-acquired pressure ulcers: results from the national Medicare patient safety monitoring system study. J Am GeriatrSoc. 2012;60(9):1603–8.
4. Padula WV, Mishra MK, Makic MB, Sullivan PW. Improving the quality of pressure ulcer care with prevention: a cost-effectiveness analysis. Med Care. 2011;49(4):385–92.
5. Tubaishat A, Anthony D, Saleh M. Pressure ulcers in Jordan: a point prevalence study. J Tissue Viability. 2011;20(1):14–9.
6. Adegoke BOA, Odole AC, Akindele LO, Akinpelu AO. Pressure ulcer prevalence among hospitalised adults in university hospitals in South-west Nigeria. Wound Practice & Research. 2013;21(3):128–34.
7. Moore Z, Johanssen E, van Etten M. A review of PU prevalence and incidence across Scandinavia, Iceland and Ireland (part I). J Wound Care. 2013;22(7):361–8.
8. Moore Z, Cowman S. Pressure ulcer prevalence and prevention practices in care of the older person in the Republic of Ireland. J Clin Nurs. 2012;21:362–71. https://doi.org/10.1111/j.1365-2702.2011.03749.x.
9. Moore Z, Johansen E, van Etten M, Strapp H, Solbakken T, Smith BE, Faulstich J. Pressure ulcer prevalence and prevention practices: a cross-sectional comparative survey in Norway and Ireland. J Wound Care. 2015;24(8):333–9.
10. Clark M, Semple MJ, Ivins N, Mahoney K, Harding K. National audit of pressure ulcers and incontinence-associated dermatitis in hospitals across Wales: a cross-sectional study. BMJ Open. 2017;7(8)
11. VanDenKerkhof EG, Friedlberg E, Harrison MB. Prevalence and risk of pressure ulcers in acute care following implementation of practice guidelines: annual pressure ulcer prevalence census 1994-2008. J Healthcare Quality. 2012;33(5):58–67.
12. Reddy M, Gill, Rochon PA. Preventing pressure ulcers: a systematic review. JAMA 2006;296:974–984.
13. Health Research & Educational Trust. Hospital acquired pressure ulcers/injuries (HAPU/I). Chicago, IL: Health Research & Educational Trust; 2017. Accessed at http://www.hret-hiin.org/.
14. Haileyesus Gedamu, Mignote Hailu A. A. Prevalence and Associated Factors of Pressure Ulcer among Hospitalized Patients. Journal of Advanced in nursing. December 2014(8).
15. Fishbein M, Ajzen I. The influence of attitudes on behavior. In: Albarracín D, Johnson BT, Zanna MP, editors. The Handbook of Attitudes: Psychology Press. p. 2005.
16. Maylor M, Torrance C. Pressure sore survey part 3: locus of control. J Wound Care. 1999;8:101–5.
17. Beeckman D, Defloor T, Schoonhoven L, Vanderwee K. Knowledge and attitudes of nurses on pressure ulcer prevention: a cross-sectional multicenter study in Belgian hospitals. Worldviews Evid-Based Nurs. 2011;8:166–76.
18. Grimshaw J, Eccles M, Tetroe J. Implementing clinical guidelines: current evidence and future implications. J Contin Educ Heal Prof. 2004;24(Suppl. 1):S31–7.
19. Ayello EA, Meaney G. Replicating a survey of pressure ulcer content in nursing textbooks. J Wound Ostomy Continence Nurs. 2003;30:266–71.
20. Hill L. Wound care nursing: the question of pressure. Nurs Times. 1992;88(12):76.
21. Moore Z, Price P. Nurses' attitudes, behaviours and perceived barriers towards pressure ulcer prevention. J Clin Nurs. 2004;13:942–51. https://doi.org/10.1111/j.1365-2702.2004.00972.x.

22. Kallman U, Suserud B. Knowledge, attitudes and practice among nursing staff concerning pressure ulcer prevention and treatment – a survey in a Swedish healthcare setting. Scand J Caring Sci. 2009;23:334–41.

23. Islam S, Sae-Sia APDW, Khupantavee APDN. Knowledge attitude and practice on pressure ulcer prevention among nurses in Bangladesh. Poster presentation in the 2nd international conference on humanities and. Soc Sci. 2010;

24. Demarré L, Vanderwee K, Defloor T, et al. Pressure ulcers: knowledge and attitude of nurses and nursing assistants in Belgian nursing homes. J ClinNurs. 2012;21:1425–34.

25. Tubaishat A, Aljezawi M, Al Qadire M, Mohammad. Nurses' attitudes and perceived barriers to pressure ulcer prevention in Jordan. Journal of wound care. 2013;22:490–7. https://doi.org/10.12968/jowc201322.

26. Uba A, Kever L. Knowledge, attitude and practice of nurses towards pressure ulcer prevention. Int J Nurs and midwifery. 2015;7(4):54–60.

27. Kaddourah B, Abu-Shaheen AK, AL Tannir M. Knowledge and attitudes of health professionals towards pressure ulcers at a rehabilitation hospital. BMC Nurs. 2016;15:17.

28. Samuriwo R, Dowding D. Nurses' pressure ulcer related judgments and decisions in clinical practice: a systematic review. International Journal of Nursing Studies. 2014;51(12):1667–85.

29. Carol Tweed & Mike Tweed. Intensive care nurses' knowledge of pressure ulcers. American J Crit Care, July 2008, Volume 17, No. 4 (online www. ajcconline.org and click).

30. Launiala A. How much can KAP survey tell us about people's knowledge, attitude, and practice? Some observations from medical anthropology research on malaria in pregnancy in Malawi. Anthropology matters Journal. 2009;11:1–13.

31. Bergstrom N, Bennet MA, Carlos CE. Treatment of pressure ulcers in adults: clinical practice guide line. Agency for health care policy and Research Publications. 1994;15:181–8.

32. Lamond D, Farnell S. The treatment of pressure sores: a comparison of novice and expert nurses' knowledge, information use and decision accuracy. J Advnurs. 2001;27:280–6.

3

To what extent has doctoral (PhD) education supported academic nurse educators in their teaching roles

Carol Bullin

Abstract

Background: A doctoral degree, either a PhD or equivalent, is the academic credential required for an academic nurse educator position in a university setting; however, the lack of formal teaching courses in doctoral programs contradict the belief that these graduates are proficient in teaching. As a result, many PhD prepared individuals are not ready to meet the demands of teaching.

Methods: An integrative literature review was undertaken. Four electronic databases were searched including the Cumulative Index to Nursing & Allied Health Literature (CINAHL), PubMed, Educational Resources Information Center (ERIC) and ProQuest. Date range and type of peer-reviewed literature was not specified.

Results: Conditions and factors that influenced or impacted on academic nurse educators' roles and continue to perpetuate insufficient pedagogical preparation include the requirement of a research focused PhD, lack of mentorship in doctoral programs and the influence of epistemic cultures (including institutional emphasis and reward system). Other factors that have impacted the academic nurse educator's role are society's demand for highly educated nurses that have increased the required credential, the assumption that all nurses are considered natural teachers, and a lack of consensus on the practice of the scholarship of teaching.

Conclusions: Despite recommendations from nursing licensing bodies and a major US national nursing education study, little has been done to address the issue of formal pedagogical preparation in doctoral (PhD) nursing programs. There is an expectation of academic nurse educators to deliver quality nursing education yet, have very little or no formal pedagogical preparation for this role. While PhD programs remain research-intensive, the PhD degree remains a requirement for a role in which teaching is the major responsibility.

Keywords: Academic nurse educators, Doctoral preparation, Scholarship of teaching, Pedagogy, Undergraduate nursing education, Literature review

Background

Professional health education has not adequately advanced in preparing health care workers to effectively meet the current and future expectations of the health care system [1]. Static curricula, lack of emphasis on pedagogy, and silo mentality are cited as barriers that have impeded changes necessary to professional education [1]. The Carnegie Foundation for the Advancement of Teaching's national study on the transformation of nursing education [2], identified that nurses must have the abilities and skills to perform in multiple settings and contexts, within situations that are unclear, contextual, and dynamic. Addressing these changes are the responsibility of those providing nursing education, specifically academic nurse educators. Teachers of nursing education require both in-depth, discipline-specific and pedagogical knowledge to effectively meet the anticipated complexities of professional nursing practice [3].

Correspondence: carol.bullin@usask.ca
College of Nursing, University of Saskatchewan, Room 4338 E-Wing, Health Sciences Building, 104 Clinic Place, Saskatoon, SK S7N 2Z4, Canada

A doctoral degree, either a doctorate of philosophy (PhD) or equivalent is currently the required academic credential for an academic nurse educator in a university setting. Interestingly, while approximately 80% of these graduates take a position in college/university teaching [4], the primary focus of PhD coursework is to develop research interests [5, 6]. Academics enter higher education with very high levels of knowledge in subjects or disciplines but no knowledge of teaching adults [7]. For this reason, few academic nurse educators are formally prepared for a teaching role [3, 8]. Skinner (as cited in Brightman) [2] best articulated the issue of the lack of formal teaching preparation in higher education:

It has been said that college teaching is the only profession for which there is no professional training, and it is commonly argues that this is because our graduate schools train scholars and scientists rather than teachers. We are more concerned with the discovery of knowledge than with its dissemination. (p.1).

Comprehending the issue around the lack of formal teaching preparation for academic nurse educators, necessitates a brief overview of both the current context of the discipline of nursing and nursing education, in addition to the historical development of academic preparation for the role of a nurse educator. This issue is common and not limited to either North America or to the discipline of nursing and nursing education [5, 9–11]. For academic nurse educators to provide quality learning experiences to nursing students, they require appropriate academic preparation that includes pedagogical knowledge, or simply stated, formal knowledge of ways to effectively communicate subject matter that fosters learning and ultimately, understanding. However, excellence in teaching is neither truly valued nor rewarded in many academic institutions [1, 12]. Academic scholarship is commonly defined strictly in terms of research. This undervaluing of teaching is also evident in nursing with the advent of the term *research* being incorporated into the scholarship of nursing. Prior to the mid-nineteenth century, teaching had been the primary focus of scholarship in higher education [13]. At this time, professional nursing faculties did not have the same emphasis on research as the broader university; however, as more nurses obtained PhDs, graduate programs were established, and programs of nursing research developed. The goal of nursing PhD programs was to prepare nurse scientists [14, 15], and as a result, teaching became a secondary activity.

Formal teaching preparation for nurses has declined significantly from 1976 in which 24% of nursing Masters' programs graduates primary area of study was education (teaching), in contrast to 5.3% in 2004 [5]. This decline was due to an increased emphasis on preparing nurses to practice at an advanced clinical levels (i.e. nurse practitioners and clinical nurse specialists). The trend in advanced practice nursing has recently resurfaced in the United States with the entry level to advanced practice shifting from the masters to a doctoral degree [16]. This shift is evident in the proliferation of Doctor of Nursing Practice (DNP) programs in the United States. For example, in 2014, there were 5290 doctoral students enrolled in 130 PhD programs as compared to 18,352 doctoral students enrolled in 219 DNP programs [16]. However, while the DNP is an advanced clinical practice degree, many graduates are taking faculty positions for which they are not prepared [4, 17, 18]. It is well documented that programs leading to the Masters or doctoral degrees in Nursing does not prepare those nurses for many of the roles and responsibilities associated with academe [8, 19, 20].

In order to advance the scholarship of teaching, the AACN [5, 9, 21] identified the need to establish best practices in teaching, while the National League for Nursing (NLN) [21, 22] highlighted the development of nursing education theory and ultimately, educational mastery. However, faculty and administrators of graduate nursing programs have focused on developing nursing research and have continued to making little effort to prepare future faculty for teaching [3, 11, 23]. Therefore, if a PhD is required of academic nurse educators for a role in teaching and the focus of PhD preparation has traditionally privileged research and developing one's role as a researcher, how will PhD preparation address the teaching component of the academic nurse educators' role? Based on the information above, it is important to understand the state of the literature regarding a PhD requirement and the extent to which a PhD supports academic nurse educators in their teaching roles.

Method

A preliminary search, not restricted to English language literature, was done to determine what literature review strategy was most appropriate to answer the aim of the study. Based on the results of this search, an integrative literature review method [24] was selected. An integrative review allows for the integration of various types of literature and research methodologies. A keyword search of the literature was undertaken as of March 2017 using Cumulative Index to Nursing and Allied Health Literature (CINAHL), PubMed, Educational Resources Information Center (ERIC) and ProQuest databases. The search terms used included: "nurse educator", "PhD", "doctoral preparation in nursing", "nursing faculty", "nursing education", "scholarship in nursing", "scholarship of teaching", "ideal nurse educator", "educators in higher education", and "value of teaching" in varying combinations. The population selected for this review were registered nurses that were either preparing or prepared, at the doctoral (i.e., PhD) level as a requirement for an academic nurse educator role in a university setting. The review process involved a search of the current literature, evaluation of the retrieved articles and synthesis of results. For inclusion in the integrative review all literature must have: 1) been available in English text, 2) focused on the experiences of academic nurse educators' required doctoral preparation (in a university setting), 3) available in peer-reviewed outlets and, 4) no date restriction. Literature that referenced nurse educators in other than university settings was not included. The peer-reviewed literature was included or excluded based on whether or not it met the inclusion criteria. The search and selection process is outlined in Fig. 1.

Results

In sum, a total of 139 peer-reviewed works were retrieved and included in this review, relative to the experience of nurse educators' in preparing or prepared, at the doctoral level for a role in academe. Most were published in the United States ($n = 126$); other countries included Canada ($n = 9$), Australia ($n = 3$), Taiwan (n = 1), Slovenia (n = 1) and, United Kingdom (n = 1). The date range is from 1990 to present. Types of peer-reviewed literature included research studies qualitative design ($n = 21$), quantitative design ($n = 8$), and mixed method design ($n = 4$); however, discussion papers and reports contributed much of the literature reviewed. A summary of these results are illustrated in Table 1 Summary of peer-reviewed literature and organized according to the themes and subthemes identified from the literature search.

A paucity of literature is available on both the formal academic preparation of, and comprehension of academic nurse educators' roles [5, 25]. The increased emphasis on the achievement of scholarship in higher

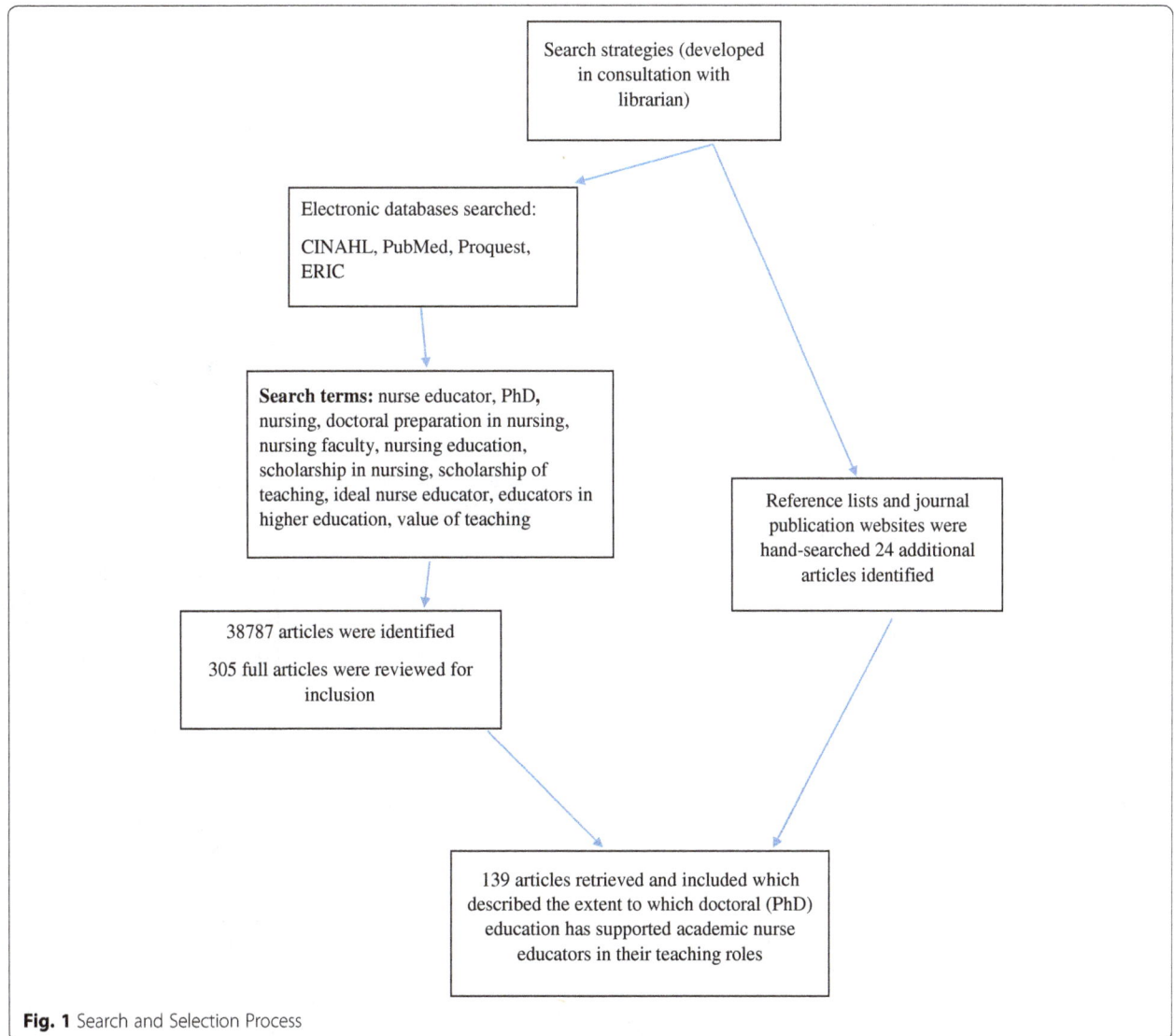

Fig. 1 Search and Selection Process

Table 1 Summary of peer-reviewed literature

Author	Year	Theme/*subtheme*	Peer-reviewed literature	Literature content
Adams [62]	2011	Theme 1: Nurse Educator Expectations	Report	Expectations for preparing future faculty
AACN [5]	2005		Report	Nursing education faculty
Anderson [37]	2008		Qualitative, semi-structured interviews ($n = 18$)	Transitioning from a clinical expert to novice educator
Austin [51]	2002		Discussion paper	Future faculty preparation
Bass [98]	2006		Book	Re-examining doctoral education
Bartels [94]	2007		Discussion paper	Role preparation for the academy (scholarship)
Benner et al. [3]	2010		Book	Transforming nursing education
Bergner et al. [110]	2010		Discussion paper	Teaching training for PhD students
Booth et al. [8]	2016		Discussion paper	Formal pedagogical preparation required for nurse educators
Bok [135]	2013		Commentary	Preparing PhD students to teach
Bogo [136]	2010		Discussion paper	Preparing doctoral students to teach
Brightman [2]	2009		Discussion paper	Teaching doctoral students \how to teach
Cooley et al. [111]	2015		Qualitative, hermeneutical, phenomenology ($n = 7$)	Facilitators & barriers to nurse educator practice development
Diekelmann [63]	2005		Discussion paper	New pedagogies to transition nursing practice
Diekelmann [39]	2003		Book	New pedagogies for health professionals
Dreifeurst et al. [112]	2016		Sequential, explanatory, descriptive survey ($n = 548$)	PhD preparation for nurse faculty
Edwardson [6]	2004		Discussion paper	Shortcomings & relevance of the PhD
Fang et al. [56]	2016		Cross sectional questionnaire ($n = 933$)	Barriers & facilitators to nurse faculty roles
Fiedler et al. [11]	2015		Qualitative, in-depth interviews ($n = 8$)	Faculty preparation education course
Findlow [124]	2012		Discussion paper	Professional academic identity in nursing
Gaff [120]	2002		Discussion paper	Doctoral preparation for a faculty career (Preparing Future Faculty Program PFF)
Ivey [19]	2007		Discussion paper	Formal pedagogical preparation of nurse educators
Ironside [92]	2006		Editorial	Pedagogical preparation for nurse educators
Ironside [95]	2005		Qualitative hermeneutical ($n = 45$)	Pedagogical preparation for nurse educators
Jackson et al. [103]	2011		Sequential, exploratory mixed methods ($n = 24$)	PhD requirement for academic nursing
Johnsen-Crawley [25]	2004		Discussion paper	Teacher preparation models
Johnson-Farmer et al. [61]	2009		Qualitative, grounded theory ($n = 17$)	Teaching excellence as a dynamic process
Kalb et al. [137]	2012		Qualitative, online survey ($n = 76$)	Developing leadership in nursing
Kwiram [46]	2006		Book	

Table 1 Summary of peer-reviewed literature *(Continued)*

Author	Year	Theme/*subtheme*	Peer-reviewed literature	Literature content
				Re-examination of doctoral education
Lancet Commissions [1]	2010		Report	Transformation of nursing education
Lewallen et al. [23]	2011		Discussion paper	Preparation of nurse educators for research & teaching roles
Lindeman [33]	2000		Discussion paper	Transforming nursing education
MacMillan [64]	2013		Report	Future of undergraduate nursing education in Canada
Meacham [90]	2002		Discussion paper	New faculty preparation
Morris et al. [52]	2012		Book	Transformative learning in nursing
NLN [108]	2007		Discussion paper	Nurse educator roles and responsibilities
Nehls et al. [47]	2016		Mixed methods, interviews and database reviews *(n = 84)*	Choosing a PhD program
Oermann et al. [35]	2016		Quantitative survey *(n = 482)*	Roles in nursing programs for PhD & DNP prepared nurses
Schriner [53]	2007		Qualitative, hermeneutical, ethnographic inquiry *(n = 7)*	Transitioning from a clinical expert to a faculty role
Schulman et al. [138]	2006		Discussion paper	Re-examining doctoral preparation
Siler et al. [20]	2001		Qualitative, hermeneutical, phenomenological *(n = 12)*	Understanding the experiences of new faculty
Tanner [96]	2002		Editorial	Advancing teaching pedagogies in nursing education
Barnes et al. [134]	2008	*Mentorship*	Qualitative, in-depth interviews *(n = 25)*	Role of doctoral advisors
Baxley et al. [131]	2014		Book	Mentorship in nursing
Bell-Elliason et al. [139]	2008		Quantitative survey *(n = 224)*	Characteristics of ideal doctoral mentors
Grossman [132]	2013		Book	Mentorship in nursing
Hall et al. [127]	2009		Discussion paper	Mentorship in the development of professional researchers
Johnson et al. [128]	2014		Quantitative, on-line survey *(n = 95)*	How mentoring prepares doctoral students for a faculty role
Noonan et al. [133]	2007		Qualitative, focus groups *(n = 16)*	Mentoring doctoral students
Paglis et al. [129]	2006		Quantitative, survey *(n = 130)*	Mentoring doctoral students as career preparation
Rose [130]	2005		Quantitative, survey *(n = 537)*	The ideal doctoral student mentor
Hoessler et al. [48]	2015	*Graduate TAs*	Mixed methods, document analysis	Graduate student teaching training
Kenney et al. [49]	2014		Qualitative *(n = 13)*	Program structures & practices of graduate training

Table 1 Summary of peer-reviewed literature *(Continued)*

Author	Year	Theme/*subtheme*	Peer-reviewed literature	Literature content
Love Stowell et al. [41]	2015		Conceptual model	Pedagogical preparation of graduate students
Parker et al. [135]	2015		Qualitative, survey (*n* = 48)	Training for graduate TAs
Agger et al. [18]	2014	*Doctoral Preparation*	Qualitative, semi-structured interviews (*n* = 15)	DNP prepared nurses in academic roles
AACN a [17]	2016		Report	Faculty vacancies – DNP not prepared for academic role
Apold [109]	2008		Discussion paper	Doctoral nursing education
Nyquist et al. [117]	2004		Discussion paper	Re-designing doctoral nursing education
Walker et al. [118]	2016		Discussion paper	Doctoral education for nurses – PhD or DNP?
Winter et al. [97] [e]	2000		Discussion paper	Evaluation criteria for practice-based doctoral degrees
Acorn et al. [77]	2013	Theme 2: Lack of consensus on scholarship	Discussion paper	Defining and describing scholarship in nursing
Allen et al. [78]	2005		Discussion paper	Differentiating scholarly teaching & the scholarship of teaching
Benigni [115]	2007		Discussion paper	The teacher-scholar
Boyer [12]	1990		Discussion paper	Domains of scholarship
CASN [70]	2013		Report	Scholarship among nursing faculty
Chalmers [68] [b]	2011		Discussion paper	Recognizing & rewarding the scholarship of teaching in higher education
Chandramohan [38]	2009		Book	Learning to teach in higher education
Cochran-Smith [36]	2003		Discussion paper	Teacher preparation in higher education
Darling-Hammond et al. [45]	2002		Secondary analysis (*n* = 300)	Teacher preparation
Fincher et al. [67]	2006		Discussion paper	Defining and describing scholarly teaching
Gardner et al. [57]	2010		Discussion paper	Teacher-scholar model
Glanville et al. [13]	2004		Discussion paper	Defining the scholarship of teaching
Glassick et al. [71]	1997		Book	Scholarship in the professoriate
Gubbins [66]	2014		Discussion paper	Developing a program of scholarship in teaching & learning
Hatch [72]	2006		Book	The practice of teaching and learning in higher education
Korthagen et al. [32]	2005		Discussion paper	Teacher-educator preparation
Kreber [79] [a]	2015		Discussion paper	Advancing the scholarship of teaching
Kreber [30] [a]	2002		Qualitative, Delphi exploratory (*n* = 11)	Consensus on scholarship of teaching
Kreber [28]	2002		Discussion paper	Excellence in teaching & scholarship of teaching should be rewarded

Table 1 Summary of peer-reviewed literature *(Continued)*

Author	Year	Theme/*subtheme*	Peer-reviewed literature	Literature content
Kreber et al. [42]	2005		Qualitative, exploratory, semi-structured interviews ($n = 31$)	How university instructors learn about teaching
Kreber et al. [58]	2000		Conceptual model	Scholarship of teaching
Kuh et al. [84]	2007		Survey ($n = 29,444$ faculty) and ($n = 65,633$ students)	Teacher-scholar model
Martinez [34]	2008		Discussion paper	Reflective exploration of new teacher educators making the transition into the academy
McKinney [7]	2006		Discussion paper	The challenges of the scholarship of teaching and learning in higher education
McKinney [80]	2013		Book	Intra/interdisciplinary scholarship of teaching and learning
Murray [43]	2005		Qualitative, in-depth semi-structured interviews ($n = 28$)	Experiences of teacher educators in the first 3 years of practice
Nicholls [29]	2005		Discussion paper	Understanding scholarship
Norris [31] [a]	2000		Discussion paper	Teacher-based knowledge and experience or university research-based knowledge and empirical theory
Oermann [44]	2014		Discussion paper	Scholarship in nursing
O'Meara et al. [69]	2005		Discussion paper	Recognition of all forms of scholarship
Rossetti et al. [27]	2009		Qualitative, Interpretive ($n = 35$)	Educational philosophy of teaching
Shulman [73]	2004		Discussion paper	The scholarship of teaching and learning
Shulman [65]	2000		Discussion paper	The future of the doctorate
Sullivan et al. [82]	2008		Discussion paper	A review of professional education
Trigwell et al. [74]	2000		Qualitative, phenomenological ($n = 20$)	A review of professional education
Vardi et al. [75] [b]	2011		Discussion paper	Promoting the scholarship of teaching & learning
Zeichner [91]	2005		Discussion paper	Teaching teachers
Austin et al. [114]	2008	Theme 3: Research versus Teaching	Discussion paper	The integration of research, teaching, & learning
Austin et al. [81]	2006		Discussion paper	Preparation in the domains of scholarship other than discovery
Brew [86]	2003		Discussion paper, conceptual model	The relationship between research and teaching
Carter et al. [87]	2011		Qualitative, focus groups ($n = 8$)	The importance of teaching
Campbell et al. [116]	2005		Discussion paper	Re-examining the PhD in Nursing
Chen [88] [d]	2015		Qualitative, interviews and document analysis ($n = 20$)	Priority of research over teaching

Table 1 Summary of peer-reviewed literature *(Continued)*

Author	Year	Theme/*subtheme*	Peer-reviewed literature	Literature content
DeCourcy [60]	2015		Discussion paper	Describing excellence in teaching
Diezmann et al. [119]	2015		Case study	Transitioning from research scientist to teacher
Fook [106]	2001		Discussion paper	Integration of theory, practice, & research
Ketefian et al. [4]	2015		Discussion paper	Trends & factors influencing doctoral education
Malcolm [89]	2014		Discussion paper	Research-teaching link in higher education
Marentic Pozarnik et al. [59] [c]	2015		Case study	Developing excellence in teaching competencies
Matthews et al. [26] [b]	2012		Quantitative, survey ($n = 522$)	Teaching & research gap implications on the scholarship of teaching and learning
Paulsen [93]	2001		Discussion paper	Relationship between research & the scholarship of teaching
Smeltzer et al. [85]	2015		Mixed methods, focus groups and surveys ($n = 554$)	Impact of teaching on research productivity
Starr et al. [40]	2015		Discussion paper	Inquiry on teaching in higher education
Schonwetter et al. [54]	2015		Cross-sectional survey ($n = 133$)	Faculty development teaching training
Van De Ven et al. [126]	2006		Discussion paper	Engaged scholarship between theory and practice
Williams [76]	2008		Discussion paper	Nursing as an academic profession
Cronin [121]	2003	*Epistemic cultures*	Discussion paper	Requirement for alternate forms of scholarship expression
Georges [125]	2003		Discussion paper	Epistemic diversity in nursing
Knorr Cetina [122]	2007		Discussion paper	Epistemic and knowledge cultures
Mork et al. [123]	2008		Ethnographic case study ($n = 35$)	Conflicts of epistemic cultures
AACN [14]	2016	Theme 4: Lack of consensus on formal education for nurse educators	Report	Academic nursing
AACN [16]	2015		Report	Academic Nursing
AACN [10]	2015		Report	Recommended preparation of nurse educators
AACN [101]	2013		Report	Advancing higher education in nursing
AACN [99]	2010		Report	Transforming nursing education
AACN [9]	2008		Report	Recommendations on educational preference for professoriate in nursing education
Austin [55]	2002		Discussion paper	Faculty preparation
Brar et al. [102]	2010		Discussion paper	Advanced nursing education beyond the Master's degree

Table 1 Summary of peer-reviewed literature *(Continued)*

Author	Year	Theme/*subtheme*	Peer-reviewed literature	Literature content
CASN [15]	2011		Report	PhD prepared faculty
Grace et al. [83]	2016		Discussion paper	Preparation of nursing scholars & leaders
Kirkman et al. [105]	2007		Discussion paper	A comprehensive review of doctorates in nursing
Loomis et al. [104]	2006		Qualitative, internet-based, exploratory survey ($n = 69$)	Decision to pursue a PhD or a DNP
Minnick et al. [107]	2010		Survey ($n = 96$)	Capacity in doctoral research nursing programs
NLN [22]	2013		Report	Doctoral preparation for nurse educators
NLN [21]	2002		Report	Recommendations for doctoral preparation of nurse educators
Nyquist [113]	2002		Discussion paper	Revising the current PhD program
Wood et al. [100] [a]	2004		Report	Doctoral nursing in Canada

Denotes country of publication
[a]Canada, [b]Australia, [c]Slovenia, [d]Taiwan, [e]United Kingdom

education, necessitates some background on areas of scholarship, the scholarship of teaching, current practices of higher education teacher preparation, and factors that have had an influence on the academic nurse educator's role. The perceived value of the scholarship of teaching varied widely across institutions, and ultimately impacted the academic nurse educator role, [26]. In order to address the purpose of the review, the results of the literature search indicated several resulting themes. These themes framed the organization of this literature review: (1) What is an effective educator? ($n = 9$); (2) What is the current practice for the formal preparation of teachers in higher education? ($n = 32$); (3) How is excellence in teaching described? ($n = 57$) and, (4) What conditions influence or have an impact on academic nurse educator preparation for the responsibilities of their roles? ($n = 55$). The following is a discussion of these resulting themes.

What is an effective educator?

An academic nurse educator is involved in practice, education and research in both baccalaureate and graduate schools of nursing [14]. The role responsibilities of the academic nurse educator identified by the AACN [14] includes articulating and demonstrating the importance of research through the production of new, nursing-specific knowledge, and identifying the link between clinical nursing practice and education, that ultimately will lead to improved health outcomes. For academic nurse educators to meet these role responsibilities, they require the skills to promote student self- development, technical competence and critical thinking ability [27]. The literature identified a lack of agreement on the definition of an effective educator instead, citing personality characteristics as measures of teaching excellence. Successful or effective teachers for example, are described as having the ability to convey concepts in a meaningful way, and to motivate and encourage critical thinking beyond discipline-specific knowledge [27, 28]. Developing those skills associated with excellence in teaching requires both formal preparation and experience. However, the current practice in higher education is to promote ongoing, informal teaching techniques and tips as the pathway to attaining excellence in teaching, rather than acknowledging the necessity for formal pedagogical knowledge [7, 29].

Students' perceptions of a teacher's performance in relation to the success of their learning experience is most often associated with teaching excellence [28]. Student ratings and peer evaluations advance the notion that excellent teachers possess expansive teaching and learning knowledge. However, excellent teachers may not be able to articulate their teaching practice in relation to educational theories [30]. The practice of emphasizing and rewarding outcomes or products in the form of publication or teaching evaluation may be ignoring the process by which faculty learn about teaching. Awards for teaching excellence are generally not made on the level of teaching knowledge [28]. Similarly, then, can one assess the quality of a nurse educator's teaching effectiveness by virtue of possessing the credential of a PhD?

According to Kreber [28], there is a fundamental difference between *expert* teachers and *excellent* or *effective* teachers. While expert teachers are unfailingly excellent teachers, excellent teachers may or may not be experts. Experts are relentless in their pursuit of new learning opportunities and reflecting on not only on their personal teaching experience, but on how educational theory explains their practice [28]. However, experienced individuals who do not engage in reflective practice are not considered expert teachers [28]. Informal teaching knowledge garnered from personal experience is inadequate as a basis in providing quality education [31]. Thus, effective teachers require a combination of discipline-specific expertise and pedagogical knowledge based on experience and educational theory [28].

In their interpretative study, Rossetti and Fox [27] illustrated the practices of effective teachers. Regardless of the disciplines across which this study was conducted, the findings are relevant to the discipline of nursing as they are central to the nature of professional nursing practice. Effective teaching practice is dependent on a teacher's formal knowledge of teaching. While nurse educators are considered experts in their area of practice, clinical expertise does not necessarily equate into teaching expertise. Most often those who come to the academy are experts in their fields or disciplines but lack pedagogical knowledge [3]. There is an important distinction between the discipline of nursing and the discipline of education; teaching is both a profession and a second discipline. Therefore, academic nurse educators must develop expertise in pedagogical practices [7, 8]. In order to provide the high quality instruction that is required for new nurses in meeting both current and future health care demands, academic nurse educators need to be highly skilled teachers.

What is the current practice for the formal preparation of teachers in higher education?

Increased societal demands for the responsibility and accountability of services provided are particularly relevant to the professional disciplines of medicine, law, nursing, and teaching [32–35]. As a result, the responsibility for educating skilled professional practitioners has been entrusted to educational institutions [36]. Providing a high quality education should be central to educators across disciplines; yet, the literature lacks in research on teacher (educator) preparation in higher education [6, 27, 29, 37–39]. In spite of the increased focus on the educational practices of teachers in the delivery of quality education, minimal attention has been afforded to higher education teacher preparation practices and

policies [36, 40, 41]. Significantly, there is a finite body of research on teaching expertise in higher education [42].

Institutional culture defines scholarship according to research and publication output, rather than teaching knowledge [34, 43, 44]. Despite the importance of preservice training needs, the pursuit of traditionally acknowledged scholarly activities are given the highest priority by the academy [45]. For example, utilizing doctoral students ill-prepared for teaching, is the current practice of teacher education in higher education. Earning income is most probably the motivator for doctoral students, rather than striving to be an effective teacher. Many graduate scholarships available to doctoral students are dependent on teaching an undergraduate class, resulting in many doctoral students learning informally about teaching through their teaching assistant (TA) experience. Graduate teaching experience does not equate with the preparation required to develop teaching proficiency [46, 47], indicating the need for doctoral students to have formal teaching education including pedagogical approaches and curriculum development [48–50]. In general, employing TAs in graduate schools is directed towards meeting departmental teaching requirements rather than towards mentoring graduate students in teaching or developing prospective professors [51]. Subsequently, the utilization of inadequately prepared TAs to deliver undergraduate education is under increasing scrutiny.

A cursory search of the Internet identified that many Canadian universities had teaching centers offering basic teaching courses to graduate students and new faculty that included an introduction to teaching program and/or workshops on teaching-specific topics [48, 49]. However, for the most part, participation in these programs are optional. While university teaching centers assist graduate students in learning to be TAs, they do not provide adequate preparation for a faculty role [47].

Due to the economic climate, advanced practice clinicians currently occupy many nursing faculty positions as educational institutions sustain the practice of devaluing academic proficiency and experience [39]. While advance practice clinicians are clinical content experts, they generally have little, if no, previous formal training in adult education [52–54]. The lack of formal teaching education for graduate nursing students and ultimately, being unprepared for a faculty role is a growing concern [25, 39, 55]. As a result, successful transition from a clinical environment into an academic culture for nurses that pursue doctoral education in their discipline, may be difficult [39, 56]. The goal in delivering effective nursing education is not simply in the nursing content knowledge itself, but rather with pedagogical knowledge that engages and informs that knowledge [52].

How is excellence in teaching described?

The increasing focus on achievement of excellence in teaching in the literature reflects the emphasis on the pursuit of scholarship in higher education. Achieving excellence in teaching requires a high level of individual commitment to move beyond what is already known and provide students with opportunities to develop their critical thinking abilities [57]. It was apparent in the current literature, that there is little documented research about understanding educators' experiences relative to how knowledge and practice are developed [58, 59]. Up to the present, the focus of the literature has been on the theoretical concepts of teaching expertise, the scholarship of teaching, and teaching excellence rather than on experiential practices [42, 60, 61]. The present review of the literature identifies a significant theme: the experiences of the teaching profession in general, and specifically, the need for further research in addressing the formal preparation needs of teachers in various disciplines [3, 20, 27, 34, 36, 43, 58, 62–64]. Several topics identified in the literature contribute to the discourse on "teaching excellence": (a) defining scholarship, (b) the scholarship of teaching, (c) pedagogical knowledge, and (d) the characteristics of effective educators. Findings from the literature for each of these sub-themes will be discussed both generally, and specifically within the discipline of nursing.

Scholarship

Shulman [65] described a scholar as a consummate professional; an individual that continuously reflects on their practice while ensuring high standards, and who is open to advancing knowledge to others. Conversely, according to Boyer [12], a scholar was an academic whose primary focus was to conduct and publish research, while the practice of imparting and/or applying knowledge became secondary. The proliferation in the 1960s and 1970s of American higher education created a demand for academic professionals, thus *narrowing* the definition of scholarship that still exists in many institutions of higher learning [66]. Consequently, scholars were defined as academics whose priority was to conduct research and publish, in which research demonstrated scholarly work. The assumption was that imparting knowledge to students simply occurred and therefore, was not deemed to be scholarship [12]. The three basic tenets of scholarship are that the work is made public, it is peer reviewed, and that it can be reproduced by others as a means to advance knowledge [65–67]. Importantly, achieving scholarship is dependent on whether others are able to understand, and are agreeable to this knowledge [65]. Therefore, it would seem imperative that the skills and abilities associated with

effective teaching and learning practices, and ultimately knowledge delivery, be a priority in the academy.

The scholarship of discovery is recognized by the academy as the optimum pathway leading to new research funds and status. However, standard criteria is lacking in assessing the achievement of scholarship due to the disagreement around the definition of scholarship in general, and specifically, in teaching [72, 73 74, 70, 75, 30, 28, 61, 6].

Discourse around the restricted interpretation and acknowledgement of scholarship in higher education emerged from the seminal works of Boyer [12] and Glassick, Taylor Huber, and Maeroff [68]. Boyer [12] disputed how scholarship was evaluated and rewarded in higher education, according to this narrow definition. As illustrated by his expanded definition of scholarship, Boyer maintained that scholarship is found in all facets of academic life – discovery, teaching and learning, integration, and application of knowledge [57, 69]. Teaching involves the process of conveying knowledge through the scholarship of discovery, the scholarship of integration and the scholarship of application [12, 57]. Boyer's model consists of four separate yet overlapping facets of scholarship. This model has been embraced by both the academy and professional organizations, and adapted to discipline-specific contexts.

According to the Canadian Association of Schools of Nursing (CASN) [70] position statement on scholarship, scholarship is defined as the creation, affirmation, amalgamation, and/or implementation of knowledge intended to advance the discipline of nursing. Specifically, discovery as inquiry leading to new knowledge (original research that advances knowledge); teaching as pedagogical inquiry (discovery, integration, and application); application as discipline-specific knowledge expertise guiding professional practice (using new and synthesized knowledge in problem solving); and integration as the synthesis of knowledge. Further, scholarship involves critical reflection, discipline-specific knowledge expertise and innovative approaches to topics of interest under study [67, 71]. These statements expand on Boyer's [12] traditional definition of scholarship that included discovery, teaching, application, and integration. The question for me, related to the scholarship of teaching, is how will academic nurse educators effectively convey knowledge to nursing students without having a solid pedagogical foundation themselves?

The scholarship of teaching

As with scholarship, the difficulty in defining the scholarship of teaching has been cited throughout the literature by scholars from all disciplines [29, 44, 58, 66, 68, 69, 72–76]. Elaborating on the relationship between teaching, scholarly teaching, and the scholarship of teaching, Fincher and Work [67], described teaching as the development and delivery of activities designed to promote learning, while scholarly teaching advances teaching by connecting teaching with learning. Student learning is the outcome of both teaching and scholarly teaching [67]. Scholarly teaching requires ongoing revision of course materials including curriculum development and integration of published research into the course content, critical reflection, and mentoring students [77, 78].

A scholarly approach to teaching involves the application of educational theory and research to practice [58], in which the focus is on process rather than the product. The scholarship of teaching involves the understanding of effective teaching and learning practices that both enhance and expand learning opportunities outside of the traditional classroom experience [67, 77]; it is not a fourth distinct form of scholarship but may involve discovery, integration, or application [67]. However, confounding the problem is that Boyer's definition of the scholarship of teaching is not clear [13, 44, 67, 77, 79].

Based on this lack of consensus, McKinney [80] emphasized the need to clearly distinguish between teaching and scholarship. She elaborated further, adding that disciplinary differences impacted on how academic activities were defined in relation to scholarly activity and scholarship. Often, scholarly teaching and the scholarship of teaching are used interchangeably. However, in reality, good teaching or teaching excellence is being practiced rather than the scholarship of teaching [67]. While teaching and scholarly teaching facilitate learning, they do not constitute scholarship [77, 78]. Because of this lack of consensus, there is disagreement both between and within disciplines about accepted standards of scholarship and related activities.

Intense competing values within in the academy are responsible for institutional structures and practices to prevail in academic communities and within academic cultures, influencing the values and rewards systems [7, 81]. As a result, the scholar's role is designated as a researcher in contemporary higher education practice [29, 82], with very little regard to the scholar's ability as an effective teacher [58, 79, 83, 84].

Boyer [12] and Glassick et al. [71] advanced the theme that in narrowly defining scholarship as it related to discovery, priority consideration and ultimately, significant value was placed on research. Consequently, a reward system defined in totality by research and research-related activities, became the accepted benchmark for achieving scholarship [72, 85]. Therefore, for teaching to be acknowledged as an accepted form of scholarship, its practice must be recognized as discovery of new knowledge [66, 74]. Firstly, if the priority of doctoral education is to prepare researchers, and scholarship is defined

in terms of research, to what degree does doctoral preparation advantage academic nurse educators in their teaching roles? Secondly, do these quantifiable measures equate into teaching excellence in nursing education?

The scholarship of teaching is commonly regarded as *"the"* indicator of excellence in teaching, perpetuating the belief that excellent teachers possess extensive pedagogical knowledge [58]; a dilemma faced by many educational institutions in addressing the relationship between teaching and research [68, 75, 86–90]. Teaching excellence is generally measured through demonstrated outputs that include teaching awards, excellent evaluations, and scholarly publications [60, 75, 91, 92]. CASN's [72] description of achieving the scholarship of teaching (in nursing) validates this practice in which the scholarship of teaching is evidenced by peer reviewed presentations, publications, grants, and other related activities. Oermann [44] argues that there needs to be a broader perspective on how the scholarship of teaching is evaluated. For example, shifting the emphasis from the traditional forms of evidence of achievement to consideration for investigations on effective learning and teaching practices that promote student learning.

Pedagogical knowledge

Pedagogical knowledge is knowledge of the principles of effective teaching and learning [58, 93]; it is an essential component of learning to teach [42]. Pedagogical knowledge includes the skill to present discipline-specific content in a way that facilitates understanding and the ability to facilitate critical thinking and self-directed learning [58].

Due to a wide variation in student learning preferences, teachers must have the ability to effectively articulate and execute alternative forms of content delivery. This ability is founded on formal knowledge of pedagogical practices [73]. Pedagogical skills are essential because given the critical enquiry level of students, teachers are required to provide effective instruction for unanticipated and unfamiliar learning situations [73]. Pedagogical content knowledge is the link between content and pedagogical knowledge [93]. In higher education, discipline-specific knowledge and pedagogical knowledge are inextricably connected [43].

The modernization of health care, rapidly increasing technologies, globalization, and the worldwide shortage of nurses implicate the necessity for changes in how nurses practice, and, more importantly, how they are educated. It is imperative that health professionals possess a high level of proficiency in both pedagogical knowledge and teaching skills to effectively meet the demands of current teaching and the health care systems in providing quality education [39, 92]. Past pedagogical practices used to prepare proficient practitioners is outdated.

As a result, contemporary teaching and advanced pedagogical theory must inform each other [3, 94–96]. Regardless of the discipline, effective educators including nurse educators, require similar formal knowledge in adult education and pedagogical theory, providing the foundation for teaching practice.

However, due to current perceptions (both organizational and individual) around the value of teaching, and resultant lack of importance placed on teaching is evident throughout institutions of higher learning. For example, while the mission of most higher education institutions is identified as teaching, scholarship, and service, scholarship (research) is generally the priority [11]. It is imperative that agreement on the value of teaching be addressed at both the institutional level and specifically, within the multiple academic communities that constitute the institution.

What conditions influence the academic nurse educator role?

A PhD requirement, perpetuation of epistemic communities, and a doctoral supervisor's mentorship role in PhD programs have the potential to impact the nurse educator's role. These will be discussed in the following section.

PhD requirement

The origin of the word "doctorate" is from the Latin verb docere "to teach." Historically, the doctorate was acknowledged on the premise that teaching was both an honor and a rare opportunity [97]. Despite etymology, doctoral programs across disciplines are generally designed to provide a research-intensive training experience [11, 98, 99]. Doctoral education is intended to produce scholars who will advance the discipline. Doctoral students are given the opportunity to develop their expertise in order to carry out original research and scholarly inquiry that leads to new discipline-specific knowledge [11, 100]. However, for future faculty to be successful in the academy, graduate programs need to expand their educational approach beyond research training, to include all role responsibilities, and significantly, to recognize the importance of teaching [62].

A PhD is the academic requirement for most tenure-track nursing faculty positions, yet most notably recognized as a research degree [101–104]. Numerous professions have responded to the demand for increased academic ranking by requiring a doctoral degree [103, 105]. For the discipline of nursing to be acknowledged and accepted on the same level as other professions is the appeal of the PhD [105]. Fook [106] identified that when professional knowledge is validated according to patriarchal criteria, those professions achieve position and status among other professions. Accordingly, those individuals with a PhD designation are considered to be privileged scholars [65].

Preparation at the doctoral level is a requisite for academic nurse educators in order to make a contribution of new knowledge the body of nursing literature and to prepare future nurses [1, 3, 94]. Most doctoral programs in the United States identify the PhD as a research degree and the advanced practice degree as a DNP [107]. Interestingly, a PhD has become the both a required and preferred credential for a teaching position in many universities. Clearly, research has taken precedent over teaching.

However, heavy teaching loads are often assigned to new faculty that have recently completed their PhDs. In general, academic nurse educators are involved with teaching and teaching related-activities for an estimated 27 h on a weekly basis [108]. Significantly, while teaching generally occupies the majority of faculty time, it is a role for which they are not adequately prepared [11, 109]. Interestingly, the first doctoral degrees earned by nurses were in education with a teaching focus [6]. Formal teaching preparation should be fundamental to doctoral training because of the emphasis on job-related teaching that many doctorally prepared individuals encounter [46, 94, 110]. Thus, if we as academic nurse educators have valid rationale for requiring a PhD, then it is the responsibility of doctoral programs to provide the knowledge and skills necessary to educate nursing students, and ultimately future nurses [2, 11, 16, 55, 111–113].

Preparing professionals to conduct academic research that contributes to new knowledge is a well-established practice throughout PhD program curricula [7, 55, 114–118]. Although original research is central to both the academy and the public, the relationship between doctoral education and actual job expectations have become largely disconnected [18, 114, 116, 117, 119, 120]. This disconnection has brought into question the overemphasis on research and ensuing lack of teaching mentorship in doctoral programs [11, 18, 114]. Most doctoral programs lack a systematic approach to preparing doctoral students as educators for the transition to the faculty role. Most doctoral curricula do not include structured teaching experiences resulting in the lack of any formal pedagogical training [11]. Because curricular content is left to the discretion of individual institutions (and based on their perception of the value of teaching) there is no real commitment or recommendation on how best to educate future nursing professoriate [11].

In acknowledging that the capacity to carry out research is not synonymous with being an effective teacher, the AACN [9] recommended the need for formal pedagogical preparation including teaching practicums in doctoral programs.. Interestingly, a task force

report [99] identified teaching as a substantial component of many PhD graduates' roles, yet simultaneously
indicated that PhD preparation was directed towards a
research career. According to Brightman [2], PhD programs do not offer formal training in teaching because
of the traditional practices perpetuated by the academic
system in which research is overvalued and teaching
undervalued; thus, the emphasis of doctoral programs is
on learning research methods and discipline-specific
knowledge. How is the capacity to conduct research
equivalent to teaching proficiency?

Epistemic cultures

It is evident from the manner in which most professional communities function, that there is a great discrepancy as to the meaning of the scholarship of
teaching and related activities. The very organization of
these professional communities which are framed
around discipline-specific theoretical knowledge, clinical
practices and related reward systems lends itself to the
perpetuation of an epistemic culture [121]. Epistemic
cultures are self-contained in relation to the regulation
of membership, policies, procedures and practices [121–
123]. For example, groups of practitioners and groups of
researchers constitute different epistemic cultures. Importantly, these practices are implicated in widening the
theory practice divide [122, 124–126].

Specific knowledge processes and practices are embedded within these groups and reinforced by organizational
and/or institutional context that results in barriers that
impede the integration of knowledge across practices.
Within epistemic communities, discipline specific knowledge is both developed and sustained by the community
members, thus facilitating isolated and limited interactions both within, and outside of the community [123,
126]. Because embedded processes and practices within
epistemic communities are reinforced by organizational
and/or institutional context, there is a great likelihood
for barriers to develop, creating a challenge for success-
ful/effective involvement and/or participation from other
professional communities [123]. This is significant in relation to the current practices of the nursing profession
in seeking collaborative status within an interdisciplinary
context.

Knorr Cetina [122] described the focus of an epistemic
culture to establish the perpetuators of knowledge construction rather than of knowledge construction itself.
For example, one of the most common practices of academic epistemic cultures is to disseminate knowledge at
conferences attended by those within the same culture
which further reinforces existing practices and preferences [121]. Ultimately, professional silos are created
and maintained, facilitating isolated professional practices and encouraging competition among these

professions, otherwise known as tribalism [1, 121]. Due
to the continued reinforcement of traditional practices
within epistemic communities, an expanded view of
teaching must be both introduced and integrated into
the broader academic community [7]. The academic
nurse educator role has been significantly impacted by
the ability of epistemic cultures to both flourish and sustain their practices across academic and nursing communities, and within PhD program curricula.
Importantly, these long standing traditions within disciplines are highly influential on the focus for graduate
studies [81].

The role of mentoring in doctoral programs

Because the mentor-mentee relationship has received increased attention in relation to its critical role in graduate education, there has been a recent proliferation of
literature on the subject. The mentor-mentee relationship has advanced from simply seeing a student through
to degree completion to actually influencing a student's
professional and personal growth [49, 127–130]. Currently however, mentoring relationships in doctoral programs most often focus on the pursuit of scientific
inquiry, the transferring of knowledge, facilitating research activities and developing research partnerships
[131]. Because mentorship impacts significantly on the
development of the doctoral student, teaching, research,
and academic role responsibilities should be included
[56] as essential components of this relationship.

A mentor is described as a successful leader who ad-
vises, coaches, role models and initiates professional
connections [132]. The mentor is considered a role
model from which the mentee mirrors their mentor's
demonstrated behaviors and practices as part of their
own professional working identity [128, 132]. This psychosocial component of mentoring contributes positively
to building the mentee's level of confidence and ultimately, competence [128]. Importantly, mentoring perpet-
uates itself, in that graduates of doctoral programs who
experienced positive mentoring relationships have the
potential for, and the willingness to, mentor others
[133].

Responsibilities attached to modeling with doctoral
students includes both initiating and facilitating informal
and formal dialogue and structured, discipline-specific
learning sessions around professional roles and responsibilities [81]. The purpose of these activities are to support the student as they develop their own identity as
both a scholar and a member of a profession [81]. Additional responsibilities include advising students, evaluating or providing feedback to colleagues, administrative
duties, and developing new technology and approaches
to teaching [55].

Barnes and Austin [134] described mentorship as the development and maintenance of an effective working relationship throughout the entirety of a student's doctoral studies. Campbell et al. [116] described mentoring as a relationship between that mentor and mentee that is individualized to meet both the professional and personal goals of the student. Necessary activities to be included throughout this relationship would be to provide advice, information and constructive feedback, to ensure high research standards, to facilitate professional networks, and to introduce the student to discipline-specific practices. According to Barnes and Austin [134], research and research-related activities are both regarded and rewarded more favorably at research universities than teaching and teaching-related activities. Granting agencies policies, and teaching and research, publishing, and applying for external funding requirements were identified as limitations to mentoring by supervisors [134]. As a result, teaching mentorship was not regarded by doctoral supervisors as a responsibility of their role.

Discussion

The requirement of a doctoral (PhD preferred) degree for academic nurse educators, the perpetuation of epistemic communities, and the lack of effective mentoring in doctoral programs, have greatly impacted the roles and responsibilities of academic nurse educators. Specifically, the need to legitimize professional knowledge, reinforcing traditional practices within professional communities, and research only mentorship, do not meet the realistic expectations of the role of the academic nurse educator in the delivery of nursing education. However, the current literature identifies these same issues [8] of which there has been no substantial change.

Several key themes were identified from the review of the literature. The expectations of academic nurse educators in that they are required to deliver a quality education to nursing students, yet most have no formal preparation. A doctoral degree (PhD preferred) is the requirement for a position as an academic nurse educator in most university schools of nursing, with the major portion of a nurse educator's workload is teaching and related activities. However, a PhD is generally research-focused with no formal, organized pedagogical courses or experiences for doctoral students. There is an inability both across and within disciplines to reach consensus on what constitutes scholarship from which standards for excellence in teaching, scholarly teaching, and the teacher-scholar vary widely. Due to this lack of consensus in interpretation, interdisciplinary collaboration will continue to struggle. Institutional emphasis and ultimately the reward system, is based on research related productivity, while teaching is perceived to be secondary. Epistemic cultures within the university (academic) community further perpetuated the research versus teaching debate. Future discussion should

consider the *recommendations* of national nursing licensing bodies versus the desired future of nursing education based on realistic expectations. Rather than making recommendations of which institutions may choose or not choose to follow, there needs to be a consistent approach to the preparation of academic nurse educators. Other related issues include the lack of consensus regarding educational preparation and incongruences between the desired future of nursing education and current graduate nursing curricula. Might graduate programs offer streams in education, research, and/or clinical practice that are designed to meet specific roles and responsibilities?

However, several practices unique to nursing are implicated in the lack of progress in the delivery of profession nursing education. For example, registered nurses in practice, with or without a bachelor's and/or master's degree in nursing, may potentially supervise undergraduate students in a clinical and/or laboratory setting. Registered nurses with a PhD should supervise graduate students, however, this does not happen in practice areas where the practice *expert* does not have a doctoral degree. While the emphasis remains on educating specified numbers of undergraduate nursing students to meet the needs of health care systems, there is not the same focus on consistent preparation of graduate nursing students at the doctoral (PhD) level; these are the very individuals that the nursing profession needs to be effective educators. A particular gap in the literature is the number of research-based studies ($n = 33$) that were identified in the literature search. It is evident that there is a lack of evidence-based research and the need for studies to be undertaken regarding the most effective preparation for academic nurse educators.

Conclusion

This paper explored the state of the literature regarding doctoral (PhD) preparation of academic nurse educators; 139 works have been synthesized to meet the aims of the literature review. Given the current doctoral (PhD) curricula both in Canada and the United States, adequate preparation for the role of academic nurse educator in effectively meeting related responsibilities remains in jeopardy.

Abbreviations
AACN: American association of colleges of nursing; CASN: Canadian association of schools of nursing; DNP: Doctor of nursing practice; EdD: Doctorate of education; NLN: National league for nursing; PhD: Doctorate of philosophy

Acknowledgements
Dr. Patrick Renihan (doctoral supervisor); Department of Educational Administration, University of Saskatchewan.

Funding
Not applicable.

Authors' contributions

The author read and approved the final manuscript.

Competing interests

The author declares that she has no competing interests

References

1. Lancet Commissions. Health Professions for a New Century: Transforming Education to Strengthen Health Systems in an Interdependent World (Global Independent Commission Report). Boston: Elsevier; 2010. www.thelancet.com/journals/lancetarticle/PIIS0140-6736(10)61854-5/.
2. Brightman HJ. The need for teaching doctoral students how to teach. Int J Doctoral Stud. 2009;4:1–11.
3. Benner P, Sutphen M, Leonard V, Day L. Educating nurses. In: A call for radical transformation. San Francisco: Jossey-Bass; 2010.
4. Ketefian S, Redmond RW. A critical examination of developments in nursing doctoral education in the United States. Revista Latino-Americana de Enfermagem. 2015;23:363–71.
5. American Association of Colleges of Nursing. Faculty Shortages in Baccalaureate and Graduate Nursing Programs (White Paper). Washington: American Association of Colleges of Nursing; 2005. http://www.aacnnursing.org/News-Information/Position-Statements-White-Papers/Faculty-Shortages.
6. Edwardson SR. Matching standards and needs in doctoral education in nursing. J Prof Nurs. 2004;20:40-6.
7. McKinney M. Attitudinal and structural factors contributing to challenges in the work of the scholarship of teaching and learning. New Dir Inst Res. 2006;129:37–50.
8. Booth TL, Emerson CJ, Hackney MG, Souter S. Preparation of academic nurse educators. Nurse Educ in Prac. 2016;19:54–7.
9. American Association of Colleges of Nursing. The Preferred Vision of the Professoriate in Baccalaureate and Graduate Nursing Programs (Position Statement). Washington: American Association of Colleges of Nursing; 2008. http://www.aacnnursing.org/News-Information/Position-Statements-White-Papers/Preferred-Vision.
10. American Association of Colleges of Nursing. Futures Task Force Final Report. Washington: American Association of Colleges of Nursing; 2015a. http://www.aacnnursing.org/Portals/42/Publications/Futures-Task-Force-Final-Report.pdf.
11. Fiedler R, Degenhardt M, Systematic EJL. Preparation for teaching in a nursing doctor of philosophy program. J Prof Nurs. 2015;31:305–10.
12. Boyer EL. Scholarship reconsidered. Priorities of the professoriate. Princeton: Carnegie Foundation for the Advancement of Teaching/Princeton University Press; 1990.
13. Glanville I, Houde S. The scholarship of teaching: implications for nursing faculty. J Prof Nurs. 2004;20:7–14.
14. American Association of Colleges of Nursing. Advancing Health Care. Transformation: A New Era for Academic Nursing. Washington: American Association of Colleges of Nursing; 2016b. http://www.aacnnursing.org/Portals/42/Publications/Futures-Task-Force-Final-Report.pdf.
15. Canadian Association of Schools of Nursing. Doctoral Nursing Education in Canada (Position Statement). Ottawa: Canadian Association of Schools of Nursing; 2011. http://www.casn.ca/wp-content/uploads/2014/10/DoctoralEducation2011.pdf.
16. Leading Excellence and Innovation in Academic Nursing (Annual Report 2015). Washington: American Association of Colleges of Nursing; 2015b. http://www.aacnnursing.org/Portals/42/Publications/Annual-Reports/AnnualReport15.pdf.
17. American Association of Colleges of Nursing. Special survey on vacant faculty positions for academic year 2016–2017. Washington: American Association of Colleges of Nursing; 2016a. http://www.aacnnursing.org/Portals/42/News/Surveys-Data/vacancy16.pdf.
18. Agger CA, Oermann MH, Lynn MR. hiring and incorporating doctor of nursing practice-prepared nurse faculty into academic nursing programs. J Nurs Educ. 2014;53:439-46.
19. Ivey J. The preparation of nurse faculty: who should teach students? Topics Adv Prac eJ. 2007;7:1–2.
20. Siler B, Kleiner C. Novice faculty: encountering expectations in academia. J Nurs Educ. 2001;40:397–403.
21. National League for Nursing. The Preparation of Nurse Educators (Position Statement). New York: 2002. http://www.nln.org/docs/default-source/advocacy-public-policy/the-preparation-of-nurse-faculty.pdf?sfvrsn=0.
22. National League for Nursing. A Vision for Doctoral Preparation for Nurse Educators. New York: 2013. http://www.nln.org/docs/default-source/about/nln-vision-series-%28position-statements%29/nlnvision-6.pdf?sfvrsn=4.
23. Lewallen LP, Kohlenberg E. (2011). Preparing the nurse scientist for academia and industry. Nurs Educ Perspect. 2011;32:22–5.
24. Whittmore R, Knafl K. The integrative review: updated methodology. J Adv Nurs. 2005;52:546–53.
25. Johnson-Crawley N. An alternative framework for teacher preparation in nursing. J Contin Educ Nurs. 2004;35:34–43.
26. Matthews KE, Lodge JM, Bosanquet A. (2012). Early career academic perceptions, attitudes and professional development activities: questioning the teaching and research gap to further academic development. Int J Acad Dev. 2012;19:112–24.
27. Rossetti J, Fox PG. Factors related to successful teaching by outstanding professors: an interpretative study. J Nurs Educ. 2009;48:11–6.
28. Kreber C. Teaching excellence, teaching expertise, and the scholarship of teaching. Innov High Educ. 2002b;27:5–23.
29. Nicholls G. The challenge to scholarship: rethinking learning, teaching and research. London: Routledge; 2005.
30. Kreber C. Controversy and consensus on the scholarship of teaching. Stud High Educ. 2002a;27:151–67.
31. Norris SP. The pale of consideration when seeking sources of teaching expertise. Am J Educ. 2000;108:167–95.
32. Korthagen F, Loughran J, Lunenburg M. Teaching teachers – studies into the expertise of teacher educators. Teach Teach Educ. 2005;21:107–15.
33. Lindeman CA. The future of nursing education. J Nurs Educ. 2000;39:5–12.
34. Martinez K. Academic induction for teacher educators. Asia Pac J Teach Educ. 2008;36:35–51.
35. Oermann MH, Lynn MR, Agger CA. Hiring intentions of directors of nursing programs related to DNP-and PhD-prepared faculty and role of faculty. J Prof Nurs. 2016;32:173–7.
36. Cochran-Smith M. Learning and unlearning: the education of teacher educators. Teach Teach Educ. 2003;19:5–28.
37. Anderson JK. An academic fairy tale. A metaphor of the work-role transition from clinician to academician. Nurse Educ. 2008;33:79–82.
38. Chandramohan B, Fallows S. Interdisciplinary learning and teaching in higher education: theory and practice. New York: Routledge; 2009.
39. Diekelmann N. Teaching the practitioners of care. New pedagogies for the health professions. Madison: The University of Wisconsin Press; 2003.
40. Starr LJ, deMartini A. Addressing the needs of doctoral students as academic practitioners: a collaborative inquiry on teaching in higher education. Can. J High Educ. 2015;45:68–83.
41. Love Stowell SM, Churchill AC, Hund AK, Kelsey KC, Redmond MD, Seiter SA, Borger NN. Transforming graduate training in STEM education. Bull Ecol Soc Am. 2015;96:317–23.
42. Kreber C, Castledon H, Erfani N, Wright T. Self-regulated learning about university teaching: an exploratory study. Teach High Educ. 2005;10:75–97.
43. Murray J. Re-addressing the priorities: new teacher educators and induction into higher education. Eur J Teach Educ. 2005;28:67–85.
44. Oermann MH. Defining and assessing the scholarship of teaching in nursing. J Prof Nurs. 2014;30:370–5.
45. Darling-Hammond L, Chung R, Frelow F. Variation in teacher preparation. J Teach Educ. 2002;53:286–302.
46. Kwiram AL. Time for reform? In: Golde CM, Walker GE, editors. Envisioning the future of doctoral education. San Francisco: Jossey- Bass; 2006. p. 144–66.
47. Nehls N, Barber G, Rice E. Pathways to the PhD in nursing: an analysis of similarities and differences. J Prof Nurs. 2016;32:163–72.

48. Hoessler C, Godden L. The visioning of policy and the hope of implementation: support for a graduate student's teaching at a Canadian institution. Can. J High Educ. 2015;45:83–101.

49. Kenney N, Watson G, Watton C. Exploring the context of Canadian graduate student teaching certificates in university teaching. Can. J High Educ. 2014;44:1–19.

50. Parker MA, Ashe D, Boersma J, Hicks R, Bennett V. Good teaching starts here: applied learning at the graduate teaching assistant institute. Can. J High Educ. 2015;45:84–110.

51. Austin AE. Preparing the next generation of faculty. J High Educ. 2002a;73:94–122.

52. Morris AH, Faulk DR. Transformative learning in nursing. New York: Springer; 2012.

53. Schreiner C. (2007). The influence of culture on clinical nurses transitioning into the faculty role. Nurs Educ Pers. 2007;28:145–9.

54. Schwetter DJ, Hamilton J, Sawatsky JV. Exploring professional development needs of educators in health sciences professions. J Dental Educ. 2015;79:113–23.

55. Austin AE (2002b). Creating a bridge to the future: preparing new faculty to face changing expectations in a shifting context. Rev Higher Educ. 2002b; 26:119-144.

56. Fang D, Benash GD, Arietti R. Identifying barriers and facilitators for PhD nursing students. J Prof Nurs. 2016;32:193–201.

57. Gardner JC, CB MG, Moeller SE. Applying the teacher scholar model in the school of business. Am J Bus Educ. 2010;3:85–9.

58. Kreber C, Cranton PA. Exploring the scholarship of teaching. J High Educ. 2000;71:476–95.

59. Marentic Pozarnik B, Lavric A. Fostering the quality of teaching and learning by developing the "neglected half" of university teachers' competencies. Cent Educ Policy Stud J. 2015;5:79–93.

60. DeCourcy E. Defining and measuring teaching excellence in higher education in the 21st century. Coll Q. 2015;18:1–6.

61. Johnson-Farmer B, Frem M. Teaching excellence: what great teachers teach us. J Prof Nurs. 2009;25:267–72.

62. Adams KA. What colleges & universities want in new faculty (report). New York; 2011. http://www.aacu.org/pff/PFFpublications/what_colleges_want/index.cfm.

63. Diekelmann, N. (2005). Keeping current: on persistently questioning our teaching practice. J Nurs Educ 2005;44:485-488.

64. MacMillan K. Proceedings of a think tank on the future of undergraduate nursing in Canada. Halifax: Dalhousie University School of Nursing; 2013.

65. Shulman LS. Inventing the future. In: Hutchings P, ed. Opening lines: Approaches to the scholarship of teaching and learning. Menlo Park: The Carnegie Foundation for the Advancement of Teaching; 2000.

66. Gubbins PO. (2014). The scholarship of teaching and learning: an opportunity for clinical faculty members in academic pharmacy and other health professions to develop a program of scholarship. Int J Scholarsh Teach Learn. 2014;8:1–16.

67. Fincher RE, Work JA. Perspectives on the scholarship of teaching. Med Educ. 2006;40:293–5.

68. Chalmers D. Progress and challenges in the recognition and reward of the scholarship of teaching in higher education. High Educ Res Dev. 2011;30: 25–38.

69. O'Meara KA, Rice RE. Faculty priorities reconsidered: rewarding multiple forms of scholarship. San Francisco: Jossey-Boss; 2005.

70. Canadian Association of Schools of Nursing. Scholarship among nursing faculty (Position Statement). Ottawa: 2013. http://www.casn.ca/wp-content/uploads/2014/10/ScholarshipInNursingNov2013ENFINALmm.pdf.

71. Glassick CE, Taylor Huber M, Maeroff GI. Scholarship assessed: evaluation of the professoriate. San Francisco: Jossey-Bass; 1997.

72. Hatch T. Into the classroom: developing the scholarship of teaching and learning. San Francisco: Jossey-Bass; 2006.

73. Shulman LS. The wisdom of practice: essays on teaching, learning, and learning to teach. San Francisco: Jossey-Bass; 2004.

74. Trigwell K, Martin E, Benjamin J, Prosser M. Scholarship of teaching: a model. High Educ Res Dev. 2000;19:155–68.

75. Vardi I, Quinn R. Promotion and the scholarship of teaching and learning. High Educ Res Dev. 2011;30:39–49.

76. Williams K. Troubling the concept of the 'academic profession' in 21st century higher education. High Educ. 2008;56:533–44.

77. Acorn S, Osborne M. Scholarship in nursing: current view. Can J Nurs Leadersh. 2013;26:24–9.

78. Allen MN, Field PA. Scholarly teaching and scholarship of teaching: noting the difference. Int J Nurs Educ Scholarsh. 2005;2:1–13.

79. Kreber C. Furthering the "theory debate" in the scholarship of teaching: a proposal based on MacIntyre's account of practices. Can. J High Educ. 2015; 45:99–115.

80. McKinney K. The scholarship of teaching and learning in and across the disciplines. Bloomington: Indiana University Press; 2013.

81. Austin AE, McDaniels M. Using doctoral education to prepare faculty to work within Boyer's four domains of scholarship. New Dir Institutional Res. 2006;129:51–65.

82. Sullivan WH, Rosin MS. A new agenda for higher education. Stanford: The Carnegie Foundation for the Advancement of Teaching; 2008.

83. Grace PJ, Willis DG, Roy C Sr, Jones DA. Profession at the crossroads: a dialogue concerning the preparation of nurse scholars and leaders. Nurs Outlook. 2016;64:61–70.

84. Kuh GD, Chen D, Nelson Laird TF. Why teacher-scholars matter. Lib Educ. 2007;(Fall):40–5.

85. Smeltzer SC, Cantrell MA, Sharts-Hopko NC, Heverly MA, Jenkinson A, Nthenge S. Assessment of impact on teaching demands on research productivity among doctoral nursing program faculty. J Prof Nurs. 2015;32:180–92.

86. Brew A. Teaching and research: new relationships and their implications for inquiry-based teaching and learning in higher education. High Educ Res Dev. 2003;22(1):3–18.

87. Carter LM, Brockerhoff-Macdonald B. The continuing education of faculty as teachers at a mid-sized Ontario university. Can J Scholarsh Teach Learn. 2011;2:1–12.

88. Chen CY. A study showing research has been valued over teaching in higher education. J Scholarsh Teach Learn. 2015;15:15–32.

89. Malcolm M. A critical evaluation of recent progress in understanding the role the research-teaching link in higher education. High Educ. 2014;67:289–301.

90. Meacham, J. Our doctoral programs are failing our undergraduate students. Lib Educ. 2002;Summer:22–27.

91. Zeichner K. Becoming a teacher educator: a personal perspective. Teach Teach Educ. 2005;21:117–24.

92. Ironside PM. Reforming doctoral curricula in nursing: creating multiparadigmatic, multipedagogical researchers. J Nurs Educ. 2006;45:51–3.

93. Paulsen MB. The relation between research and the scholarship of teaching. New Dir Teach Learn. 2001;86:19–29.

94. Bartels JE. Preparing nursing faculty for baccalaureate-level and graduate-level nursing programs: role preparation for the academy. J Nurs Educ. 2007;46:154–8.

95. Ironside PM. Teaching thinking and reaching the limits of memorization: enacting new pedagogies. J Nurs Educ. 2005;44:441–9.

96. Tanner CA. Learning to teach: an introduction to teacher talk; new pedagogies for nursing. J Nurs Educ. 2002;41:95–6.

97. Winter R, Griffiths M, Green K. The 'academic' qualities of practice: what are the criteria for a practice-based PhD? Stud High Educ. 2000;25:25–37.

98. Bass H. Developing scholars and professionals: the case of mathematics. In: Golde CM, Walker GE, editors. Envisioning the future of doctoral education. San Francisco: Jossey-Bass; 2006. p. 101–19.

99. American Association of Colleges of Nursing. Future of the Research-Focused Doctoral Program in Nursing: Pathways to Excellence (Report). Washington: 2010. http://www.uab.edu/nursing/home/images/AACN_doctoral_task_force_report.pdf.

100. Wood MJ, Giovannetti P, Ross-Kerr JC. The Canadian PhD in nursing (discussion paper). Ottawa: 2004. http://www.casn.ca.

101. American Association of Colleges of Nursing. Moving the Conversation Forward: Advancing Higher Education in Nursing (Annual Report). Washington: 2013. http://www.studylib.net/doc/18908165/2013-annual-report—american-association-ofcolleges-of-nursing.

102. Brar K, Boschma G, McCuaig F. The development of nurse practitioner preparation beyond the Master's level: what is the debate about? Int J Nurs Educ Scholarsh. 2010;7:1–15.

103. Jackson D, Peters K, Andrews S, Salamonson Y, Halcomb, EJ. "If you haven't got a PhD, you're not going to get a job": the PhD as a hurdle to continuing academic employment in nursing. Nurse Educ Today. 2011;31: 340-4.

104. Loomis JA, Willard B, Cohen J. Difficult Professional Choices: Deciding Between the PhD and the DNP in Nursing. Online J Issues Nurs. 2006;28:1-16. http://www.doctorsofnursingpractice.org/wp-content/uploads/2014/08/Loomis2006_001.pdf.

105. Kirkman S, Thompson D, Watson R, Stewart S. Are all doctorates equal or are some "more equal than others"? An examination of which ones should be offered by schools of nursing. Nurse Educ Prac. 2007;7:61–6.

106. Fook J. Linking theory, practice, and research. Crit Soc Work. 2001;2001:1–4.

107. Minnick AF, Norman LD, Donaghey B, Fisher LW, IM MK. Defining and describing capacity issues in US doctoral nursing research programs. Nurs Outlook. 2010;58:36–43.

108. National League for Nursing. How nurse educators spend their time. Nurs Educ Perspect. 2007;28:296–7.

109. Apold S. The Doctor of Nursing Practice: Looking back, moving forward. J Nurse Pract. 2008;4:101–7.

110. Bergner J, Lin L, Tepalagui NK. Teacher training for PhD students: recommendations for content and delivery. eJ Bus Educ Scholarsh Teach. 2015;9:61–9.

111. Cooley SS, DeGagne JC. Transformative experience: developing competence in novice nursing faculty. J Nurs Educ. 2015;55:96–100.

112. Dreifeurst KT, AM MN, Weaver MT, Broome ME, Burke Drauker C, Fedko AS. Exploring the pursuit of doctoral education by nurses seeking or intending to stay in faculty roles. J Prof Nurs. 2016;32:202–12.

113. Nyquist JD. The PhD: A tapestry of change for the 21st century. Change. 2002;34:13–20.

114. Austin AE, Connolly MR, Colbeck CL. Strategies for preparing integrated faculty: the Center for the Integration of research, teaching, and learning. New Dir Teach Learn. 2008;113:69–81.

115. Benigni V. Developing the teacher scholar…a call for the new professoriate. The graduate teaching academy. Journalism Mass Commun Educator. 2007; 61:358–60.

116. Campbell SP, Fuller AK, Patrick DA. Looking beyond research in doctoral education. Front Ecol Environ. 2005;3:153–60.

117. Nyquist JD, Woodford BJ, Rogers DL. Re-envisioning the PhD: a challenge for the twenty first century. In: Wulff DH, Austin AE, editors. Paths to the professoriate: strategies for enriching the preparation of future faculty. San Francisco: Jossey-Bass; 2004. p. 194–216.

118. Walker K, Duff J, Campbell S. Cummings E. Doctoral education for nurses today: the PhD or professional doctorate? Aus J Adv Nurs. 2016;34:60–9.

119. Diezmann C, Watters JJ. The knowledge base of subject matter experts in teaching: a case of a professional scientist as a beginning teacher. Int J Sci Math Educ. 2015;13:1517–37.

120. Gaff JG. The disconnect between gradiuate education and the realities of faculty work: A review of recent research. Lib Educ. 2002;88:6-13.

121. Cronin B. Scholarly communication and epistemic cultures. J Acad Librariansh. 2003:1–24.

122. Knorr Cetina K. Culture in global societies: knowledge cultures and epistemic cultures. Interdiscip Sci Rev. 2007;32:361–75.

123. Mork BE, Aanestad M, Hanseth O, Grisot M. Conflicting epistemic cultures and obstacles for learning across communities of practice. Knowl Process Manag. 2008;15:12–23.

124. Findlow S. Higher education change and professional academic identity in newly'academic disciplines' & the case of nurse education. High Educ. 2012; 63:117–33.

125. Georges JM. An emerging discourse toward epistemic diversity in nursing. Adv Nurs Sci. 2003;26:44–52.

126. Van De Ven AH, Johnson PE, Knowledge. For theory and practice. Acad Manag Rev. 2006;31:802–21.

127. Hall LE, Burns LD. Identity development and mentoring in doctoral education. Harvard. Educ Rev. 2009;79:49–70.

128. Johnson TC, Keller RH, Linnhoff S. Mentoring in doctoral programs and preparedness of early career marketing educators. Acad Edu Leadersh J. 2014;18:15–22.

129. Paglis LL, Green SG, Bauert T. Does advisor mentoring add value? A longitudinal study of mentoring and doctoral student outcomes. Res Higher Educ. 2006;47:451–76.

130. Rose GL. Group differences in graduate students concepts of the ideal mentor. Res High Educ. 2005;46:53–80.

131. Baxley SM, Ibitayo KS, Bond ML. Mentoring Today's nurses. Sigma Theta Tau International: Indianapolis; 2014.

132. Grossman SC. Mentoring in nursing: a dynamic and collaborative process. New York: Springer Publishing Company; 2013.

133. Noonan MJ, Black R, Ballinger R. Peer and faculty mentoring in doctoral education: definitions, experiences, and expectations. Int J Teach Learn High Educ. 2007;19:251–62.

134. Barnes BJ, Austin AE. The role of doctoral advisors: a look at advising from the advisor's perspective. Innov High Educ. 2008;33:297–315.

135. Bok D. We must prepare ph.D. students for the complicated art of teaching. Chron High Educ. 2013;(November 11):1–7.

136. Bogo M. Doing' teaching. Preparing doctoral students to become stewards of their disciplines through teaching. In: Forum; 2010.

137. Kalb KA, O'Conner-Von SK, Schipper LH, Watkins AK, Yetter DM. Educating leaders in nursing: faculty perspectives. Int J Nurs Educ Scholarsh. 2012;9:1–13.

138. Shulman LS, Golde CM, Conklin Bueschel A, Garabedian KJ. Reclaiming education's doctorates: A critique and a proposal. Educ Res. 2006;April: 25–32.

139. Bell-Ellison B, Dedrick RF. What do doctoral students value in their ideal mentor? Res High Educ. 2008;49:555–67.

4

Lessons learnt in recruiting disadvantaged families to a birth cohort study

Amit Arora[1,2,3,4*], Narendar Manohar[1], Dina Bedros[5], Anh Phong David Hua[5], Steven Yu Hsiang You[5], Victoria Blight[6], Shilpi Ajwani[2,5], John Eastwood[7,8,9,10] and Sameer Bhole[2,5]

Abstract

Background: Dental decay in early childhood can be prevented by a model based on shared care utilising members of primary care team such as Child and Family Health Nurses (CFHNs) in health promotion and early intervention. The aims of this study were to identify the facilitators and barriers faced by CFHNs in recruiting research participants from disadvantaged backgrounds to a birth cohort study in South Western Sydney, Australia.

Methods: Child and Family Health Nurses recruited mothers-infants dyads ($n = 1036$) at the first post-natal home visit as part of Healthy Smiles Healthy Kids Study, an ongoing birth cohort study in South Western Sydney. The nurses ($n = 19$) were purposively selected and approached for a phone based in-depth semi-structured interview to identify the challenges faced by them during the recruitment process. Interviews were audio-recorded, subsequently transcribed verbatim and analysed by thematic analysis.

Results: The nurses found the early phase of parenting was an overwhelming stage for parents as they are pre-occupied with more immediate issues such as settling and feeding a newborn. They highlighted some key time-points such as during pregnancy and/or around the time of infant teething may be more appropriate for recruiting families to dental research projects. However, they found it easier to secure the family's attention by offering incentives, gifts and invitations for free oral health services. The use of web-based approaches and maintaining regular contact with the participants was deemed crucial for long-term research. Cultural and linguistic barriers were seen as an obstacle in recruiting ethnic minority populations and the need for cultural insiders in the research team was deemed important to resolve the challenges associated with conducting research with diverse cultures. Finally, nurses identified the importance of inter-professional collaboration to provide easier access to recruiting research participants.

Conclusions: This study highlighted the need for multiple time-points and incentives to facilitate recruitment and retention of disadvantaged communities in longitudinal research. The need for cultural insiders and inter-professional collaboration in research team are important to improve research participation.

Keywords: Oral health, Longitudinal research, Cohort study, Nurses, Children, Early childhood caries

Background

Dental caries (tooth decay) is one of the most common multifactorial chronic disease affecting children [1]. When it occurs in children aged less than 6 years, it is referred to as Early Childhood Caries (ECC) which is defined as the "presence of one or more decayed (non-cavitated or cavitated lesions), missing (due to caries), or filled tooth surfaces in any primary (baby) tooth" [2]. ECC is a serious oral health problem which is widespread in many populations across the world and especially prevalent in socially disadvantaged groups [3, 4]. The most recent Australian National Child Oral Health Survey 2012–2014 reported that over 34% of 5–6-year-olds had one or more decayed, missing (due to caries) and filled primary teeth [5]. The problem of ECC is not limited to Australia, as similar findings have also been observed internationally [6].

The effects of ECC extend beyond the primary dentition and have significant comorbidities – increased likelihood

* Correspondence: a.arora@westernsydney.edu.au
[1]School of Science and Health, Western Sydney University, 24.2.97 Campbelltown Campus, Locked Bag 1797, Penrith, NSW 2751, Australia
[2]Sydney Dental Hospital and Oral Health Services, Sydney Local Health District, Surry Hills, NSW, Australia
Full list of author information is available at the end of the article

to have poor oral health in adulthood; stress on the child's family; repeated prescription of antibiotics, severe pain, sepsis, and sleep loss; increased financial burden; poor quality of life; and often a burden on the healthcare system as in severe cases or in non-compliant children treatment under a general anaesthetic is necessary [7]. There is ample evidence to show that preventive oral health messages provide a proven health benefit [8]. The success of oral health promotion interventions require appropriate health behaviours to be established early in life; hence, there is a need to focus on preventative advice to pregnant women [9] and parents of young children [4, 10]. However, visits to an oral health professional in early childhood are often limited [11] and most visits are either to a general medical practitioner or to a Child and Family Health Nurse (CFHN) [12, 13].

In the recent years, most Australian states and territories support an early childhood oral health program that links oral health professionals with general health professionals [14, 15]. Several developments have taken place in NSW since the mid-2000s in integrating the shared care model for oral health promotion. Since 2007, early childhood oral health training has been available to all health professionals including CFHNs [12] and more recently, the Midwifery Initiated Oral Health program has been introduced in South Western Sydney and Western Sydney [9, 16]. These recent developments are major achievements in early intervention strategies and utilising the shared care model approach is prudent for improving oral health outcomes.

Longitudinal research is an important approach in uncovering potential solutions for ECC. Prospective cohort studies, although time consuming and expensive to implement, offer good scientific evidence in understanding the disease mechanisms, however, recruitment and retention of research participants may be problematic and can significantly impact the study findings. Insufficient recruitment could make a study underpowered and study sample attrition could affect the validity of the study findings. The ability of a study to establish and maintain its participants increases the validity of the study as it reduces problems associated with selection bias and non-response [17]. Numerous obstacles pose as a threat to recruitment and retention of research participants. These may include issues such as lack of cultural sensitivity towards participants, lack of trust with healthcare system, concerns of participants being a "guinea pig", limited literacy skills of participants, and personal commitments of research participants [18–22].

The literature on challenges with recruiting and retaining research participants is primarily from the United States [18–22], with limited information from Australia, particularly South Western Sydney as this is an ethnically diverse region with high levels of social disadvantage [23]. Furthermore, birth cohort studies are rare in dentistry and to the best of our knowledge none of the longitudinal dental research projects have discussed the challenges in recruiting research participants. The aims of this study therefore, were to identify the facilitators and barriers faced by CFHNs in recruiting research participants from disadvantaged backgrounds to a birth cohort study in South Western Sydney.

Methods

Study background

This qualitative study is nested within an ongoing birth cohort study, 'Healthy Smiles Healthy Kids' (HSHK), investigating the relationship between early childhood feeding patterns, oral health and obesity among preschool children in South Western Sydney [24]. For this project, CFHNs recruited mother-infant dyads at the first post-natal home visit at 4 to 6 weeks, as this is the primary point of community-based health professional contact for newborn children and their carers/parents [12, 13]. A total of 1500 mothers who gave birth to infants between October 2009 and February 2010 in public hospitals located under the catchment of the former Sydney South West Area Health Service (now separated as Sydney and South-Western Sydney Local Health Districts) were approached to be a part of this study. At the first post-natal visit, CFHNs explained the project to the mothers and obtained a written informed consent. If requested, the nurses were able to arrange for interpreter services for non-English speaking parents and language appropriate written materials were provided for the major ethnic groups living in this region (i.e. Vietnamese, Arabic, Assyrian, Cambodian, Cantonese, Hindi, Mandarin, and Samoan).

Study sample

Nurse Unit Managers in the former South-Western Sydney Area Health Service were contacted to obtain details of the CFHNs who could represent all geographical sectors of South Western Sydney. The CFHNs ($n = 21$) were purposively selected and invited to participate in this qualitative study. Selection was based on ethnicity, years of experience, and geographical location. They were given an information pack that provided details of the nested study, a written consent form, and a participation information statement. All nurses initially agreed to participate but two could not be contacted for an interview despite repeated attempts and were therefore excluded. It has previously been outlined that for qualitative research with a homogenous sample such as in this study, six to eight interviews are sufficient to reach data saturation [25]. This study involved interviewing a larger number of participants ($n = 19$), with a wide variation in participant characteristics in order to enrich our data quality [26].

In-depth interviews

In-depth semi-structured interviews were conducted by two researchers (DB and AA) to record views of CFHNs on the facilitators and barriers they encountered in recruiting research participants for the HSHK study. The interviews were phone-based as the study sample was geographically dispersed [27]. The researchers used an interview guide (Table 1) that covered topics relevant to the recruitment process. The development of inter-view guide was informed by a comprehensive review of the literature to identify key areas of interest [18–22]. The draft interview guide was piloted with two CFHNs. Each interview lasted about 30–45 min and we continued inter-viewing CFHNs until no new topics emerged i.e. data reached saturation. All interviews were audio-recorded and transcribed *verbatim*. Interview debriefing between the two researchers (DB and AA) was consistently under-taken to evaluate the data collection, summarise the main findings and prepare for subsequent interviews.

Data analysis

To enhance the rigour and credibility of our research, four researchers (AA, APDH, SYHY, DB) were involved in every phase of data analysis, including transcript coding, data dis-play and interpretation. The four researchers coded the transcripts individually: two using manual coding, and two using NVivo 9 (QSR International, Cambridge, MA, USA) software, and the findings were compared. A consensus was then agreed upon between the four researchers and advice was sought from a fifth coder (NM) when disagree-ments arose. The codes were then examined through an iterative process and regrouped into four broad themes. A thematic analysis approach was used, as this method has been shown to be effective in "identifying, analysing and reporting patterns within qualitative data" [28].

Ethics

Ethics approvals for this study were obtained from the former Sydney South West Area Health Service – RPAH Zone (ID number X08–0115), Liverpool Hospital, University of Sydney, and Western Sydney University. All participants signed a written consent form to be a part of this study. This research has been conducted in full accordance with the World Medical Association Declaration of Helsinki. Written consent was obtained from all study participants.

Results

Table 2 shows the characteristics of the study participants. Most of the CFHNs were aged 40 years or older, had a postgraduate diploma or a Masters degree and had over 10 years of professional work experience. Four themes emerged from the data. These were: participant's concern of receiving overwhelming information during early stages of parenthood, strategies to improve research participa-tion, cultural barriers and involvement with research, and the emphasis for inter-professional collaboration.

Theme one: Overwhelming information during early stages of parenthood

The majority of nurses reported that one of the difficulties in recruiting participants was that parents felt overwhelmed with information, particularly during the first visit thus making the recruitment challenging.

> *"We get around to giving them all the other information then we tell them to be part of a research study I think they've had enough."* (Nurse #2)

The nurses believed that one of key reasons for fam-ilies to not join research projects in early stages of par-enting is due to the fact that many parents have other important issues on their minds during the first few weeks of the baby's birth. Matters directly related to child well-being play a major significance in the early stages of parenting compared to other matters. Further-more, the nurses were worried that they did not want to

Table 1 Semi-Structured interview questions

- What are some facilitating factors you found in recruiting families with newborn children?
- What barriers did you find recruiting families of newborn children?
- What do you think can be done to improve the recruitment process?
- How can we motivate potential participants that are not interested to participate in the study?
- Is there anything we can change to make the program more successful, especially for people in disadvantaged areas?
- Can you explain if the study recruitment caused any problems for you?

Table 2 Demographic characteristics of the study participants (*n* = 19)

Characteristic	N
Age (in years)	
30–39	3
40–49	9
50+	7
Highest education qualification	
Bachelors	4
Postgraduate Diploma	9
Masters	6
Nursing experience (years)	
1–9	7
10–19	9
20–29	3

add additional stress and commitments to the families during the initial stages of parenthood.

"They (parents) still have sleeping/settling issues or breastfeeding or bottle feeding issues and they may not necessarily be taking it in at that point." (Nurse #7)

"Probably it's not very appropriate on the first visit because we have to give them so many other things. When we first see them in the first 2 weeks they're not ready, their head's not really there and they can't take in too much information." (Nurse #14)

They also reported that families that were undergoing difficult circumstances prioritise and focus their time on other significant issues before undertaking more obligations.

"We only see two families a day with children from zero to 3 years of age and up to 20 percent of them have significant mental health issues. They are so overwhelmed that they want to talk about other stuff." (Nurse #9)

Theme two: Strategies to improve research participation
The nurses thought that early days of infancy are tough periods to recruit families for research projects. However, they highlighted that it may be wise to recruit mothers during pregnancy or around the time of infant teething.

"For a dental project, we could involve families when the baby is four or five months old. That's when the mums usually ask about teeth as the baby starts drooling and shows some signs of teething" (Nurse #1)

The nurses highlighted that the families were more inclined to participate in research studies if there were incentives for them.

"They (families) are keen if there is something free they are getting out of it" (Nurse #5)

The nurses reported that incentives could include anything from free telephone helpline on health education to free goods. In particular, they reported that things that were relevant to new parents are of importance as they would enjoy receiving it.

"Participants found out that they get health information and freebies such as sipper cup, teething ring, free toothpaste, toothbrushes and dental care - they are happy for that!" (Nurse #8)

The nurses highlighted that strategies need to be put into place to retain participants for long-term research. In general, it was suggested that getting multiple contact details of the families was crucial for research in disadvantaged areas. It was further suggested that linking the research to their hospital records will be a useful way to retain participants.

"You should take two numbers. Maybe even two mobile numbers as these days both parents have mobile numbers, or maybe say grandmother's number. This way you can send them reminders and could keep in contact with them even if they move homes or change numbers." (Nurse #17)

"You should link it to their medical and /or dental records. That way you could possibly keep updates if they move homes or change numbers". (Nurse #11)

Some nurses even suggested that sending newsletters to participants or perhaps creating a website for the research would be useful so that participants can keep themselves updated and be more involved with the project.

"You know a lot of times research fails as it becomes tough to maintain the interest of the participants. I think sending newsletters say every 3-6 months giving them updates and/or maybe creating a website keeps them engaged". (Nurse #14)

Theme three: Cultural barriers and involvement with research
The nurses found that the difficulties in recruiting participants were largely due to interpretational and cultural barriers. It was noted that the information on research should be communicated in a clear and concise manner so that it could be easily understood by participants of linguistically diverse backgrounds. The nurses recognised that the cohort study could potentially benefit a lot of families especially those from ethnic minorities.

"The document needs to be clear, simple and short. There are quite a few people who need interpreting." (Nurse #13)

"It would be good to have them in other languages... It seems to be working with a lot of Chinese or Indian families" (Nurse #10)

Some nurses pointed out that it is important to resolve 'cross-cultural differences' in research projects. They believed that it might be easier to recruit and retain participants if members of the research team are from the same cultural background to that of the research participants.

They believed that this might assist in gaining trust of the participants.

> *"It is a new environment for them (migrants), and some of them are so reliant on their families back home. I think it is good they know the research team and if they are from similar cultural background, they may see them as more trustworthy. Not just feel that I am trying to sell anything to them!"* (Nurse #5)

A few nurses highlighted that migrants are reluctant to participate in research due to the mistrust in health care system. They felt that migrants from developing countries had bad experiences in their home country and lose the trust in the health care system.

> *"They (new migrants) are unaware of the health care system in Australia. It's very different from their home country and a lot of them believe the system is corrupt. They think they are being treated as guinea pigs."* (Nurse #11)

The nurses also noticed a general trend during recruitment of participants for the research study. They reported that at times it became difficult for them to convince families of ethnic minority groups to be a part of the research as they didn't realise the benefit of research.

> *"Usually it takes a lot longer to convince non-English speaking families and some of my lower side families (low socio-economic) do not see the personal benefit."* (Nurse #15)

Theme four: The emphasis for inter-professional collaboration

The nurses recognised the issue that young children do not visit an oral health professional unless they are in pain and there was a need for oral health promotion at an early stage. The nurses were happy to collaborate in the research study as dental disease in young children affected their working lives. However, there was a strong case for the need to arrange more appropriate time to facilitate recruitment and reduce the burden on nurses. The nurses stressed the fact that they have overwhelming amount of paperwork that needs to be completed at the first post-natal visit and that sharing information about research adds more to their workload.

> *"At the first visit, we (the nurses) have so much stuff to do. It is really a challenge to recruit at the first visit as we don't get enough time to talk about everything".* (Nurse #8)

Some nurses found that the process of recruiting parents was a lot of work, as they had to discuss the research study with the family and take an informed consent. Although this was a daunting task, they reported that good working relationship between the researchers and nurses helped them to align their interest in promoting the program more effectively.

> *"Dr X that came to our meeting, he was very convincing to me. It gave me lots of enthusiasm to keep going with it."* (Nurse #12)

The nurses also highlighted the fact collaboration between researchers, oral health professionals, CFHNs, made the access and recruitment of the research participants easier. They suggested that future longitudinal research projects should also consider other avenues for recruiting research participants. These could include recruiting women during pregnancy, in mothers groups, through community organisations, or involving medical doctors and lactation consultants. These multiple recruitment avenues will only be possible if health professionals work collaboratively.

> *"The parenting groups was quite a good audience... they're a good opportunity to get as many clients as possible"* (Nurse #9)

> *" Perhaps the program could be targeted through the GP practices and medical centres. They all turn up to the doctors at some point."* (Nurse #16)

> *"During the first six weeks of the baby, it is tough for mums. I think getting the parents involved before the child is born is a good way to involve families or may be approach community organisations for the migrants"* (Nurse #2)

Finally, the nurses suggested that it will be useful to keep them updated with the research findings as they would feel a greater sense of accomplishment and encourages future collaborative work.

Discussion

The CFHN is an integral member of the primary health care team in Australia as they provide support and guidance to mothers of young children on a number of health related issues including oral health. This qualitative study provides insights on the facilitators and barriers faced by CFHNs in recruiting disadvantaged families to a birth cohort study in South Western Sydney. In particular, the CFHNs recognise that dental caries is major problem in disadvantaged communities and there is need for inter-professional collaboration to promote oral health in young children. While our research aimed to identify the means by which CFHNs can efficiently and effectively connect with disadvantaged families, we found several challenges associated with communicating the importance of oral health to parents, particularly in ethnic minorities.

Some research participants in the cohort study were concerned with the amount of health information they had to absorb in the first few months of the child's birth [29–31]. This nested study reiterated that this element created difficulty for the nurses to recruit families, as some parents were at a stage where their minds were not prepared to handle the supplementary material, causing much of it to be overlooked. When using clinicians for recruitment in research projects, other researchers [32–34] experienced similar challenges to those found in our study. Reported challenges were tension between providing care for families at a crucial time and recruiting for research, clinician's lack of time, forgetting to mention the study to participants, and not prioritising recruitment. However, using clinicians is still a commonly used approach to recruit research participants in public health research. The nurses reported that finding alternate ways to recruit families should also be considered for such research projects. Other researchers have recruited disadvantaged families early-on during pregnancy [16, 35, 36], through medical practices [37], community health clinics [38], community groups [39, 40], or kindergartens [41].

The nurses in the study reported that future research projects could possibly use web-based approaches such as websites to recruit and retain participants. This is highlighted in a recent review on the effectiveness of web-based approaches to recruit research participants [42]. The review concluded that web-based approaches such as Facebook, Twitter, and Google adverts were effective in recruiting research participants, however, there were no significant differences in retaining participants to research studies [42]. Robinson and colleagues [43, 44] reviewed strategies to retain study participants and concluded that good organisational and communication skills of the researchers, sending out study reminders, highlighting the benefits of the study to participants, effective contact and/or scheduling strategies, community involvement, reimbursements, and incentives (financial and non-financial) were key factors for minimising attrition in research. Some of these strategies were also reported in our interviews. In particular, the nurses highlighted the importance of having multiple contact details of the participants and/or linking the research with medical and/or dental records. Other researchers have reported on the use of electronic medical records in longitudinal research is beneficial [45, 46].

Research demonstrates that digital access and use among lower income and disadvantaged groups in Australia is related to a range of broader social determinants of health, such as education, income, housing tenure, and social connections [47]. This creates a digital divide whereby people from low socioeconomic backgrounds are less likely to use smartphones and have access to the internet [47]. However, according to the Australian digital inclusion index [48], this digital divide is narrowing. Further, there is conflicting evidence that demonstrates not all low income earners are digitally disadvantaged; Choi and DiNitto [49] reported that low income people used technology despite their social disadvantage and in Australia nearly nine out of 10 people own a smartphone [50].

In this study, the CFHNs perceived that participation in dental research increased when study participants were offered incentives to take part in research. The nurses found that it was easier to secure the attention of families by offering valuable oral health information and incentives such as free sipper cups, toothpaste, toothbrushes, health promotion books, home visits and free oral health services. Many studies have illustrated that the use of incentives is an effective means to improve participation as it demonstrates a respect for the participant's time and commitment [21, 46]. Robinson and colleagues [43, 44] recently highlighted the importance of financial incentives, non-financial incentives and reimbursements for retention of research participants. Mcsweeney and colleagues [21] reported that incentives were important for acknowledging and respecting the time and effort contributed by parents and their children. However, Baxter and colleagues [17] suggested that incentives should be carefully chosen. In the HSHK study, we decided to use incentives that were deemed appropriate for the study purposes such as oral health advice leaflets, teething ring, sipper cup, toothpaste, toothbrushes, and free oral health services to maintain interest of the participants.

The nurses observed that cultural barriers played a significant role when recruiting participants from culturally and linguistically diverse backgrounds. It was imperative for the nurses to connect with families on a level that was respectful to cultural norms and beliefs. It was advantageous for the nurses to utilise interpreters in order to build trust with the participants at the time of recruitment. Many studies have highlighted upon the importance of eliminating potential linguistic barriers by using bilingual study personnel and translated forms [17–19, 21]. The CFHNs perceived that the ethnic minority families' lack of trust in the health care system was as a barrier to participate in health research. The perceptions of trust and mistrust of scientific investigators, of government, and of academic institutions has been a central barrier to recruitment of minority populations, particularly African migrants [19, 21, 39].

In this study, the nurses highlighted that it may easier to recruit and retain participants if members of the research team involved in recruitment are from the same cultural background to that of the research participants. Research conducted by Lee and colleagues [51] noted that communicating in native language of the study participants demonstrated respect from the study team and ensured that study participants fully understand the research to give an informed consent. Furthermore, evidence from health and social science research highlights the importance of being a cultural insider [52, 53] as they share similar social background, culture and language to that of the local people. It is suggested that cultural insiders have better insights when describing the social and cultural characteristic of the group with whom they undertake research as they are better placed to build rapport and gain trust of the participants [54]. Some researchers have suggested the use of community leaders in recruiting participants from ethnic minority communities as a way to resolve 'power-differences' between the practitioner and the patient [39, 51]. Therefore, it is important that culturally competent approaches and appropriate means of communication is utilised to improve recruitment. Although cultural insiders and community leaders are crucial in research, it is imperative to note that CFHNs operate from the concept of 'cultural safety' that emerged in the 1980s which focuses on the patient feeling safe, respected and listened to [55]. If a cultural safety approach is used, it is not necessary to utilise recruiters who share the same cultural background as participants. It redefines the patient-practitioner relationship so that it shifts the power, responsibility, and authority to lie with the patient receiving care [56, 57].

In the current study, the nurses emphasised the importance for inter-professional collaboration for successful research recruitment. Casamassimo and colleagues have highlighted the importance of inter-disciplinary research framework for improving oral health outcomes in children [58]. In recent years, most Australian states and territories support an early childhood oral health program that links oral health professionals with general health professionals [14, 15]. Since 2007, early childhood oral health training has been available to all health professionals including CFHNs [12] and more recently, the Midwifery Initiated Oral Health program has been introduced in South Western Sydney and Western Sydney [9, 16]. Furthermore, the introduction of the Medicare Benefits Schedule Primary Care Items for Healthy Kids Checks and Child Immunisation has also promoted communication between health professionals [59]. These recent developments utilising the shared care model, are major achievements in oral health promotion.

Strengths and limitations

This study had a number of strengths that are worth reporting. Firstly, we used a qualitative approach to obtain perception of CFHN's on recruitment of disadvantaged families to a longitudinal research project. The flexibility of the research design gives an opportunity for further investigation if required and fosters simultaneous data collection and analysis [26]. Secondly, the study had a high response rate thus achieving a 90% response rate. A sample of 19 research participants was enough to reach data saturation, that is all the dimensions of interest were explored and no new information would have been collected from interviewing more participants [60]. A potential limitation of this study was that the interviews were limited to the CFHNs in South Western Sydney; therefore, the findings may not be generalisable to all of New South Wales or Australia.

Implications

Dental decay is one of the most common chronic childhood diseases. The results of this qualitative study reinforce the importance of a model of shared care involving members of the primary care team such as CFHN in health promotion and early intervention for preventing ECC. Recruiting disadvantaged families to longitudinal research projects is often difficult and so involving CHFNs at this stage might be advantageous since mothers are more receptive to their advice. This study highlighted that participant recruitment for research projects need to be aimed at appropriate time-points with the use of incentives. Further, web-based approaches aimed at participant recruitment were identified by CFHNs may be more innovative and effective; and regular contact with disadvantaged families another possible strategy for maximising retention. If we are to decrease health disparities among disadvantaged populations in Australia, we must find plausible solutions for dealing with the "trust" element, which in essence, is a key barrier in research participation. Gaining the trust of the culturally and linguistically diverse population groups may be possible by including cultural insiders in the research team.

Conclusions

The CHFNs found the early phase of parenting was an overwhelming stage for parents as they are preoccupied with more immediate issues such as settling and feeding a newborn. Other time-points such as during pregnancy and/or around the time of infant teething may be more appropriate for recruiting families to dental research projects. However, they found it easier to secure the family's attention by offering incentives, gifts and invitations for free oral health services. The use of web-based approaches and maintaining regular contact with the participants were identified as possible strategies for continual engagement with participants. Cultural and linguistic barriers were seen as an obstacle in recruiting ethnic minority populations. However, the need for cultural insiders in the research team was deemed important to resolve the challenges associated with conducting research with diverse cultures. Finally, nurses identified the importance of inter-professional collaboration to provide easier access to recruiting research participants.

Abbreviations
CFHN: Child and Family Health Nurses; HSHK: Healthy Smiles Healthy Kids; NSW: New South Wales

Acknowledgements
We would like to thank Ms. Trish Clark (Nurse Unit Manager) and the Child and Family Health Nurses who recruited families to this birth cohort study. We would like to thank staff from the former Sydney South West Area Health Service, Sydney Local Health District, and South Western Sydney Local Health District for their commitment to the study. We would like to thank the families who are a part of the Healthy Smiles Healthy Kids study for their continued commitment to this ongoing cohort study.

Funding
This study was supported by Australian National Health and Medical Research Council Grants (1033213, 1069861, 1134075), NSW Health, Sydney Local Health District, Western Sydney University, Oral Health Foundation, and Australian Dental Research Foundation. The funding bodies assist with providing funds to support the cost of running the Healthy Smiles Healthy Kids Project and provide salary support to AA and NM. They do not have any influence on design of the study, data collection, analysis, and interpretation of data and in writing the manuscript.

Authors' contributions
AA, VB, JE, SA, and SB conceived the study. AA and DB conducted the interviews. AA, NM, DB, APDH, and SYHY performed the analysis and prepared the first draft of the manuscript. SA, SB, JE and VB critically revised the manuscript for intellectual content. All authors approved the final manuscript as submitted and agree to be accountable for all aspects of this work.

Competing interests
The authors declare that they have no competing interests.

Author details
[1]School of Science and Health, Western Sydney University, 24.2.97 Campbelltown Campus, Locked Bag 1797, Penrith, NSW 2751, Australia. [2]Sydney Dental Hospital and Oral Health Services, Sydney Local Health District, Surry Hills, NSW, Australia. [3]Discipline of Paediatrics and Child Health, Sydney Medical School, Westmead, NSW, Australia. [4]Collaboration for Oral Health Outcomes Research, Translation, and Evaluation (COHORTE) Research Group, Ingham Institute for Applied Medical Research, Liverpool, NSW, Australia. [5]Faculty of Dentistry, The University of Sydney, Surry Hills, NSW, Australia. [6]Child and Family Health Nursing, Primary & Community Health, South Western Sydney Local Health District, Narellan, NSW, Australia.

[7]Department of Community Paediatrics, Sydney Local Health District, Croydon Community Health Centre, Croydon, NSW, Australia. [8]Sydney Medical School, The University of Sydney, Sydney, NSW, Australia. [9]School of Women's and Children's Health, UNSW Australia, Kensington, NSW, Australia. [10]School of Medicine, Griffith University, Gold Coast, QLD, Australia.

References
1. Centre for Oral Health Strategy. Early childhood oral health guidelines for child health professionals. 2nd ed. Sydney: NSW Health; 2009.
2. Kawashita Y, Kitamura M, Saito T. Early childhood caries. Int J Dent. 2011; 2011: Article ID 725320.
3. Hallett KB, O'Rourke PK. Social and behavioural determinants of early childhood caries. Aust Dent J. 2003;48:27–33.
4. Arora A, Schwarz E, Blinkhorn AS. Risk factors for early childhood caries in disadvantaged populations. J Investig Clin Dent. 2011;2:223–8.
5. Ha DH, Roberts-Thomson KF, Arrow P, Peres KG, Do LG. Children's oral health status in Australia. In: Do LG, Spencer AJ, editors. Oral health of Australian children: the National Child Oral Health Study 2012–14. Adelaide: University of Adelaide Press; 2016. p. 2012–4.
6. Pitts N, Chadwick B, Anderson T. Report 2: dental disease and damage in children. Child dental health survey 2013 - England, Wales and Northern Ireland. Leeds: National Health Service; 2015.
7. Casamassimo PS, Thikkurissy S, Edelstein BL, Maiorini E. Beyond the dmft: the human and economic cost of early childhood caries. J Am Dent Assoc. 2009;140:650–7.
8. de Silva AM, Hegde S, Akudo Nwagbara B, Calache H, Gussy MG, Nasser M, et al. Community-based population-level interventions for promoting child oral health. Cochrane Database Syst Rev. 2016; https://doi.org/10.1002/14651858.CD009837.pub2.
9. George A, Johnson M, Blinkhorn A, Ellis S, Bhole S, Ajwani S. Promoting oral health during pregnancy: current evidence and implications for Australian midwives. J Clin Nurs. 2010;19:3324–33.
10. Morrow JW, Keels MA, Hale KJ, Thomas HF, Davis MJ, Czerepak CS, et al. Preventive oral health intervention for pediatricians. Pediatrics. 2008; 122:1387–94.
11. Slack-Smith LM. Dental visits by Australian preschool children. J Paediatr Child Health. 2003;39:442–5.
12. Arora A, Bedros D, Bhole S, Do LG, Scott J, Blinkhorn A, et al. Child and family health nurses' experiences of oral health of preschool children: a qualitative approach. J Public Health Dent. 2012;72:149–55.
13. Goldfeld S, Wright M, Oberklaid F. Parents, infants and health care: utilization of health services in the first 12 months of life. J Paediatr Child Health. 2003;39:249–53.
14. Maher L, Phelan C, Lawrence G, Dawson A, Torvaldsen S, Wright C. The early childhood oral health program: promoting prevention and timely intervention of early childhood caries in NSW through shared care. Health Promot J Austr. 2012;23:171–6.
15. National Oral Health Promotion Clearing House. Oral health promotion for infants, preschool and school children Adelaide: The University of Adelaide; 2011 [cited 2017 7 May].
16. Johnson M, George A, Dahlen H, Ajwani S, Bhole S, Blinkhorn A, et al. The midwifery initiated oral health-dental service protocol: an intervention to improve oral health outcomes for pregnant women. BMC Oral Health. 2015;15:2.
17. Baxter J, Vehik K, Johnson SB, Lernmark B, Roth R, Simell T. Differences in recruitment and early retention among ethnic minority participants in a large pediatric cohort: the TEDDY study. Contemp Clin Trials. 2012;33:633–40.
18. Ford DY, Grantham TC, Whiting GW. Culturally and linguistically diverse students in gifted education: recruitment and retention issues. Except Child. 2008;74:289–306.
19. Diaz VA, Mainous AG 3rd, McCall AA, Geesey ME. Factors affecting research participation in African American college students. Fam Med. 2008;40:46–51.
20. Goode PS, FitzGerald MP, Richter HE, Whitehead WE, Nygaard I, Wren PA, et al. Enhancing participation of older women in surgical trials. J Am Coll Surg. 2008;207:303–11.
21. McSweeney JC, Pettey CM, Fischer EP, Spellman A. Going the distance: overcoming challenges in recruitment and retention of black and white women in multisite, longitudinal study of predictors of coronary heart disease. Res Gerontol Nurs. 2009;2:256–64.

22. Jacobs EA, Rolle I, Ferrans CE, Whitaker EE, Warnecke RB. Understanding African Americans' views of the trustworthiness of physicians. J Gen Intern Med. 2006;21:642–7.

23. Australian Bureau of Statistics. Socio-economic Indexes for Areas (SEIFA): 2006: Australian Bureau of Statistics; 2008 [cited 2017 15 March]. Available from: http://www.ausstats.abs.gov.au/ausstats/subscriber.nsf/0/72283F45CB86E5FECA 2574170011B271/$File/2039055001_socio-economicindexesforareas(seifa)- technical paper_2006.pdf. Accessed 15 Mar 2017.

24. Arora A, Scott J, Bhole S, Do L, Schwarz E, Blinkhorn A. Early childhood feeding practices and dental caries in preschool children: a multi-centre birth cohort study. BMC Public Health. 2011;11:28. https://doi.org/10.1186/1471-2458-11-28.

25. Kuzel AJ. Sampling in qualitative inquiry. In: Crabtree BF, Miller WL, editors. Doing qualitative research. 2nd ed. Thousand Oaks: SAGE Publications; 1999. p. 33–46.

26. Patton MQ. Qualitative research and evaluation methods 4th ed. Thousands Oaks: SAGE Publications; 2015.

27. Chapple A. The use of telephone interviewing for qualitiative research. Nurse Res. 1999;6:85–93.

28. Braun VCV. Using thematic analysis in psychology. Qual Res Psychol. 2006;3:77–101.

29. Arora A, McNab MA, Lewis MW, Hilton G, Blinkhorn AS, Schwarz E. 'I can't relate it to teeth': a qualitative approach to evaluate oral health education materials for preschool children in new South Wales, Australia. Int J Paediatr Dent. 2012;22:302–9.

30. Arora A, Nguyen D, Do QV, Nguyen B, Hilton G, Do LG, et al. 'What do these words mean?': A qualitative approach to explore oral health literacy in Vietnamese immigrant mothers in Australia. Health Educ J. 2014;73:303–12.

31. Arora A, Liu MN, Chan R, Schwarz E. 'English leaflets are not meant for me': a qualitative approach to explore oral health literacy in Chinese mothers in southwestern Sydney, Australia. Community Dent Oral Epidemiol. 2012;40:532–41.

32. Miller WR, Bakas T, Buelow JM, Habermann B. Research involving participants with chronic diseases: overcoming recruitment obstacles. Clin Nurse Spec. 2013;27:307–13.

33. Sygna K, Johansen S, Ruland CM. Recruitment challenges in clinical research including cancer patients and caregivers. Trials. 2015;16:428.

34. Newington L, Metcalfe A. Factors influencing recruitment to research: qualitative study of the experiences and perceptions of research teams. BMC Med Res Methodol. 2014;14:10.

35. Wigen TI, Espelid I, Skaare AB, Wang NJ. Family characteristics and caries experience in preschool children. A longitudinal study from pregnancy to 5 years of age. Community Dent Oral Epidemiol. 2011;39:311–7.

36. Manca DP, O'Beirne M, Lightbody T, Johnston DW, Dymianiw D-L, Nastalska K, et al. The most effective strategy for recruiting a pregnancy cohort: a tale of two cities. BMC Pregnancy Childbirth. 2013;13:75.

37. Dela Cruz GG, Rozier RG, Slade G. Dental screening and referral of young children by pediatric primary care providers. Pediatrics. 2004;114:e642–e52.

38. Warner ET, Glasgow RE, Emmons KM, Bennett GG, Askew S, Rosner B, et al. Recruitment and retention of participants in a pragmatic randomized intervention trial at three community health clinics: results and lessons learned. BMC Public Health. 2013;13:192.

39. Dancy BL, Wilbur J, Talashek M, Bonner G, Barnes-Boyd C. Community-based research: barriers to recruitment of African Americans. Nurs Outlook. 2004;52:234–40.

40. Hillier FC, Batterham AM, Nixon CA, Crayton AM, Pedley CL, Summerbell CD. A community-based health promotion intervention using brief negotiation techniques and a pledge on dietary intake, physical activity levels and weight outcomes: lessons learnt from an exploratory trial. Public Health Nutr. 2012;15:1446–55.

41. Gao X, Lo ECM, McGrath C, Ho SMY. Innovative interventions to promote positive dental health behaviors and prevent dental caries in preschool children: study protocol for a randomized controlled trial. Trials. 2013;14:118.

42. Lane TS, Armin J, Gordon JS. Online recruitment methods for web-based and mobile health studies: a review of the literature. J Med Internet Res. 2015;17:e183.

43. Robinson KA, Dennison CR, Wayman DM, Pronovost PJ, Needham DM. Systematic review identifies number of strategies important for retaining study participants. J Clin Epidemiol. 2007;60:757. e1-. e19.

44. Robinson KA, Dinglas VD, Sukrithan V, Yalamanchilli R, Mendez-Tellez PA, Dennison-Himmelfarb C, et al. Updated systematic review identifies substantial number of retention strategies: using more strategies retains more study participants. J Clin Epidemiol. 2015;68:1481–7.

45. Effoe VS, Katula JA, Kirk JK, Pedley CF, Bollhalter LY, Brown WM, et al. The use of electronic medical records for recruitment in clinical trials: findings from the lifestyle intervention for treatment of diabetes trial. Trials. 2016;17:496.

46. Ruffin MT, Nease DE. Using patient monetary incentives and electronically derived patient lists to recruit patients to a clinical trial. J Am Board Fam Med. 2011;24:569–75.

47. Newman LA, Biedrzycki K, Baum F. Digital technology access and use among socially and economically disadvantaged groups in South Australia. J Community Inf. 2010;6(2).

48. Thomas J, Barraket J, Ewing S, MacDonald T, Mundell M, Tucker J. Measuring Australia's digital divide: the Australian digital inclusion index 2016. Melbourne: Swinburne University of Technology; 2016.

49. Choi NG, DiNitto DM. TThe Digital Divide Among Low-Income Homebound Older Adults: Internet Use Patterns, eHealth Literacy, and Attitudes TowardComputer/Internet Use J Med Internet Res. 2013;15(5):e93 doi: https://doi.org/10.2196/jmir.2645.

50. Deloitte Touche Tohmatsu Limited. Mobile Consumer Survey 2016 Sydney: 2016.

51. Lee SK, Sulaiman-Hill CR, Thompson SC. Overcoming language barriers in community-based research with refugee and migrant populations: options for using bilingual workers. BMC Int Health Hum Rights. 2014;14:11.

52. Suwankhong D, Liamputtong P. Cultural insiders and research fieldwork: case examples from cross-cultural research with Thai people. Int J Qual Methods. 2015;14:1–7.

53. Manohar N, Liamputtong P, Bhole S, Arora A. Researcher positionality in cross-cultural and sensitive research. In: Liamputtong P, editor. Handbook of research methods in health social sciences. Singapore: Springer Singapore; 2017. p. 1–15.

54. Liamputtong P. Performing qualitative cross-cultural research. Cambridge: Cambridge University Press; 2010.

55. Ramsden IM. Cultural safety and nursing education in Aotearoa and Te Waipounamu. Wellington: Victoria University of Wellington; 2002.

56. Greenwood S, Wright T, Nielsen H. Conversations in context: cultural safety and reflexivity in child and family health nursing. J Fam Nurs. 2006;12:201–24.

57. Gerlach AJ. A critical reflection on the concept of cultural safety. Can J Occup Ther. 2012;79:151–8.

58. Casamassimo PS, Lee JY, Marazita ML, Milgrom P, Chi DL, Divaris K. Improving Children's oral health: an interdisciplinary research framework. J Dent Res. 2014;93:938–42.

59. Australian Government Department of Health and Aging. Medicare Benefit Schedule primary care items: healthy kids check–fact sheet. Canberra: Commonwealth of Australia; 2010 [cited 2017 7 May].

60. Liamputtong P. Qualitative research methods. 4th ed. South Melbourne: Oxford University Press; 2013.

5

Proportion of medication error reporting and associated factors among nurses

Abebaw Jember[1*], Mignote Hailu[1], Anteneh Messele[2], Tesfaye Demeke[3] and Mohammed Hassen[1]

Abstract

Background: A medication error (ME) is any preventable event that may cause or lead to inappropriate medication use or patient harm. Voluntary reporting has a principal role in appreciating the extent and impact of medication errors. Thus, exploration of the proportion of medication error reporting and associated factors among nurses is important to inform service providers and program implementers so as to improve the quality of the healthcare services.

Methods: Institution based quantitative cross-sectional study was conducted among 397 nurses from March 6 to May 10, 2015. Stratified sampling followed by simple random sampling technique was used to select the study participants. The data were collected using structured self-administered questionnaire which was adopted from studies conducted in Australia and Jordan. A pilot study was carried out to validate the questionnaire before data collection for this study. Bivariate and multivariate logistic regression models were fitted to identify factors associated with the proportion of medication error reporting among nurses. An adjusted odds ratio with 95% confidence interval was computed to determine the level of significance.

Result: The proportion of medication error reporting among nurses was found to be 57.4%. Regression analysis showed that sex, marital status, having made a medication error and medication error experience were significantly associated with medication error reporting.

Conclusion: The proportion of medication error reporting among nurses in this study was found to be higher than other studies.

Keywords: Medication error, Medication error reporting, Federal Level Governmental Hospital, Nurse

Background

Medication therapy is the most common intervention prescribed for healthcare consumers [1] and safe medication administration represents one of the routine, highly complex and essential nursing care responsibilities [2]. Medication administration is amongst the potentially hazardous nursing tasks in hospitals because of liability to errors [3]. The reporting of error incidents and specific phases of healthcare delivery such as the safe use of medications can improve the safety of patients [4].

A single medication error (ME) may prolong hospital stay or even end up in death. This affects the quality and continuity of the healthcare services [5] by affecting patient safety which is an important indicator of healthcare quality and encompasses various nursing care procedures. Executing a ME has been seen to be psychologically devastating to the nurse and harmful to the patient [6].

Globally, MEs present a substantial contribution to ill health, and even death and are listed as one of the five medical error categories classified by the American Institute of Medicine [7]. Out of estimated patients' deaths of 6000 to 20,000 each year from medical errors in Taiwan, 10% of medical lawsuits were because of MEs where the majority of the errors were grossly underreported [8]. A prospective cross-sectional study conducted in an intensive care unit of a specialized hospital in Ethiopia showed a ME of 51.8% [9].

* Correspondence: abebaw5360@gmail.com
[1]Department of Medical Nursing, School of Nursing, College of Medicine and Health Sciences, University of Gondar, Gondar, Ethiopia
Full list of author information is available at the end of the article

Nevertheless how huge or insignificant the incidence, it is difficult to have a general concept of MEs in less developed and developing countries due to inefficient documentation and error-reporting systems and insufficient research in the area [7]. Analysis and appreciation of the root causes of MEs allows developing complex medication error prevention mechanisms [10] which improve patient safety.

Literature review

A medication error is any preventable event that may cause or lead to inappropriate medication use or patient harm [11]. Medication error is a global issue where 5% of the MEs are deadly and almost 50% are preventable [12]. Medication error reporting is one of the major issues in today's health care and prevention is linked to accurate reporting of errors [7]. Voluntary reporting is indispensable to appreciate the extent and impact of MEs [13]. Nurses' interception of 86% of the MEs was presented in a descriptive cross-sectional study conducted in one large medical center hospital in southern Taiwan with sample size of 597 nurses using self-administered questionnaires and the significance of error reporting was given a weight as intercepting [8]. Moreover, consideration of nurses' perceived barriers to medication error reporting (MER) is a crucial step to strengthen medication safety [8] and it was shown in a study that more than 90% of healthcare consumers believe that errors should be reported [3].

Incidence and prevalence of medication errors

Medication errors which are made during prescription, dispensing and administration [14] are common and preventable causes of patient harm [15]. Precise figure of the incidence and prevalence of MEs is difficult to obtain because the rate varies from study to study [7]. Studies showed a range of rate of serious patient injuries due to medication errors as 1 to 2% [16], 9 to 13% [2], 29% [17], and as high of 51.8% [9], and estimated 30.5% deaths per year in a survey in the United States of America (USA) were attributable to MEs [15]. A study conducted in Southern Iran with the purpose of determining the frequency of MEs in an emergency department of a teaching hospital revealed that 96.5% of patients had experienced at least one medication error, making the rate of errors 3.5 per patient [18]. A descriptive survey of 300 nurses working in hospitals affiliated to Iran University of Medical Sciences using stratified multistage sampling disclosed a mean of 19.5 medication errors that the nurses acknowledged within 3-months period however the mean of error reporting was only 1.3 of error cases [19, 20].

Factors related to medication error reporting

A focus group study on barriers to MER in Canada identified barriers as an individual, organizational and cultural [21]. According to a descriptive cross-sectional study with sample size of 799 nurses conducted in Jordan, the proportion of medication error reporting was relatively high among female nurses than male nurses [7]. Twenty-six percent of nurses in a study conducted in Israel indicated that all MEs in their wards were reported and 46% of the nurses showed self-reporting of MEs. The nurses emphasized on a personal barrier to non-reporting such as ME experiences and error reporting experiences [22].

A perception that incidence reports do not result in significant changes or benefits and errors that did not result in harm were among the factors that affected the attitude of nurses to report medication errors [23, 24]. Perceived barriers which affect attitude of nurses to report medication errors were fear of adverse consequences from reporting and being subjected to disciplinary actions, fear of being blamed, fear of reaction from the nurse manager, from peers and fear of loss of jobs [6–8, 19, 25]. Other barriers for not reporting MEs include nurses not being aware that an error had occurred, process of reporting (detailed paperwork, time constraints, not understanding incident reporting process), forgetting to make a report when the ward is busy, lack of time for reporting and lack of awareness of the importance of reporting [19, 23, 26].

Two-thirds (66.7%) of nurses involved in a study conducted in two state hospitals in Turkey who stated that they involved in medication errors in the preceding 6 months had not reported the errors. The reported reasons (social factors) for not reporting MEs included fear of consequences, fear of a culture of blame and the need to cover up for the colleague involved [27].

Modifiable barriers to MER for nurses reported in different studies as organizational factors were revealed as lack of feedback to the reporter, lack of a readily available MER system, lack of information on how to report a ME, no positive feedback for giving medication correctly, too much emphasis on ME as a quality indicator of nursing care and motivational factors (such as no encouragement by management, fear of loss of professional registration), lack of organizational leadership and support [3, 8, 19, 25, 28]. Similarly taking medical responsibility and fear of distrust from patients were barriers of medication error reporting [29].

Encouraging administrative attitudes and responses to MER were appreciated in a study to enhance nurses' voluntary reporting [30]. It is indicated in the literature that strategies should be implemented to establish reporting mechanisms to reduce medication errors at national as well as international levels [31]. Establishing structured protocols on drug administration and adopting a nonpunitive approach to reporting medication errors were shown to decrease medication errors and improve patient safety [32]. Proportion of medication error reporting by nurses might be affected by multiple factors such as socio-demographic, social, attitude of nurses, and organizational factors [7, 8, 12, 19] (Fig. 1 indicates the factors involved in medication error reporting).

Health care systems in most developing countries suffer from serious deficiencies in quality, equity, efficiency and financing [33]. The quality of care is evaluated in the light of the provider's technical standards and clients' expectations. Medication administration is among the routine and highly complex nursing care activities which plays a great role in patient care and outcome. Medication safety and medication errors are important concerns for healthcare consumers, health-care professionals, researchers and policy makers worldwide.

Nurses are more prone to making medication errors because of the increasing demands and pressures placed on them. Critical incidents must be detected and reported and turned into positive situations, from which lessons are learned and used to design better patient care practices and systems. So far nurses are at the front line of defense to intercept and report medication errors, yet the errors are severely under-detected and under-reported in practice.

Medication errors affect the quality of health care delivery. Improving patient safety and learning from errors relies on voluntary error reporting which gives the complete picture of medication errors. Thus, exploration of the proportion of nurses reporting medication errors and associated factors is important to inform service providers, program implementers and policy makers to improve the quality of the healthcare service.

Aim

The aim of this study was to assess the proportion of medication error reporting and to explore the relationships among the barriers; socio-demographic factors, organizational factors, social factors, and attitude of nurses.

Incident reporting represents more appropriate information about incidents and can detect preventable events if it is supported within the clinical settings. However, many of the incidents are not reported or are simply not recognized and yet it has been shown in the literature that nurses predominantly report incidents compared to other healthcare professionals [34]. Conversely, studies have demonstrated under-reporting of MEs among nurses [35].

Methods

An institution based quantitative cross-sectional study was conducted at three Federal Ministry of Health level governmental hospitals located in the nation's capital Addis Ababa from March 6 to May 10, 2015. There are four hospitals under the FMoH; Alert, St. Peter, St. Paul and Amanuel. Amanuel Mental Specialized Hospital is the only referral mental hospital in the country which delivers counseling and treatment for patients. St. Paul's Millennium Medical College Hospital delivers medical services for an annual average of 200,000 patients. St. Peter's TB Specialized Hospital has been giving services related to tuberculosis treatment. Alert Hospital was excluded because of protocol issues.

Sample size determination

A single population proportion formula was used to calculate the sample size:

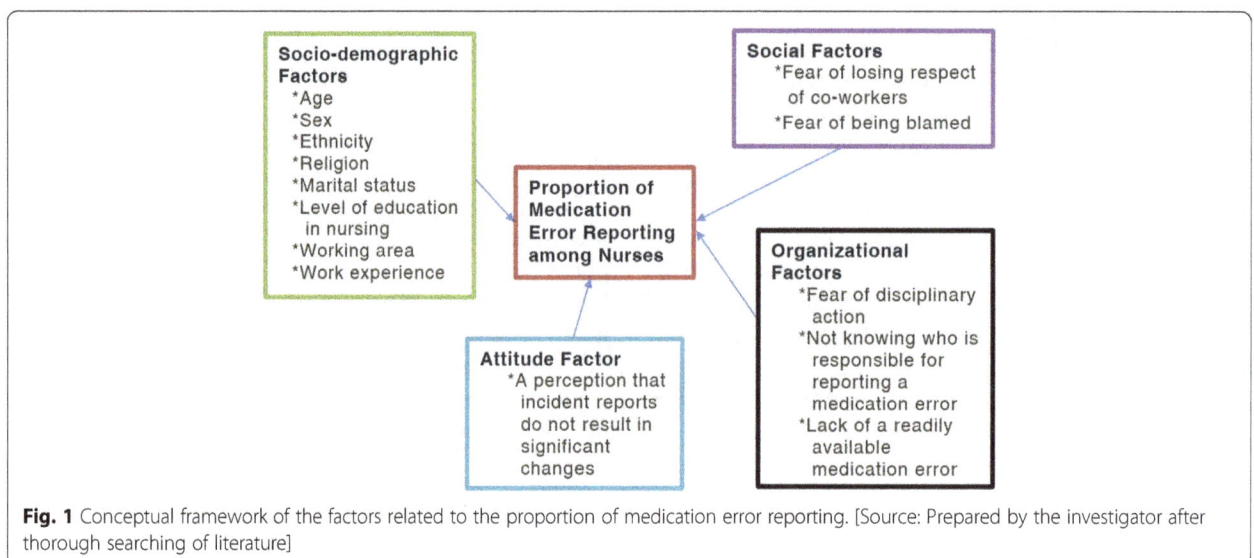

Fig. 1 Conceptual framework of the factors related to the proportion of medication error reporting. [Source: Prepared by the investigator after thorough searching of literature]

$$n = \frac{Z^2\alpha_{/2}\,p(1-p)}{d^2}$$

Where: n = minimum sample size required for the study.

z = score for 95% confidence interval (z = 1.96).

p = prevalence of medication error reporting (50%).

d = tolerable error (d = 5%).

Since the proportion of medication error reporting in Ethiopia is unknown, 50% prevalence of medication error reporting was taken:

$$n_o = \frac{(1.96)^2\,0.5(1-0.5)}{0.05^2}$$

$$n_o = \frac{0.9604}{0.0025} = 384.16 \approx 385$$

For possible non-response, the sample size was increased by 10%, thus comprising 38.416 respondents the final sample size became *423*.

Sampling procedure

Stratified sampling technique was used to allocate the sample proportionally to each FMoH level governmental hospital and then the study participants who had work experience of six months and above were selected from the list of all nurses using simple random sampling technique; a lottery method (Fig. 2).

Data collection tool and procedure

Data were collected by three nurses who were diploma holders using structured self-administered English-version questionnaire. The data collection tool was adopted from two studies conducted in Australia by Evans [3] and in Jordan by Mrayyan et al. [7] with the authors' permissions and face and content validity were established by two expert nurse advisors. The tool was composed of five parts. The first part contained socio-demographic characteristics of nurses. The second part of the questionnaire was related to error incidence. The third part related to medication error reporting was used to estimate the proportion of medication error reporting. The fourth and fifth parts were used to collect data regarding the attitudes of nurses on medication error reporting and perceived organizational culture and reality of dealing with errors respectively (Additional file 1).

Data quality control

Data quality was assured by conducting a pretest among 22 (5%) nurses at Zewditu hospital and appropriate modifications were made after analyzing the pre-test result before the actual data collection. The questionnaire

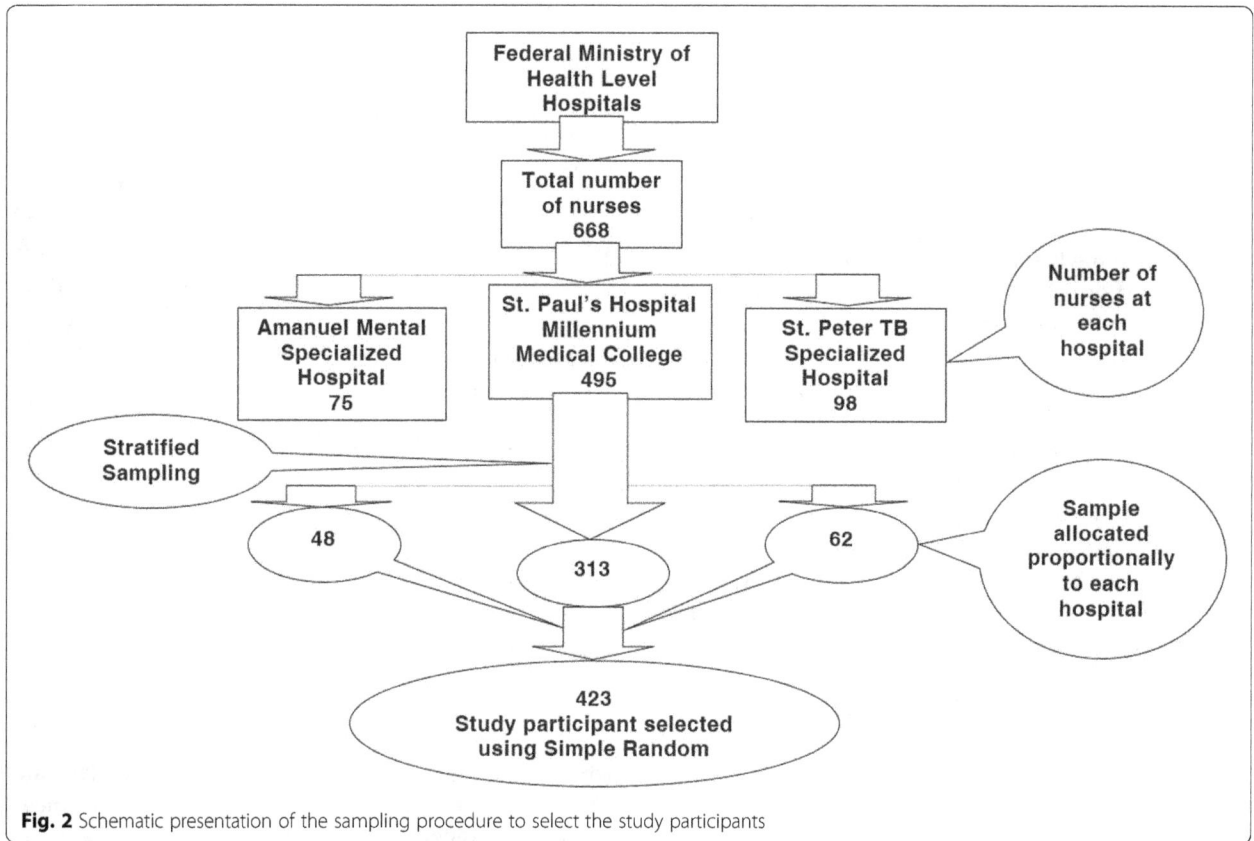

Fig. 2 Schematic presentation of the sampling procedure to select the study participants

was coded before data collection and cross-checked for consistency and completeness every day.

Data management and analysis

The returned questionnaires were checked for completeness, cleaned and the data were entered into EPI Info-7 and then exported to SPSS (Statistical Package for the Social Sciences) version 20.0 for analysis. Frequencies and cross tabulations were used to summarize descriptive statistics and tables were used for data presentation. Binary logistic regression was used to identify factors associated with medication error reporting and then the variables were checked for significant association using *p*-value, odds ratio and 95% confidence interval.

Result

Socio-demographic characteristics

Out of 423 proposed study participants, 403 participated in the study giving a response rate of 95.27%. Six (1.41%) of the returned questionnaires were found to be incomplete and excluded and the rest 20 (4.72%) of nurses chose not to participate in the study. 397 (93.85%) of study participants' responses were analyzed. The majority (53.7%) of respondents were male. The mean (+ standard deviation) age of the respondents was 28.37 (+ 5.55) years. 307 (77.3%) respondents were Orthodox Christian followed by Protestant 48 (12.1%), 208 (52.4%) of the respondents were Amhara in their ethnic background and 291 (73.3%) of the participants were single. On the other hand, 154 (38.8%) of the respondents worked in internal medicine wards and level of education of 237 (59.7%) of the participants was Bachelor of Science in Nursing. Moreover, 182 (45.8%) of the respondents served 1–3 years in the nursing profession (Table 1).

Proportion of medication error reporting

The proportion of medication error reporting among nurses in this study was found to be 57.4% (*n* = 288). Out of the total participants (*n* = 397), relatively high (74.5%) proportion of medication error reporting was found among female nurses as compared to male nurses (42.7%). A high proportion (70.8%) of medication error reporting was disclosed by married participants than participants who are single (52.6%). On the other hand, 277 (69.8%) of the participants perceived that medication errors should be reported as they occur. Moreover, (70.7%) of the nurses who did not make errors themselves reported medication errors.

Factors associated with medication error reporting

In bivariate logistic regression analysis sex, marital status, having made a medication error, medication error experience, and working area were associated with medication error reporting. However, in multivariate analysis

sex, marital status, having made a medication error and medication error experience were associated with medication error reporting (Table 2).

Table 1 Demographic characteristics of nurses at federal level teaching hospitals, Addis Ababa 2015 (*n* = 397)

Variables	n (%)
Sex	
Male	213 (53.7)
Female	184 (46.3)
Age	
19–29	312 (78.6)
30–39	52 (13.1)
40–49	21 (5.3)
50–59	12 (3.1)
Ethnicity	
Amhara	208 (52.4)
Oromia	93 (23.4)
SNNPR	60 (15.1)
Tigray	20 (5.0)
Others[a]	16 (4.0)
Religion	
Orthodox	307 (77.3)
Protestant	48 (12.1)
Muslim	36 (9.1)
Catholic	6 (1.5)
Marital Status	
Single[b]	291 (73.3)
Married	106 (26.7)
Level of education in nursing	
BSc	237 (59.7)
Diploma	160 (40.3)
Working area	
Internal medicine ward	154 (38.8)
Surgical ward	73 (18.4)
Emergency room	63 (15.9)
Psychiatry	47 (11.8)
Intensive care unit	31 (7.8)
Pediatric ward	29 (7.3)
Service year in the nursing profession	
< 1	54 (13.6)
1–3	182 (45.8)
4–5	67 (16.9)
6–10	62 (15.6)
> 10	32 (8.1)

[a]Others: Benishangul-Gumuz, Harari, Gambella
[b]Single includes divorced and widowed

Table 2 Bivariate and multivariate logistic regression analysis of factors associated with proportion of medication error reporting among nurses at selected Federal Ministry of Health level hospitals, Addis Ababa 2015 ($n = 397$)

Variables	Medication error reporting practice		Odds Ratio (95% CI)	
	Yes	No	Crude	Adjusted
Sex				
Male	91	122	1.00	1.00
Female	137	47	0.256 (0.167–0.393)	0.273 (0.165–0.450)*
Marital status				
Single	153	138	1.00	1.00
Married	75	31	0.458 (0.284–0.739)	0.454 (0.251–0.821)*
Medication error experience				
Yes	94	104	1.00	1.00
No	134	65	0.438 (0.292–0.659)	0.445 (0.274–0.722)*
I made medication errors				
Yes	170	145	1.00	1.00
No	58	24	0.485 (0.287–0.820)	0.426 (0.230–0.789)*
Should errors be reported				
Yes	132	145	1.00	1.00
No	96	24	0.228 (0.137–0.377)	0.151 (0.082–0.277)*
Error reporting leads to beneficial and constructive activity				
Yes	197	159	1.00	1.00
No	31	10	0.400 (0.190–0.840)	0.881 (0.334–2.322)
Working area: Intensive care unit				
Yes	39	24	1.00	1.00
No	8	23	4.672 (1.804–12.101)	4.471 (0.502–13.307)
Religion: Protestant				
Yes	165	142	1.00	1.00
No	34	14	0.478 (0.247–0.927)	0.672 (0.296–1.525)

*Statistically significant at $P < 0.05$

The proportion of medication error reporting was high among female nurses as compared to male nurses. Female nurses were 72.7% times more likely to report medication errors than male nurses (AOR = 0.273; 95% CI = 0.165–0.450). Similarly, marital status was an important predictor of medication error reporting. Nurses who are married were 54.6% times less likely to report medication errors as compared to those who are single (AOR = 0.454; 95% CI = 0.251–0.821).

Having a medication error experience was found to be another important determinant of medication error reporting. Nurses who had no medication error experience were 55.5% times more likely to report medication errors than those who had medication error experiences (AOR = 0.445; 95% CI = 0.274–0.722). The odds of medication error reporting among nurses who have not made errors themselves was 57.4% times higher as compared to those nurses who had previously made medication errors (AOR = 0.426; 95% CI = 0.230–0.789).

Discussion

The proportion of medication error reporting among nurses was found to be 57.4%. This finding is slightly higher as compared to studies in Jordan 42.1% [7], Australia 41.9% [3] and California, USA 28.9% [6]. The possible differences could be related to the differences in organizational medication error reporting systems and differences in the time frame that the studies are bounded.

In this study medication error experience of nurses was significantly associated with medication error reporting. Nurses who had previous experiences of medication errors and their reporting processes that errors made by others were 55.5% less likely to report error incidents than those who did not have error experiences and those nurses who had previously made medication errors were 57.4% less likely to report error incidents than those who did not make medication errors. This result is consistent with the result from Israel [22] and South Korea [26] that ME and having made errors hindered nurses from reporting MEs. However, this result was inconsistent with other results from Taiwan [8], Southern Taiwan [29] and Saudi Arabia [25]. The difference may be related to the severity of medication errors since minor errors are less likely to be reported, even though it was difficult to determine the effect of medication errors experienced regarding severity.

Most of the participants (69.8%) perceived that errors should be reported as they occur for the safety of patients and this was consistent with the study from the United Kingdom [23] however lower than the study from Taiwan (87.7%) [8]. The possible difference may be due to the lack of a readily available practice system of medication error reporting.

In this study, the proportion of female nurses who reported medication errors was higher than the male nurses and was statistically significant. The result was similar with that of the study from Jordan [7]. In contrast to other studies, marital status in this study was statistically significant with error reporting (AOR = 0.454; 95% CI = 0.251–0.821) showing that nurses who are married were 54.6% less likely to report medication errors. This might be related to barriers like fear of disciplinary actions since it was put in second place as perceived barrier to reporting by nurses though not statistically significant.

Conclusion
The proportion of medication error reporting among nurses in this study was found to be high. Medication error experience, having made a medication error, sex of participants and marital status were significantly associated.

Limitation
Causes of medication errors were not studied in this research. Knowing the causes of medication errors gives a complete picture of medication errors. Therefore, it would be better if the study was triangulated. Response bias and recall bias were not reduced.

Recommendation
To Federal Ministry of Health
It is recommended that the Federal Ministry of Health identify and address gaps in medication error identification and reporting regarding the establishment of the reporting system to improve patient safety.

To the respected hospitals
The respective hospitals efforts will be significant in identifying and addressing gaps in medication error reporting among nurses and creating a conducive environment for the establishment and maintenance of efficient reporting system. A condition in which reported errors are changed into opportunities to learn from them.

To the respected nurses
Nurses' contribution to the documentation of errors and reporting is an important input for the smooth provision of quality care and improved patient outcome.

To researchers
Further investigation, qualitative in nature, should be made in order to have a complete picture of medication errors in Ethiopia.

Abbreviations
FMoH: Federal Ministry of Health; ME: Medication error; MER: Medication error reporting; MoH': Ministry of Health; USA: United States of America

Acknowledgements
We would like to express our deepest and heartfelt gratitude to the University of Gondar for funding the research work. Our gratitude further goes to the respective hospitals, Amanuel Mental Specialized Hospital, St. Paul's Hospital Millennium Medical College, and St. Peter's TB Specialized Hospital, and the nurses who chose to participate in this study.

Funding
This work was supported by the University of Gondar by funding the expenses of the research work.

Authors' contributions
AJF: Theorized the research problem, designed the study, conducted field work, analyzed the data and revised the manuscript. MHG: Involved in the supervision of the field work, revision of the research design, data analysis and revision of the manuscript for publication. AMB: Involved in the supervision of the field work, revision of the research design, data analysis and revision of the manuscript for publication. TDA: Involved in the supervision of the field work, revision of the research design, data analysis and revision of the manuscript for publication. MHS: Contributed in the revision of the research design, statistical analysis, and preparation of the manuscript. All authors read and approved the final manuscript.

Ethics approval and consent to participate
Ethical clearance and approval was obtained from Ethical Review Committee of School of Nursing, College of Medicine and Health Sciences, University of Gondar and permission was obtained from the Ethical Review Committees of each respective hospital.
Consent form was put as a first page of each questionnaire, and included the name of the researcher, the purpose of the study, and a number of ethically based instructions. Participants were assured that their involvement in the study was after having been informed about the study without undue influence and could withdraw from the study at any time without the need to give reason. The privacy of the participants was maintained while they fill the questionnaire and confidentiality of the participants was maintained by keeping anonymity and keeping the data only accessible by the investigator. Although there may not be immediate and direct benefits for the participants, nurses were informed of the benefits from the nursing knowledge gained through the process. The participants were informed that there were no financial benefits for participating in the research, no potential harms that impact on employment, or social status, the utilization of the gathered data to be used only for the intended research,

and the publication of the results of the study in a reputable journal with no identifiable information that links to the participants.

Competing interests

The authors declare that they have no competing interests.

Author details

[1]Department of Medical Nursing, School of Nursing, College of Medicine and Health Sciences, University of Gondar, Gondar, Ethiopia. [2]Unit of Community Health Nursing, School of Nursing, College of Medicine and Health Sciences, University of Gondar, Gondar, Ethiopia. [3]Department of Pediatric and Child Health Nursing, School of Nursing, College of Medicine and Health Sciences, University of Gondar, Gondar, Ethiopia.

References

1. Wakefield DS, Wakefield BJ, Uden-Holman T, Borders T, Blegen M, Vaughn T. Understanding why medication administration errors may not be reported. Am J Med Qual. 1999;14(2):81–8.
2. Anselmi ML, Peduzzi M, dos Santos CB. Errors in the administration of intravenous medication in Brazilian hospitals. J Clin Nurs. 2007;16(10): 1839–47.
3. Evans SM. Attitudes and barriers to incident reporting: a collaborative hospital study. Qual Saf Health Care. 2006;15(1):39–43.
4. Gaal S, Verstappen W, Wensing M. Patient safety in primary care: a survey of general practitioners in the Netherlands. BMC Health Serv Res. 2010;10(1):21.
5. Zeleke A, Chanie T, Woldie M. Medication prescribing errors and associated factors at the pediatric wards of Dessie referral hospital, Northeast Ethiopia. Int Arch Med. 2014;7(1):18.
6. Ulanimo VM, O'Leary-Kelley C, Connolly PM. Nurses' perceptions of causes of medication errors and barriers to reporting. J Nurs Care Qual. 2007;22(1):28–33.
7. Mrayyan MT, Shishani K, Al-Faouri I. Rate, causes and reporting of medication errors in Jordan: nurses? Perspectives. J Nurs Manag. 2007;15(6):659–70.
8. Chiang H-Y, Pepper GA. Barriers to nurses' reporting of medication administration errors in Taiwan. J Nurs Scholarsh. 2006;38(4):392–9.
9. Agalu A, Ayele Y, Bedada W, Woldie M. Medication administration errors in an intensive care unit in Ethiopia. Int Arch Med. 2012;5(1):15.
10. Montesi G, Lechi A. Prevention of medication errors: detection and audit. Br J Clin Pharmacol. 2009;67(6):651–5.
11. Banning M. Medication errors: professional issues and concerns. Nurs Older People. 2006;18(3):27–32.
12. Nuckols TK, Bell DS, Liu H, Paddock SM, Hilborne LH. Rates and types of events reported to established incident reporting systems in two US hospitals. Qual Saf Health Care. 2007;16(3):164–8.
13. Halbesleben JRB, Wakefield BJ, Wakefield DS, Cooper LB. Nurse burnout and patient safety outcomes nurse safety perception versus reporting behavior. West J Nurs Res. 2008;30(5):560–77.
14. Keers RN, Williams SD, Cooke J, Ashcroft DM. Prevalence and nature of medication administration errors in health care settings: a systematic review of direct observational evidence. Ann Pharmacother. 2013;47(2):237–56.
15. Haw C, Stubbs J, Dickens GL. Barriers to the reporting of medication administration errors and near misses: an interview study of nurses at a psychiatric hospital. J Psychiatr Ment Health Nurs. 2014;21(9):797–805.
16. Nebeker JR, Barach P, Samore MH. Clarifying adverse drug events: a Clinician's guide to terminology, documentation, and reporting. Ann Intern Med. 2004; 140(10):795–801.
17. Donchin Y, Gopher D, Olin M, Badihi Y, Biesky M, Sprung CL, et al. A look into the nature and causes of human errors in the intensive care unit. Qual Saf Health Care. 2003;12(2):143–7.
18. Vazin A, Zamani Z, Hatam N. Frequency of medication errors in an emergency department of a large teaching hospital in southern Iran. Drug Healthc Patient Saf. 2014;6:179–84.

19. Joolaee S, Hajibabaee F, Peyrovi H, Haghani H, Bahrani N. The relationship between incidence and report of medication errors and working conditions. Int Nurs Rev. 2011;58(1):37–44.
20. Hajibabaee F, Joolaee S, Peyravi H, Alijany-Renany H, Bahrani N, Haghani H. Medication error reporting in Tehran: a survey. J Nurs Manag. 2014;22(3): 304–10.
21. Hartnell N, MacKinnon N, Sketris I, Fleming M. Identifying, understanding and overcoming barriers to medication error reporting in hospitals: a focus group study. BMJ Qual Saf. 2012;21(5):361–8.
22. Kagan I, Barnoy S. Factors associated with reporting of medication errors by Israeli nurses. J Nurs Care Qual. 2008;23(4):353–61.
23. Sanghera IS, Franklin BD, Dhillon S. The attitudes and beliefs of healthcare professionals on the causes and reporting of medication errors in a UK intensive care unit. Anaesthesia. 2007;62(1):53–61.
24. Kingston M, Evans S, Smith B, Berry J. Attitudes of doctors and nurses towards incident reporting: a qualitative analysis. http://www.mja.com.au/public/issues/181_01_050704/kin10795_fm.html [Internet]. 2004 [cited 2015 Jun 20]; Available from: https://digital.library.adelaide.edu.au/dspace/handle/2440/9952.
25. Almutary HH, Lewis PA. Nurses' willingness to report medication administration errors in Saudi Arabia. Qual Manag Health Care. 2012;21(3): 119–26.
26. Kim KS, Kwon S-H, Kim J-A, Cho S. Nurses' perceptions of medication errors and their contributing factors in South Korea: nurses' perceptions of medication errors. J Nurs Manag. 2011;19(3):346–53.
27. Güneş ÜY, Gürlek Ö, Sönmez M. Factors contributing to medication errors in Turkey: nurses' perspectives. J Nurs Manag. 2014;22(3):295–303.
28. Handler SM, Perera S, Olshansky EF, Studenski SA, Nace DA, Fridsma DB, et al. Identifying modifiable barriers to medication error reporting in the nursing home setting. J Am Med Dir Assoc. 2007;8(9):568–74.
29. Lin Y-H, Ma S. Willingness of nurses to report medication administration errors in southern Taiwan: a cross-sectional survey. Worldviews Evid-Based Nurs. 2009;6(4):237–45.
30. Institute of Medicine (US) Committee on Quality of Health Care in America. In: Kohn LT, Corrigan JM, Donaldson MS, editors. To Err is Human: Building a Safer Health System [Internet]. Washington (DC): National Academies Press (US); 2000. [cited 2018 Mar 9]. Available from: http://www.ncbi.nlm.nih.gov/books/NBK225182/.
31. Brady A-M, Malone A-M, Fleming S. A literature review of the individual and systems factors that contribute to medication errors in nursing practice. J Nurs Manag. 2009;17(6):679–97.
32. Petrova E, Baldacchino D, Camilleri M. Nurses' perceptions of medication errors in Malta. Nurs Stand. 2010;24(33):41–8.
33. Assefa F, Mosse A, Hailemichael Y. Assessment of clients' satisfaction with health service deliveries at Jimma University specialized hospital. Ethiop J Health Sci. 2011;21(2):101.
34. Bohomol E, Ramos LH, D'Innocenzo M. Medication errors in an intensive care unit. J Adv Nurs. 2009;65(6):1259–67.
35. Mayo AM, Duncan D. Nurse perceptions of medication errors: what we need to know for patient safety. J Nurs Care Qual. 2004;19(3):209–17.

6

Factors affecting the cultural competence of visiting nurses for rural multicultural family support in South Korea

Min Hyun Suk[1], Won-Oak Oh[2]* and YeoJin Im[3]

Abstract

Background: With the recent growth of multicultural families in the Korean society, the importance of the role of qualified visiting nurses in the delivery of culturally sensitive health care has grown dramatically. As the primary health care provider for multicultural families enrolled in public community-based health care centers, the cultural competence of visiting nurses is an essential qualification for the provision of quality health care for multicultural families, especially in rural areas. Cultural competence of visiting nurses is based on their cultural awareness and empathetic attitude toward multicultural families. This study aimed to examine the levels of cultural competence, empowerment, and empathy in visiting nurses, and to verify the factors that affect the cultural competence of visiting nurses working with rural multicultural families in South Korea.

Methods: Employing a cross-sectional descriptive study design, data from 143 visiting nurses working in rural areas were obtained. Data collection took place between November 2011 and August 2012. The measurement tools included the modified Korean version of the Cultural Awareness Scale, the Text of Items Measuring Empowerment, and the Interpersonal Reactivity Index to measure the level of empathy of visiting nurses. Analyses included descriptive statistics, a t-test, an ANOVA, a Pearson correlation coefficient analysis, and a multiple linear regression analysis.

Results: The cultural competence score of the visiting nurses was 3.07 on a 5-point Likert scale (SD = 0.30). The multiple regression analysis revealed that the cultural competence of visiting nurses was significantly influenced by experience of cultural education, empathy, and scores on the meaning subscale of the empowerment tool ($R^2 = 10.2\%$).

Conclusions: Institutional support to enhance visiting nurses' empowerment by assuring the significance of their job and specific strategies to enhance their empathy would be helpful to improve the cultural competence of visiting nurses. Additionally, regular systematic education on culturally sensitive care would be helpful to enable visiting nurses to provide culturally sensitive care for multicultural families.

Keywords: Cultural competence, Cultural diversity, Empowerment, Empathy, Community health

Background

Cultural competence indicates the awareness and incorporation of knowledge about individuals and groups of people into specific standards, policies, practices, and attitudes by incorporating the patient's views, personal value base and beliefs [1]. Cultural competence in nursing reflects the nurse's ability to provide individualized culturally sensitive patient care with a respect and an openness to the patient's social or cultural background [2]. In a multicultural society, the cultural competence of health care professionals can be a reflection of their ability to provide sensitive care for clients with diverse social or cultural backgrounds. This may include an understanding of patients' cultural heritage, respect for patients' health beliefs, and an understanding of how other cultural issues may affect the level of care provided [3]. As one of the representative multicultural societies, the equal access to health care and the qualified culturally competent care for those with different cultural and ethnic background have been consistently emphasized in

* Correspondence: wooh@korea.ac.kr
[2]College of Nursing, Korea University, 145 Anam-ro, Seongbuk-gu, Seoul 02841, South Korea
Full list of author information is available at the end of the article

the United States. Culturally competent health care enhances health outcomes through the development of positive relationships between health care providers and clients, and it can reduce ethnic disparities in health care [4, 5].

South Korea has rapidly changed into a multicultural society in the recent decade. The major cause of these rapid changes is international marriage, majority of which have occurred between Korean males residing in rural areas and foreign females immigrants from Vietnam, the Philippines, and China. International marriages accounted for 8.7% of all Korean marriages in 2014 [6]. As most of the multicultural families reside in rural areas, and the productive industries are concentrated in the urban areas in Korea, they have a relatively low socioeconomic status as compared to families comprising members with identical cultural backgrounds. In addition to economic vulnerabilities, new concerns such as lack of access to health care, especially in multicultural families living in rural areas, as well as the high possibility of receiving less optimal qualified health care mainly because of a language barrier in specific health care situations have emerged.

With the social agreement on the need to support multicultural families, especially immigrant women and their children, the "Center of Family Support for Marriage Immigrants" program was initiated in South Korea in 2006, to help them enhance their cultural adaptation by overcoming language barriers and maximizing health care access. This program was then extended to the "multicultural family support system" with an aim to meet the health care needs of families with different cultural backgrounds and to provide them comprehensive health care support by introducing a new health care workforce at the national level.

Visiting nurses, as nursing professionals engaged in working in community public health care centers, provide services for the vulnerable population throughout the life span, including care for elderly persons living alone and young infants and toddlers in low income families. The care of visiting nurses typically includes disease prevention and ensures that community residents engage with direct and indirect health care services, including chronic disease management. Since 2007, they have emerged as professionals who provide health care for multicultural families in the primary health care setting.

In this regard, the visiting nurses' culturally competent care for multicultural families to overcome their lack of access to health care and to ensure quality health care has become critical. Nurses' cultural competence influences their ability to provide individualized health care for families with various cultural backgrounds. As a significant attribute of cultural competence, empathy is

recognized as one of the factors that strengthens the cultural competencies of health care providers [7, 8] and it is considered a critical predictor of successful cultural integration. Empathy is a basic component of cultural competence, which is expressed through their caring and comprehensive attitude with a consideration on patients' individual experiences [9, 10]. Empathy in visiting nurses refers to the capability of the health care provider to understand clients' situations, perspectives, and feelings, and also helps them to communicate and act with multicultural families in a positive manner by actively mediating the attributes of cultural competence [10, 11]. Health care providers' respectful and careful understanding of clients with different cultural backgrounds is a critical prerequisite in culturally competent care. Therefore, culturally competent care is significantly associated with the empathetic ability of nurses, and nurses' cultural competence may be revealed through their empathetic communication with the family.

Further, when nurses provide competent care for patients with culturally diverse backgrounds, empowerment is an important attribute in their nursing practice that may influence the provision of culturally competent nursing care [12]. Empowerment may enhance nurses' cognitive resources and improve their confidence through autonomy [13, 14]. By promoting their own sense of power and heightened motivation, nurses are able to provide competent care and empower others. Thus, empowering the cultural competence of health care providers may also be helpful in the provision of improved health care services for vulnerable populations, such as multicultural families.

In spite of the growing need for health care providers' cultural competence in community health care, there is a serious lack of thorough investigation on the cultural competence of visiting nurses at the domestic and international level. Recent studies on cultural competence in nursing have focused on assessing cultural competence and examining the predictors of the same at an early stage. Additionally, previous domestic studies on multicultural families have identified the current health care status and the health care needs of multicultural families.

Given that the significance of empowerment and empathy of visiting nurses in building their ability to provide cultural competent care for multicultural families, a study to investigate the factors affecting visiting nurses' cultural competence by including empowerment and empathy would be meaningful to plan strategies for working with multicultural families. Therefore, the present study aimed to examine the levels of cultural competence, empowerment, and empathy in visiting nurses, who are primary health care professionals for multicultural families in the rural areas of South Korea, and to verify the factors that affect the cultural competence of visiting nurses.

Methods
Design and sample
A cross-sectional descriptive study design was used. The target population of this study was Korean visiting nurses. The accessible population was a group of visiting nurses who were enrolled in 23 public health centers situated in Gyeongbuk province, the 2nd largest district except for the metropolitan areas in S. Korea, where 15.5% of multicultural families resided in 2012. Inclusion criteria were being enrolled in a public community health care center and being responsible for the health care services for the residents in the corresponding area. Those in charge of office work in the community health care centers were excluded.

We used G power 3.0 analysis to calculate the most reasonable sample size to secure a reliable interpretation of the study results and to prevent immoderate data collection. Using a constant that was most suitable for a multiple regression analysis (effect size .15, a significance level .05, a power .95), a minimum sample of 107 participants was required. Considering a 20% data wastage rate, we collected data from 156 visiting nurses, and the data from 143 participants was finally used after excluding 13 incomplete or incorrectly responded questionnaires.

Data collection and ethical considerations
All the data collection procedures in this study conformed to the Declaration of Helsinki. The study posed a low or not more than a minimal risk to the study participants. Data collection was conducted with the approval of the head of the relevant public health care centers, from November 2011 to August 2012. We consider the characteristics of multicultural society in South Korea have not been changed dramatically compared to 5 years ago. This is based on our statistics that the cases of international marriage, which is the main unique characteristic factor to shape the multi-cultural society in our society, has not been increased because of the consolidated restriction on international marriage policy since 2011.

With the cooperation of the team manager for visiting nurses, the research team attended the training center for visiting nurses in the public health care centers. After securing permission of the directors who manage and educate visiting nurses at such centers, we attached a public notice for recruiting participants for this study.

The visiting nurses who expressed willingness to join in this study were enrolled. Informed written consent was obtained from all participants following an explanation of the purpose, methods, risks, and benefits of the study and the rights of participants, such as voluntary participation, and provision of the researchers' contact information provided. Additionally, the participants were informed that they could withdraw from the study at any time. After completing the self-reported questionnaire, they returned it to the research team member in person. Moreover, the confidentiality of the information obtained was guaranteed by all data collectors and investigators by using code numbers rather than personal identifiers and by keeping the questionnaires locked in the corresponding author's cabinet.

Measures
Demographic characteristics
To investigate the demographic characteristics of visiting nurses, we used a 7-item questionnaire that included age, marital status, education years, experience as a visiting nurse, and experience of education on culturally competent care.

Cultural competence
Cultural competence was assessed using the modified Korean version [15] of the Cultural Awareness Scale (CAS) [16] was used. The CAS was selected as it measures comprehensive perception on the cultural competence of the nurses, such as an awareness of the differences in culture, personal values, beliefs, and biases of the self and others, rather than asking about specific knowledge or ability related to the specific cultural areas. Additionally, the items of the measurement tool were adequate for the Korean situation of the newly introduced multicultural society, owing to which nurses' cultural competence would be at an early stage of development.

After excluding the items related social welfare area and those which were not fit for the Korean situation, a total 12 items were answered on a 5-point Likert scale. It includes three dimensions: "Awareness of the differences in culture," "Awareness of personal values, beliefs and biases of the self," and "Awareness of the values, beliefs and biases of others." Higher scores reflect higher cultural competence. The internal consistency coefficient, as measured by the Cronbach's alpha, was .73 in the study by Min & Lee [15], and .74 in the present study.

Empowerment
The level of empowerment of visiting nurses was measured using the revised Korean version [17] of the Text of Items Measuring Empowerment (TIME), developed by Spreitzer [18]. This measurement focuses on the nurses' psychosocial empowerment rather than their practice outcomes. We selected this measure because the level of psychosocial empowerment of nurses can enhance their motivation to provide culturally competent care in their daily practice. Additionally, the

translated version was suitable enough to use with a Korean sample. A 5-point Likert scale is used to assess each of the 12 items that cover four subscales ("meaning," "competence," "self-determination," and "impact"), with three questions in each subscale. Higher scores reflect higher levels of empowerment. The Cronbach's alpha of the Korean version was .899 in Nam and Park's study [17] and .870, 850, and .890 for the subscales in the present study.

Empathy

The Korean translation [19] of the Interpersonal Reactivity Index (IRI) used in Davis' study [20] was used to assess the level of empathy among visiting nurses. It was originally developed to measure empathetic abilities and interpersonal interactions of nursing students. We selected the IRI as it could reflect the visiting nurses' empathy and sensitive interpersonal relationships in caring for patients with different cultural backgrounds in the Korean society. The index uses a 5-point Likert scales ranging from "Don't agree" (1) to "Strongly agree" (5) for each of the 28 items. These items cover the following four subscales: "Perspective taking," "fantasy," "empathic concern," and "personal distress." Content and face validity were assessed by seven health care professionals, including professors in nursing science, doctoral students in nursing, nurse managers, and staff nurses. Two items that did not accurately convey the intended meaning were corrected as a result of this process. The Cronbach's alpha in a previous study [19] was .84 and .71 in the present study.

Data analysis strategy

Data analysis was performed using PASW software (version 19.0). Percentages, means, and standard deviations (SDs) were calculated for participants' demographic characteristics. In addition, means, SDs, and possible ranges of cultural competence, empowerment, and empathy scores were also calculated. Differences in cultural competence scores by demographics were analyzed by either t-tests or ANOVA. Pearson correlation coefficients were computed to examine the relationships among these variables. Finally, each variable that was significantly correlated with scores in cultural competence and the two main research variables (empathy, empowerment) were included in a stepwise multiple linear regression model to verify the factors affecting the cultural competence of visiting nurses.

Results

Data from the 143 participants were finally analyzed after excluding 13 incomplete questionnaires from the sample of 156 visiting nurses.

Demographic characteristics and differences in cultural competence by demographics

The demographic characteristics of the sample have been reported in Table 1. The mean age of visiting nurses was 39.44 years (SD = 7.66) and most participants ($n = 114$, 80.3%) were married. The average years of experience as a visiting nurse was 30.12 months (SD = 25.62). Most (79%) had completed a 3-year nursing college qualification and 18.2% had obtained a bachelor's degree from a nursing school. In total, 90.9% of visiting nurses reported an experience of caring for multicultural families. Overall, 20.3% indicated that they had received training or education on diverse cultural issues that may be helpful when caring for multicultural families.

Significant differences in visiting nurses' cultural competence scores were revealed between those that had undergone education on multicultural nursing and those that had not ($t = 2.53$, $p = .012$), with the former exhibiting higher cultural competence scores (Table 2).

Cultural competence, empowerment, and empathy in visiting nurses

The average cultural competence score among visiting nurses was 36.84 (SD = 3.61), with an item mean of 3.07 (SD = 0.30) (Table 3). The subscales showing the highest scores were awareness of personal values, beliefs, and biases of the self (Mean = 3.15, SD = 0.42) and awareness of the differences in culture (Mean = 2.98, SD = 0.45), respectively.

The average empowerment score of visiting nurses was 44.95 (SD = 6.47), with an item mean of 3.75 (SD = 0.54). The subscale with the highest item mean was meaning (Mean = 4.24, SD = 0.66), followed by competence (Mean = 4.01, SD = 0.63), self-determination (Mean = 3.76, SD = 0.80), and impact (Mean = 2.97, SD = 0.88), respectively. The average empathy score of the participants was 150.21 (SD = 10.15), with an item mean of 3.58 (SD = 0.36) on a 5-point Likert scale.

Correlations among primary variables

Correlations among cultural competence, empowerment, and empathy have been presented in Table 4. The total mean score of cultural competence in visiting nurses were positively correlated with the meaning ($r = .17$, $p = .016$) and competence ($r = .16$, $p = .022$) subscales of empowerment. The higher the mean scores on the meaning subscales of empowerment were, the higher were the mean scores on the "awareness of differences in culture" subscale of cultural competence ($r = .16$, $p = .018$). Further, positive correlations were found between the cultural competence subscale of awareness of personal values, beliefs, and biases of the self and the empowerment subscales of meaning ($r = .16$, $p = .025$) and competence ($r = .14$, $p = .042$). Although there was no significant

Table 1 Demographic Characteristics of Subjects ($N = 143$)

Characteristics	Categories	n (%)	Mean ± SD
Age (years)	< 30	32 (22.4)	
	30–40	43 (30.1)	39.44 ± 7.66
	> 40	68 (47.6)	
Marital status	Unmarried	29 (19.7)	
	Married	114 (80.3)	
Total experience as a nurse (years)	≤ 3	18 (12.6)	
	3–10	76 (53.2)	9.73 ± 5.84
	> 10	49 (34.2)	
Experience as a visiting nurse (months)	≤ 12	24 (16.8)	
	13–24	35 (24.5)	30.12 ± 25.62
	≥ 25	84 (58.7)	
Education	College	113 (79.0)	
	University	26 (18.2)	
	Master	4 (2.8)	
Experience of caring multicultural family	Yes	130 (90.9)	
	No	13 (9.1)	
Experience of cultural education	Yes	29 (20.3)	
	No	114 (79.7)	

Table 2 Differences in Cultural Competency by Demographic Characteristics ($N = 143$)

Characteristics	Categories	Cultural competence		
		Mean (SD)	t/F	p
Age (years)	< 30	36.56 (3.33)	0.48	0.621
	30–40	36.74 (4.09)		
	> 40	37.15 (3.36)		
Marital status	unmarried	36.44 (4.09)	1.10	0.271
	married	37.17 (3.53)		
Total experience as a nurse (years)	≤ 3	37.77 (3.31)	2.04	0.132
	3–10	36.22 (3.82)		
	> 10	36.57 (3.25)		
Experience as a visiting nurse (months)	≤ 12	37.44 (2.93)		
	13–24	35.96 (3.12)	2.48	0.087
	≥ 25	37.10 (3.94)		
Education	College	36.89 (3.61)		
	University	37.14 (3.75)	1.06	0.348
	Master	35.07 (3.14)		
Experience of caring for multicultural families	Yes	36.82 (3.66)		
	No	37.20 (2.64)	0.36	0.722
Experience of cultural education	Yes	38.12 (3.20)	2.53	0.012[*]
	No	36.54 (3.64)		

*Significant at $p < .05$

Table 3 Descriptive Statistics for the Study Variables (N = 143)

	Mean	SD	Item mean	Item SD	Range
Cultural competence (total)	36.84	3.61	3.07	0.30	60–31
Differences in culture	11.93	1.82	2.98	0.45	20–8
Personal values, beliefs and biases of selves	9.46	1.27	3.15	0.42	15–6
Values, beliefs, and biases of others	15.45	1.91	3.09	0.38	25–13
Empowerment (total)	44.95	6.47	3.75	0.54	59–29
Meaning	12.71	1.98	4.24	0.66	15–8
Competence	12.03	1.90	4.01	0.63	15–8
Self-Determination	11.29	2.39	3.76	0.80	15–5
Impact	8.92	2.65	2.97	0.88	15–3
Empathy	150.21	10.15	3.58	0.36	163–81

correlation between the overall cultural competence score and empathy, there was a significant positive correlation between the cultural competence subscale of awareness of personal values, beliefs, and biases of the self and overall empathy ($r = .15$, $p = .035$).

Finally, empathy was found to have a significant positive correlation with empowerment ($r = .21$, $p = .003$), meaning ($r = .19$, $p = .006$), and competence ($r = .26$, $p = .002$).

Factors affecting the cultural competence of visiting nurses
The variables included in the multiple regression analysis used to identify the factors affecting the cultural competence of visiting nurses were empowerment, empathy, and

the experience of education on cultural issues, which was the demographic variable showing a statistically significant difference in cultural competence scores. As cultural education experience was measured through a yes/no question, this was entered as a dummy variable in the multiple regression analysis.

Multicollinearity and residual analyses were conducted prior to the multiple regression analysis. All tolerance parameter estimates were over 0.1, and they ranged from 0.63–0.96. The values of the variance inflation factors (VIFs) were 1.04–1.70, which may have ruled out any issues associated with problems of multicollinearity among the variables included in the multiple regression. A subsequent residual analysis revealed a Durbin-Watson value of

Table 4 Correlation Coefficients of the Study Variables (N = 143)

	CC	CC-D	CC-P	CC-O	Emp	Emp-Mean	Emp-Comp	Emp-Self	Emp-Imp	Empathy
Cultural Competence (CC)	1									
Differences in culture (CC-D)	0.71 (<.000)**	1								
Personal values, beliefs and biases (CC-P)	0.68 (<.000)**	0.28 (<.000)**	1							
Values, beliefs, and biases of others (CC-O)	0.76 (<.000)**	0.20 (0.003)**	0.35 (<.000)**	1						
Empowerment (Emp)	0.12 (0.081)	0.09 (0.203)	0.11 (0.129)	0.07 (0.315)	1					
Meaning (Emp-Mean)	0.17 (0.016)*	0.16 (0.018)*	0.16 (0.025)*	0.06 (0.421)	0.65 (<.000)**	1				
Competence (Emp-Comp)	0.16 (0.022)*	0.08 (0.269)	0.14 (0.042)*	0.13 (0.055)	0.74 (<.000)**	0.54 (<.000)**	1			
Self-determination (Emp-Self)	0.08 (0.231)	0.05 (0.502)	0.09 (0.193)	0.05 (0.452)	0.81 (<.000)**	0.38 (<.000)**	0.48 (<.000)**	1		
Impact (Emp-Imp)	0.02 (0.783)	0.00 (0.959)	0.03 (0.688)	0.21 (0.837)	0.69 (<.000)**	0.11 (0.107)	0.25 (0.000)**	0.45 (<.000)**	1	
Empathy	0.03 (0.663)	0.02 (0.770)	0.15 (0.035)*	0.06 (0.396)	0.21 (0.003)*	0.19 (0.006)*	0.26 (0.002)**	0.11 (0.120)	0.14 (0.051)	1

*Significant at $p < .05$
**Significant at $p < .01$

1.89, which verified the independence among residuals. All 143 observed values were included, as the Cook's D values were less than 0.1 for all participants.

In the subsequent multiple regression analysis that was conducted to identify the relative influences of the study variables, experience of cultural education, empathy, and the meaning subscale of empowerment were found to have a significant influence on the cultural competence of visiting nurses. The R square of the regression model was 10.2%, and it was 4.3% for cultural education experience, 3.85% for empathy, and 2.1% for meaning. These figures have been presented in Table 5.

Discussion

This study investigated the cultural competence of visiting nurses in Korea and identified the factors that affect this trait by including the variables of empowerment and empathy.

First, we could verify that the visiting nurses were primarily responsible for providing care to multicultural families in the rural area in which the present study was conducted. Specifically, over 90% of the visiting nurses in this study had experienced the provision of care for multicultural families. In spite of the rapid growth of multicultural families in the recent decade, there has been rudimentary level of governmental support for health care professionals in providing culturally sensitive care for multicultural families, which was evidenced by the finding that only about 20% of the visiting nurses had received training on culturally sensitive care.

In other countries with a large multicultural population, such as the United States, cultural diversity training is integrated with the nursing curriculum and forms a part of their clinical nursing practice [21, 22]. Such a system helps to ensure that health care professionals have adequate cultural competence and cultural sensitivity to successfully work with multicultural families and communities [23]. In Korea, a developing multicultural society, there has been a lack of preparation for the various challenges associated with multiculturalism and this is also true for the application of health care and the nursing curriculum in general.

Therefore, it will be important that such gaps in the system be addressed and that cultural diversity issues are discussed and acted upon. A systematic review reported that educational programs to improve nurses' culturally

competent care have a positive influence on nurses' cultural competence [24]. Therefore, a well-designed education program aimed to enhance the cultural competence of visiting nurses, and which is suitable enough to reflect the Korean cultural context, should be introduced as early as possible.

Although a direct comparison of study results may be limited due to the shortage of studies on multicultural issues, the mean cultural competence scores among visiting nurses in this study were above the median level, which was higher than those among nurses in tertiary level university hospitals [25] and undergraduate nursing students in Korea [26] but were lower than those in undergraduate freshmen and faculty members in US nursing schools [27]. Considering that nurses' cultural competence is reflected in their ability to provide qualified health care to clients with various cultural backgrounds [12], it was significant to find that levels of empowerment among visiting nurses in this study were above the median value. However, as compared to scores on the meaning and competence subscales of empowerment, those on the impact subscale of this measure were relatively low. This means that although nurses may easily perceive the importance of providing health care to families and are relatively confident in doing so, they tend to downplay the importance of their specific role in health care outcomes, possibly due to their unstable position as an employee. Additional institutional support aimed at providing increased job security for visiting nurses might help enhance their empowerment.

It is significant to note the present findings of empathy scores above the median level. Empathy allows visiting nurses to create interactions based on mutual respect and through the acceptance of alternative lifestyles and the reduction of bias [28, 29]. Nurses with high level of cultural competence are able to use interpersonal communication, relationship skills, and behavioral flexibility to work effectively in cross-cultural situations [30].

In regard to correlation among study variables, there was no significant correlation between empowerment and cultural competence, which resembles the results reported by Bauce, Kridli, and Fitzpatrick [12]. Given that empowerment may be an important contributor to professional nursing practice and may influence the provision of culturally competent care [12], strategies to enhance nurses' empowerment, which subsequently may

Table 5 Factors Affecting Cultural Competence ($N = 143$)

Variables	B	S.E.	β	Adjusted R^2	Cumulative R^2	t (p)	F (p)
Experience of cultural education	2.67	0.82	0.17	0.043	0.043	6.99 (.009)**	7.61 (<.001)**
Empathy	0.04	0.02	0.02	0.038	0.081	6.45 (.012)*	
Empowerment (meaning)	2.17	0.17	0.17	0.021	0.102	4.75 (.031)*	

*Significant at $p < .05$
**Significant at $p < .01$

strengthen culturally sensitive care, need to be developed. Instrument development to measure nurses' empowerment in regard to their culturally competent care would also be helpful for further investigation.

Further, contrary to previous studies, we could not find a significant correlation between empathy and cultural competence in this study. This may have occurred owing to the use of the IRI to assess empathy, as it focuses on the broad aspects of nursing, and not the aspects of perception, attitude, and specific skills of culturally competent care in nurses. Development of a sensitive instrument to measure nurses' empathy in the Korean culture is therefore necessary. Nonetheless, empathy was finally verified as one of the factors influencing the cultural competence of visiting nurses in our regression model.

As an important finding, we identified the three significant factors affecting the cultural competence of visiting nurses in this study, namely, cultural education experience, empathy, and perceived work role meaning (a subcategory of empowerment). First, improved cultural competence among health care providers has a positive effect on patient care by creating interactions that are based on respect and that incorporate the health beliefs, practices, and cultural and linguistic needs of culturally diverse clients. Considering the current lack of training on cultural issues available to visiting nurses, the introduction of culture-related education is an urgent issue in Korea's new multicultural society. For multicultural families in rural areas, considered as one of the vulnerable sections of the populations in terms of health care access and quality, careful investigations into their current health care status and future health needs are also required in order to provide effective health care. Additionally, the development and implementation of strategies to enhance empathetic attitudes and levels of empowerment among visiting nurses, especially those related to the importance of their own roles as health care providers, are required to improve the cultural competence of visiting nurses.

In spite of the significant research findings of this study that identified the factors that affect cultural competence among visiting nurses, there were some limitations in this study.

First, the population in this study included a limited location of Korean rural areas in 2011/2012. Although we calculated the sample size based on G power analysis to secure reliable interpretation of the study results, and the study location was wide enough to ensure the selection of study participants with a suitable effect size, a nationwide study would be beneficial to confirm the present results. Given the dynamic nature of migration and research in this area, it is important to acknowledge the findings relate one point in time.

Second, the regression model in this study reported a relatively low R square value. This indicates that an additional study would require to incorporate other variables that may also influence cultural competence, such as individual knowledge on cultural issues, linguistic competence, ideas on patient centeredness, and/or degree of understanding of the health care system [31, 32]. Additionally, it would be beneficial to use other cultural competence measurements after assessing the psychometric properties of the Korean translated version of the tools.

Conclusions

Cultural education experience, empathy, and perceived work role meaning as a subcategory of empowerment were found to have a significant influence on the cultural competence of visiting nurses. Considering the rapid social changes leading to a culturally-diverse health care environment, it is critical to develop appropriate educational programs for visiting nurses, who are the foremost nursing profession caring for culturally diverse patients in the rural community. In this context, practical and efficient educational protocols should include methods to foster the self-awareness of visiting nurses on their potential biases toward the patient with different cultural backgrounds. Additionally, attention should be paid on the improvement of the nurses' empathetic and accepting attitude by enhancing their understanding of different health care customs. Second, efforts to enhance the mutual communication between visiting nurses and patients are required. Active involvement of the health care system to decrease language barriers, such as commercialization of phone or in-person interpreters, needs to be designed. Finally, we need to reinforce the general empowerment of visiting nurses, which would subsequently enable them to provide competent nursing care for culturally diverse patients.

Abbreviations
CC: Cultural competence; CC-D: Cultural competence-differences in culture; CC-O: Cultural competence-values, beliefs, and biases of others; CC-P: Cultural competence-personal values, beliefs and biases; Emp: Empowerment; Emp-Comp: Empowerment-competence; Emp-Imp: Empowerment-impact; Emp-Mean: Empowerment-meaning; Emp-Self: Empowerment-self-determination; SD: Standard deviation

Acknowledgements
None

Funding
None

Authors' contributions
MH conceived the study, coordinated the overall activity. WO participated in the design of the study and carried out the statistical analysis. YJ participated in the design of the study and drafted the manuscript. All authors read and approved the final manuscript.

Competing interests

The authors declare that they have no competing interests.

Author details

[1]Department of Nursing, CHA University, 30 Beolmal-lo, Bundang-gu, Seongnam-shi, Gyeongghi-do 13496, South Korea. [2]College of Nursing, Korea University, 145 Anam-ro, Seongbuk-gu, Seoul 02841, South Korea. [3]College of Nursing Science, Kyung Hee University, 26 Kyungheedae-ro, Dongdaemun-gu, Seoul 02447, South Korea.

References

1. Donald B, Davis P, Coleman HLK. Multicultural counseling competencies: assessment, evaluation, education and training, and supervision. In: Sodowsky GR, Kuo-Jackson PY, Loya GJ, editors. . Thousand Oaks: Sage Publications; 1997. p. 3–41.
2. Papadopoulos I, Tilki M, Lees S. Promoting cultural competence in healthcare through a research-based intervention in the UK. Divers Health Care. 2004;1(2):107–16.
3. Giger J, Davidhizar RE, Purnell L, Harden JT, Phillips J, Strickland O, et al. American academy of nursing expert panel report: developing cultural competence to eliminate health disparities in ethnic minorities and other vulnerable populations. J Transcult Nurs. 2007;18(2):95–102.
4. Brach C, Fraserirector I. Can cultural competency reduce racial and ethnic health disparities? A review and conceptual model. Med Care Res Rev. 2000; 57:181–217. https://doi.org/10.1177/1077558700574009.
5. Callister LC. What has the literature taught us about culturally competent care of women and children. MCN Am J Matern Child Nurs. 2005;30(6):380–8.
6. Korean Statistical Information. Title of subordinate. In: International marriage migrants tables for Korea; 2014. http://www.index.go.kr/potal/main/EachDtlPageDetail.do?idx_cd=2430. Accessed 16 June 2015.
7. Looi JC. Empathy and competence. Med Journal Aust. 2008;188(7):414–6.
8. Peek EH, Park CS. Effects of a multicultural education program on the cultural competence, empathy and self-efficacy on nursing students. J Korean Acad Nurs. 2013;43(5):690–6. https://doi.org/10.4040/jkan.2013.43.5.690.
9. Egan G. The skilled helper. Pacific Grove: Brooks/Cole Publishing Company; 1994.
10. McCoy JA. Is empathy a fundamental substrate for cultural competence?. Chicago: American College of Surgeons 92nd annual clinical congress; 2006.
11. Chung RC, Bemak F. The relationship of culture and empathy in cross-culture counseling. J Counsel Dev. 2002;80(2):154–9.
12. Bauce K, Kridli SA, Fitzpatrick JJ. Cultural competence and psychological empowerment among acute care nurses. J Cult Compet Nurs and Healthcare. 2014;4(2):27–38. https://doi.org/10.9730/ojccnh.org/v4n2a3.
13. Dawson L, Lighthouse S. Assessment of self-efficacy for cultural competence in prescribing. The J Nurs Pract. 2010;6(1):44–8. https://doi.org/10.1016/j.nurpra.2009.02.012.
14. Zimmerman MA, Israel BA, Schulz A, Checkoway B. Further explorations in empowerment theory: an empirical analysis of psychological empowerment. Am J Community Psychol. 1992;20(6):707–27.
15. Min SH, Lee MY. A exploratory study about the cultural competence of university students – focused on the cultural awareness. J Adolesc Wel. 2009;11(1):183–206.
16. Cuevas MC. Cultural competence, cultural awareness, and attitudes of social work students. Austin: University of Texas; 2002.
17. Nam KH, Park JH. A study on the relationship of empowerment with job satisfaction and organizational commitment perceived by nurses. J Korean Nurs Adm Acad Soc. 2002;8(1):137–50.
18. Spreitzer GM. Psychological empowerment in the workplace. Acad Manag J. 1995;38(5):1442–65.
19. Park SH. Empathy. Won Mi Sa: Seoul; 1994.
20. Davis MH. Measuring individual differences in empathy: evidence for a multi-dimensional approach. J Pers Soc Psychol. 1983;44(1):113–26. https://doi.org/10.1037/0022-3514.44.1.113.
21. Bednarz H, Schim S, Doorenbos A. Cultural diversity in nursing education: perils, pitfalls, and pearls. J Nurs Educ. 2010;49(5):253–60. https://doi.org/10.3928/01484834-20100115-02.
22. Pacquiao D. The relationship between cultural competence education and increasing diversity in nursing schools and practice settings. J Transcult Nurs. 2007;18(1 Suppl):28S–37S. https://doi.org/10.1177/1043659606295679.
23. Bagnardi M, Bryant L, Colin J. Banks multicultural model: a framework for integrating multiculturalism into nursing curricula. J Prof Nurs. 2009;25(4):234–9. https://doi.org/10.1016/j.profnurs.2009.01.010.
24. Horvat L, Horey D, Romios P, Kis-Rigo J. Cultural competence education for health professionals. Cochrane Database Syst Rev. 2011;10 https://doi.org/10.1002/14651858.CD009405.
25. Chae DH, Park YH, Kang KH, Lee TH. A study on factors affecting cultural competency of general hospital nurses. J Korean Acad Adm. 2013;18(1):76–86. https://doi.org/10.11111/jkana.2012.18.1.76.
26. Kim DH, Kim SE. Cultural competence and factors influencing cultural competence in nursing students. J Korean Aca Psychiatri Ment Health Nurs. 2013;22(3):159–68. https://doi.org/10.12934/jkpmhn.2013.22.3.159.
27. Sargent SE, Sedlak CA, Martsolf DS. Cultural competence among nursing students and faculty. Nurse Edu Today. 2005;25(3):214–21.
28. Hoffman ML. Empathy and moral development: implications for caring and justice. New York, NY: Cambridge University Press; 2000.
29. Mercer SW, Reynolds WJ. Empathy and quality of care. Br J Gen Pract. 2002; 52(Suppl):S9–12.
30. Stanhope M, Lancaster J. Public health nursing; population-centered health care in the community. 7th ed. Mosby Elservior: Missouri; 2008.
31. Saha S, Beach MC, Cooper AC. Patient centeredness, cultural competence, and healthcare quality. J Nati Med Assoc. 2008;100(11):1275–85.
32. Taylor RA, Alfred MV. Nurses' perceptions of the organizational supports needed for the delivery of culturally competent care. Wes J Nurs Res. 2010; 32(5):591–609. https://doi.org/10.1177/0193945909354999.

7

Perceptions of perioperative nursing competence: a cross-country comparison

Brigid M. Gillespie[1,2,3*] , Emma B. Harbeck[3,4], Karin Falk-Brynhildsen[5], Ulrica Nilsson[5] and Maria Jaensson[5]

Abstract

Background: Throughout many countries, professional bodies rely on yearly self-assessment of competence for ongoing registration; therefore, nursing competence is pivotal to safe clinical practice. Our aim was to describe and compare perioperative nurses' perceptions of competence in four countries, while examining the effect of specialist education and years of experience in the operating room.

Methods: We conducted a secondary analysis of cross-sectional surveys from four countries including; Australia, Canada, Scotland, and Sweden. The 40-item *Perceived Perioperative Competence Scale-Revised* (PPCS-R), was used with a total sample of 768 respondents. We used a factorial design to examine the influence of country, years of experience in the operating room and specialist education on nurses' reported perceived perioperative competence.

Results: Regardless of country origin, nurses with specialist qualifications reported higher perceived perioperative competence when compared to nurses without specialist education. However, cross-country differences were dependent on nurses' number of years of experience in the operating room. Nurses from Sweden with 6–10 years of experience in the operating room reported lower perceived perioperative competence when compared to Australian nurses. In comparing nurses with > 10 years of experience, Swedish nurses reported significantly lower perceived perioperative competence when compared to nurses from Australia, Canada and Scotland.

Conclusion: Researchers need to consider educational level and years of experience in the perioperative context when examining constructs such as competence.

Keywords: Perioperative nursing, Competence, Cross-national, Survey, Patient safety

Background

Throughout many countries, professional bodies rely on yearly self-assessment of competence for ongoing registration [1]. Thus the issue of nursing competence is a fundamental aspect of safe clinical practice. Competence is described as a combination of skills, knowledge, attitudes, values and abilities that contribute to effective performance [2]. Assessment of clinical competence is therefore crucial in identifying areas where additional professional development and education are required [3]. Nurses' perceptions of their competence is an integral component of their professional self-image [4] and may affect role and teamwork performance, job satisfaction, recruitment and retention.

Nurses in countries with distinctly different healthcare systems report similar shortcomings in their work environments associated with the quality of hospital care [5, 6]. Previous research has described differences in nursing practice across countries relative to nurses' perceptions of professional roles and clinical responsibilities [7–9]. Describing where differences occur across countries is important. Although nurses perform similar roles, there is variation in how the tasks within these roles are operationalised [10]. In addition, government and statutory regulations determine nurses' scope of practice within these roles [1]. There are also variations in models of care, educational training and certification requirements differs widely among countries [10]. These earlier studies demonstrate the power of international comparisons, cross-cultural research, which

* Correspondence: b.gillespie@griffith.edu.au
[1]School of Nursing & Midwifery, Griffith University, Gold Coast, QLD, Australia
[2]Gold Coast Hospital and Health Service, Gold Coast, QLD, Australia
Full list of author information is available at the end of the article

offers opportunities to promote international harmonisation in nursing [9, 10].

While previous research has examined differences in nursing practice and healthcare contexts across generalist areas of nursing [11, 12], there is limited research that examines whether such differences exist relative to the specialised area of perioperative practice. In perioperative nursing, these specialisations include nurse anaesthetist, anaesthetic assistant, circulating, instrument, post-anaesthetic care unit roles [10]. Although clinical practices are circumscribed across countries, there is little data to describe cross-country differences relative to self-reported competence in the context of nurse education and years of perioperative experience. Previous work undertaken in the Australian context with samples ranging from 134 to 1178 nurses suggests that education and years of perioperative experience are predictors of perceived competence [13, 14]. However, there have been few, if any, cross-national studies undertaken to describe these relationships. While practice standards may be similar across developed countries, clinical practice and educational preparation is likely to differ from country to country. In this study, we hypothesised that there would be interaction effects between country and years of experience, and country and specialist qualifications, relative to perioperative nurses' perceived competence.

Methods

Design

A secondary analysis of cross-sectional surveys from four countries including; Australia, Canada, Scotland, and Sweden was undertaken using the Perceived Perioperative Competence Scale-Revised (PPSC-R) [15]. The aim of the primary analysis in the Australian context was to refine the PPCS-R to make a more parsimonious scale. The aims of the primary research in the Canadian and Scottish contexts was to compare differences in perceptions of competence among nurses and perioperative technicians. The aim of the primary study undertaken in Sweden was to test the PPSC-R in the Swedish context using confirmatory factor analysis. Demographic data related to gender, years of perioperative experience in the operating room (OR) and specialist qualifications were collected. 'Specialty education' is defined as education that is gained beyond that acquired in a baccalaureate or diploma level nursing course [13]. Specialist qualifications included graduate certification qualifications (e.g., CNOR, EBN), diplomas, masters, and professional and research doctorate degrees.

Participants, settings and sampling

The Australian sample was drawn from 575 RNs practising in the OR departments of 3 large metropolitan hospitals in Queensland. The Canadian sample was drawn from 301 RNs working in the OR departments of 3 large inner city hospitals in Toronto, Ontario. The United Kingdom (UK) sample of 203 perioperative nurses and practitioners was drawn from 3 NHS Trusts in eastern Scotland, spanning from Aberdeen to Larbert. The Australian, Canadian and UK samples were drawn using convenience methods. A census sample of 2902 nurses who were members of the Swedish Association of Health Professionals as either OR nurses or Registered Nurse Anaesthetists (RNA) were emailed independently through the Association. Survey data across samples was collected from 2011 to 2016.

Measures

Across the four countries, the PPSC-R [15] was used to measure perceived competence. The iterative development and validation of the 40-item PPCS-R is based on a series of earlier qualitative and quantitative studies [3, 13, 15–18]. The PPCS-R uses a 5-point Likert response option, with scores ranging between 40 to 200 and higher scores indicating greater levels of reported perceived competence [15]. The PPCS-R comprises 6 factors that indicate different dimensions of perioperative competence: *Foundational knowledge and skills; Leadership; Collaboration; Proficiency; Empathy; and Professional development* [15]. The total PPCS-R score is based on the sum of all 40 items in each of the 6 factors.

During testing, the PPCS-R demonstrated robust psychometric properties in census sample of Australian perioperative nurses ($n = 1122$). In this sample, the results of the final exploratory factor analysis (EFA) with the 6 factors accounted for 58.3% of the total variance, and Cronbach's alpha (α) ranged from .81 to .89 [15]. The PPCS-R has been used in the Australian and Canadian contexts, and the internal consistency (α) for the PPCS–R was .96 and .97 respectively [9, 19]. In the current study, the PPCS-R was used as the dependant variable for the analyses. More recently, the PPSC-R was translated into Swedish and validated in a national census of 2, 902 nurses who practised in circulating/instrument and nurse anaesthetist roles [20]. Confirmatory factor analysis (CFA) supported the factor structure of the PPSC-R using the six latent factors and indicated an acceptable model fit for the Swedish sample.

Statistical analysis

IBM SPSS Statistics version 22 was used to analyses the data. Descriptive and inferential analyses were used. Descriptive statistics were used to measure variable dispersion across the sample. The types of analyses used were determined by the level of the data (i.e., categorical or continuous) and its distribution. Respondents' composite PPCS–R and subscale scores (for the six domains) were measured as continuous variables while gender, primary role, specialty qualifications and years of OR experience were analysed as categorical variables. Cronbach's alpha (α) was used to determine the internal consistency of the PPCS–R.

Inferential analyses included 4 (country: Australia, Canada, Scotland and Sweden) × 3 (years of experience in the OR: 0–5 years, 6–10 years and > 10 years) × 2 (specialist and non-specialist qualification) factorial Analysis of Variance (ANOVA). We used an alpha level of 0. 05 to determine statistical significance. Partial eta squared (η_p^2) was used as an indication of effect size. Traditionally η_p^2 values of 0.01, 0.06 and 0.14 represent small, medium and large effect sizes [21]. Levene's test for homogeneity of variances was used to assess equality of variances across groups. When this assumption was non-significant ($p > .05$), equal variances were assumed and a Bonferroni correction was used to assess significance for multiple comparisons. When homogeneity was violated $p < .05$, and equal variances were not assumed and the Games-Howell correction was used to assess significance.

Results

Survey data across the four countries was collected from 2011 to 2015. Response rates were as follows; Australia 30.6% (176/575), Canada 76.5% (134/175), Scotland 71. 1% (214/301), and Sweden 38.5% (1033/2679). Across the four countries, the combined sample of 1557 cases was reduced to a final sample of 768. The Swedish sample had 1033 cases of data and this was disproportionate to the other 3 samples sizes. Thus we used a stratified random sample of 250 cases was selected from the original sample. The 250 cases were stratified by nursing role, resulting in 125 OR nurses and 125 RNAs. However, across the samples 6 cases were also removed due to missing data. The sample demographics for the 4 countries are provided in Table 1. Internal consistency was examined for the current sample with Cronbach's alpha ranging from 0.94 for Sweden, 0.96 for Scotland and 0.97 for both Australian and Canadian samples.

Descriptive results of total PPCS-R scores for each country relative to years of OR experience and specialist qualification are detailed in Table 2. There was a significant main effect of specialist education $F (1,706) = 4.0$, $p = .047$ ($\eta_p^2 = .01$). A main effect is the effect of one the independent variable i.e., specialist education on the dependent variable PPC-R, ignoring all other independent variables. Overall, respondents who had specialist qualifications reported higher PPC ($M = 163.1$, $Std\ error = 1.3$, 95% CI 160.6–165.6) than those without specialist education ($M = 159.5$, $Std\ error = 1.3$, 95% CI 156.9–162.0).

There were also significant main effects for Country $F(3,706) = 6.5$, $p < .001$ ($\eta_p^2 = .03$), and years of OR experience $F(2,706) = 58.5$, $p < .001$ ($\eta_p^2 = .14$). However, these were qualified by a significant interaction between these variables $F(6,706) = 2.5$, $p = .022$ ($\eta_p^2 = .02$), as shown in Fig. 1. This interaction effect represents the combined effects of independent variables i.e., country

Table 1 Cross country sample demographic results

	Australia	Canada	Scotland	Sweden	Total Sample
n (%)	175 (22.8)	132 (17.2)	212 (27.6)	249 (32.4)	768
Gender					
Male	21 (12.0)	14 (10.6)	24 (11.3)	38(15.3)	97 (12.6)
Female	154 (88.0)	118 (89.4)	188 (88.7)	211 (84.7)	671 (87.4)
Nursing role					
EN	0 (0.0)	14 (10.6)	4 (1.9)	0 (0.0)	18 (2.3)
RN/OR practitioner	131 (74.9)	118 (89.4)	192 (90.6)	0 (0.0)	441 (57.4)
Clinical nurse/manager	44 (25.1)	0 (0.0)	16 (7.5)	0 (0.0)	60 (7.8)
RNA	0 (0.0)	0 (0.0)	0 (0.0)	125 (50.2)	125 (16.3)
OR nurse	0 (0.0)	0 (0.0)	0 (0.0)	124 (49.8)	124 (16.2)
Specialist qualification					
Yes	51 (29.1)	103 (78.0)	96 (45.3)	58 (23.3)	460 (59.9)
No	124 (70.9)	29 (22.0)	116 (54.7)	191 (76.7)	308 (40.1)
Years in the OR					
0–5 years	64 (36.6)	38 (28.8)	59 (27.8)	50 (20.1)	211 (27.5)
6–10 years	33 (18.9)	26 (19.7)	42 (19.8)	60 (24.1)	161 (21.0)
> 10 years	78 (44.5)	68 (51.5)	111 (52.4)	139 (55.8)	396 (51.5)

Abbreviations: EN = enrolled nurse, RN = registered nurse, RNA = registered nurse anaesthetist, OR nurse = operating room (i.e., circulating/instrument/anaesthetic roles)

Table 2 PPSC-R scores across countries relative to specialist education and years of experience in the OR

Country	Variable	Mean	Std. error	95% CI
Australia				
	Specialist qualification			
	Yes	166.2	3.3	159.7–172.6
	No	161.4	1.9	157.7–165.1
	Years of experience in the OR			
	0–5 years	148.1	4.0	140.2–156.0
	6–10 years	170.1	3.3	163.6–176.6
	> 10 years	173.1	2.2	168.8–177.5
Canada				
	Specialist qualification			
	Yes	166.3	2.1	162.1–170.5
	No	157.9	4.0	150.0–165.9
	Years of experience in the OR			
	0–5 years	144.3	4.9	134.6–154.0
	6–10 years	166.9	3.9	159.2–174.6
	> 10 years	175.2	2.7	170.0–180.5
Scotland				
	Specialist qualification			
	Yes	164.9	2.0	160.9–168.8
	No	163.3	2.2	159.0–167.6
	Years of experience in the OR			
	0–5 years	152.0	2.6	146.9–157.1
	6–10 years	163.5	3.1	157.5–169.5
	> 10 years	176.7	2.0	172.8–180.6
Sweden				
	Specialist qualification			
	Yes	156.3	2.8	150.9–161.8
	No	154.7	2.0	150.8–158.5
	Years of experience in the OR			
	0–5 years	144.9	2.7	139.5–150.2
	6–10 years	162.2	3.0	156.3–168.0
	> 10 years	158.7	2.6	153.5–163.8

and years of OR experience, on the dependent variable, PPC-R. Post hoc multiple comparisons were run by splitting analyses via years of experience in the OR (0–5 years, 6–10 years and > 10 years), which resulted in three one-way ANOVAs with country as the independent variable. There were no significant country differences in respondents with 0–5 years of OR experience $F(3,193) = 1.23$, $p = .300$. However, country differences did occur in total reported PPC for respondents with 6–10 years of experience $F(3,152) = 4.33$, $p = .006$ ($\eta_p^2 = .08$) and those with > 10 years of experience in the OR, $F(3,373) = 14.9$, $p < .001$ ($\eta_p^2 = .11$).

Pairwise comparisons between the countries for respondents with 6–10 years of experience in the OR show that in general, Australian nurses reported higher PPC when compared to the Swedish nurses only, $t = -3.6(91)$, $p = .001$. There were no significant differences between nurses in any other countries. For those with > 10 years of experience, nurses from Sweden reported significantly lower PPC when compared to nurses from Australia $t = -3.7(211)$, $p < .001$, Canada $t = -5.8$ (162.9), $p < .001$ and UK $t = -5.2(236)$, $p < .001$ respectively. No other significant differences were observed, between nurses with > 10 years' experience, in reported PPC. Means, standard error and 95% confidence intervals are shown in Table 2.

Discussion

In this secondary analysis of cross-national data, we examined the influence of specialist education and years of experience across a four-country sample in reported nurses perceived perioperative competence (PPC). Across the combined sample, 54% of survey respondents had over a decade of perioperative experience. Concomitantly, respondents reporting greater levels of PPC had more years of perioperative experience; thus the effect of years of experience follows the expected trend [13, 15, 22–24], with the exception of Sweden and to a lesser extent, Australia. In this study, 29% and 23% of Australian and Swedish nurses respectively reported having specialist qualifications. Our findings also suggest a decline in PPC for nurses from Sweden and Australia who had 6–10 years of perioperative experience and for nurses with 10 years or more perioperative experience; nurses from Sweden reporting lower PPC when compared to the other country samples. We suggest that these differences in self-reported competence may also be attributed to cultural interpretation. It may be that humility, self-control and frugality are more highly valued traits in Swedish culture. The Swedish word "lagom" meaning *less is more, just enough*, describes the basis of Swedish national psyche which is characterised by consensus, equity, and using a balanced and moderate approach [25]. Thus, we recommend caution in interpretation of these results as the lower levels of PPC among the Swedish sample are not necessarily indicative of diminished clinical mastery, performance or achievement.

Across the entire cross-national sample in this study, nearly 60% of perioperative nurses reported having a specialist qualification, with the highest numbers of nurses from Canada (78%) and Scotland (45%). Our findings suggest that there was an effect of specialist education, where nurses regardless of country of origin with specialist qualifications, reported higher levels of PPC when compared to nurses with undergraduate or vocational qualifications. Similar results have been described in a litany of earlier research on the influence

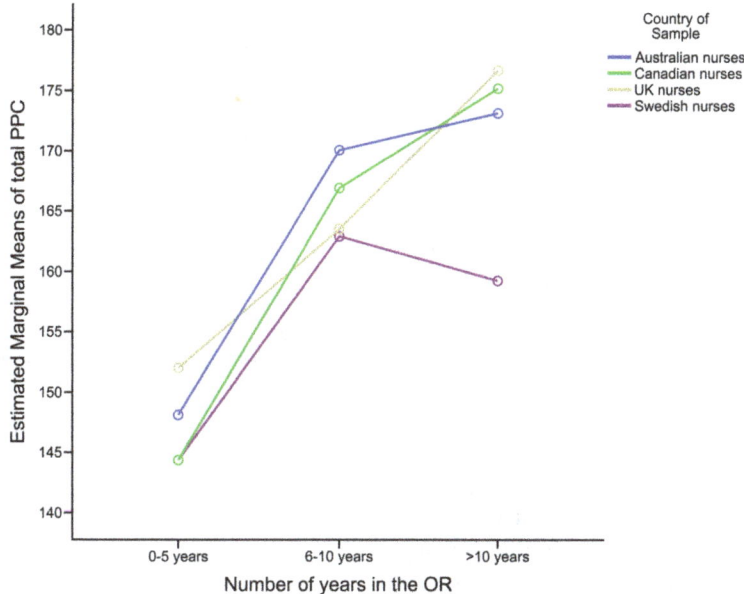

Fig. 1 Interaction plot based on s PPSC-R scores showing main effects for country and years of OR experience

of specialist or specialty education relative to self-reported competence [13, 15, 23, 26, 27]. Undoubtedly, there is likely diversity of educational programs offered at both the undergraduate and specialist levels among the cross-national samples in this study; thus, direct comparisons may be difficult to draw. For instance, in Australia, there is a range of postgraduate programs available to perioperative nurses, while in Canada, perioperative nurses are required to write a perioperative certification exam. In the UK, there are limited opportunities for nurses to extend their skills formally, while in Sweden, perioperative nurses are required to undertake postgraduate studies. Our results suggest the increases in PPC were consistent across all groups. Seminal cross-national and multisite research [5, 6, 28] confirms a logical connection between the level of nursing education, clinical judgement and patient outcomes.

There may be other reasons, not accounted for in our study to explain cross-country differences noted herein. First, while role may contribute significantly to clinical performance, it is unclear how or why it may affect perceived perioperative competence. In our study, small sample sizes and the differences in role identification across countries precluded analysis based on role categories. Second, the likely cultural differences in the conceptual interpretation of individual words or statements in the scale may have indirectly influenced our results. Finally, organisational macro-management strategies based on professional rewards may have a positive impact on nurse competence. For instance, competency-based management approaches that accurately assess a nurse's performance, skills and abilities have the potential

to increase nurses' understanding of their strengths and weaknesses [29]. Such approaches have led to increases in nurses' engagement with learning and the pursuit of additional qualifications that increase their expertise. The PPCS-R scale has potential to be used by front-line perioperative nurses as a tool to stimulate reflection on their clinical practice. This information can be used to assist perioperative nurse educators in tailoring their professional development programs to address strengths and weaknesses identified by front-line nurses.

Limitations and strengths
Although the PPC-R has been psychometrically evaluated in English [15] and Swedish [20], and has demonstrated robust properties, we acknowledge some limitations. First, most samples were drawn from convenience samples and only one sample from Sweden was population-based. Second, the response rates across all countries and samples ranged from 30% to 76%, while reasonable, may be difficult to generalise beyond the immediate sample. Third, the differences in the PPC-R sum scores between countries may reflect methodological differences between studies, such as when the conditions of data collection differed (surveyed at hospital versus emailed). Additionally as no random samples were drawn, differences may also be due to a population bias. This is one of the most frequent and most problematic shortcomings in cross-cultural studies [30]. Fourth, using years of experience as a categorical variable with pre-defined groupings is common in the literature; however this can result in reduced statistical power and increased risk of type two error [31]. Due to the secondary data analysis design of the current sample,

questionnaire data used for the sample only provided experience as a categorical variable for examination. As we found an effect of years of experience, future research should examine the how much variance can be explained by years of experience as a continuous variable. Fifth, these results were based on secondary analyses of the primary data collected several years earlier, and may not account for changes over time. Finally, the results of this cross-country comparison are based on self-assessment rather than on observed behaviours. Yet, self-reported measures are cost effective and provide opportunity for self-reflection.

Conclusion

To our knowledge, this is the first study to describe cross-country comparisons relative to perioperative nurses' perceived competence based on country, years of experience and specialty education. Our results also suggest that researchers need to take into account education qualifications and years of experience in the perioperative context when examining constructs such as competence. Cross-country comparative research contributes significantly to the body of knowledge about a specific country as well as providing information on important factors researchers need to consider when evaluating eclectic constructs such as competence in nursing samples. As such, our results may contribute to the examination of population norms for researchers who may want to evaluate perceived competence.

Acknowledgements
The research team gratefully acknowledge the willingness of survey participants.

Funding
No funding was received for this study.

Authors' contributions
BMG conceived of the study. EH, UN, MJ and KF-B assisted in the refinement of study design and method development. BMG and EH performed the analysis. BMG and UN, MJ and KF-B assisted in recruitment. BG drafted the manuscript. All authors assisted in interpretation, and revised the manuscript critically for important intellectual content. All authors participated in the design and coordination of the study, read, and approved the final manuscript. BG as the primary and corresponding author of this study agrees to be accountable for the accuracy and integrity of the work, therefore any questions should be directed to BG.

Ethics approval and consent to participate
Ethics approval to conduct this current study was not required as approval to use the results drawn from the surveys conducted in Australia, Canada and Scotland is covered in the original ethics applications: Survey data is kept "indefinitely for scholarly priority" in accordance with the Australian *National Health & Medical Research Guidelines* (2007). Access to the Swedish sample was provided by the Swedish Association of Health Professionals. Formal approval from an ethics committee in Sweden was not required as no intervention was used and no sensitive information obtained (*Ethics approval According to Swedish national legislation*

[Law 2003: 460] on ethics testing of human-related research, Swedish Constitution 2003: 460, Stockholm, http://www.riksdagen.se/sv/Dokument-Lagar/Lagar/Svenskforfattningssamling/Lag-2003460-om-etikprovning_sfs-2003-460/ Accessed: 10–11-2017). In all studies, participants' consent was implied by the return of the survey form.

Approval to conduct the primary studies was given by the following Human Research Ethics Committees and Boards:

- Human Research Ethics Committee, Griffith University (NRS/17/11/HREC and NRS/36/07/HREC);
- The Human Research Ethics Committees of the Gold Coast Hospital (2007/72), the Princess Alexandra Hospital (2007/154), and the Royal Brisbane & Women's Hospital, Queensland Australia (2007/138);
- The Research Ethics Board covering the United Health Network, inclusive of Toronto General, Mt. Sinai and Sunnybrook hospitals, Toronto Canada;
- The University of Dundee Ethics Committee, Scotland (UREC 11021);
- Three National Health Service Trusts including Grampian, Forth Valley, and Tayside hospitals, southeast Scotland.

Competing interests
The authors declare that they have no competing interests.

Author details
[1]School of Nursing & Midwifery, Griffith University, Gold Coast, QLD, Australia. [2]Gold Coast Hospital and Health Service, Gold Coast, QLD, Australia. [3]National Centre of Research Excellence in Nursing, Griffith University, Gold Coast, QLD, Australia. [4]Menzies Health Institute Queensland, Griffith University, Gold Coast, QLD, Australia. [5]Faculty of Medicine and Health, School of Health Sciences, Örebro University, Örebro, Sweden.

References
1. ANMC: National Competency Standards for the Registered Nurse. In.; 2006.
2. Australian Nursing & Midwifery Council: National Competency Standards for the registered nurse. In Canberra: ANMC; 2006: 8.
3. Watson R, Stimpson A, Topping A, Porcock D. Clinical competence assessment in nursing: A systematic review. J Adv Nurs. 2002;39(5):421–31.
4. Hedenskog C, Nilsson U, Jaensson M. Swedish-registered nurse Anesthetists' evaluation of their professional self. J Perianesth Nurs. 2017;32:106–11.
5. Aiken LH, Clarke SP, Sloane DM, Aochalski JA, Busse R, Clarke H, Giovannetti P, Hunt J, Rafferty AM, Shamain J. Nurses' reports on hospita care in five countries. Health Aff. 2001;20(3):43–53.
6. Aiken LH, Sloane DM, Bruyneel L, Van den Heede K, Griffiths P, Busse R, Diomidous M, Kinnunen J, Kózka M, Lesaffre E et al.: Nurse staffing and education and hospital mortality in nine European countries: a retrospective observational study. Lancet 2014(0).
7. Edwards PA, Davis CR. Internationally educated nurses' perceptions of their competence. J Contin Educ Nurs. 2006;37(6):265–9.
8. Safadi R, Jaradeh M, Bandak A, Froelicher E. Competence assessment of nursing graduates of Jordanian universities. Nurs Health Sci. 2010;12:147–54.
9. Gillespie B, Chaboyer W, Lingard S, Ball S. Perioperative nurses' perceptions of competence: implications for migration. XXX(XXX): ORNAC Journal; 2012.
10. Meeusen V, van Zundert A, Hoekman J, Kumar C, Rawal N, Knape H. Composition of the anaesthesia team: a European survey. Eur J Anaesthesiol. 2010;27:773–9.
11. Meretoja R, Koponen L. A systematic model to compare nurses' optimal and actual competencies in the clinical setting. J Adv Nurs. 2012;68(2):414–22.
12. Cowan D, Wilson-Barrett NI. A European survey of general nurses' self assessment of competence. Nurse Educ Today. 2007;27:452–8.

13. Gillespie B, Chaboyer W, Wallis M, Werder H. Education and experience make a difference: results of a predictor study. AORN J. 2011;94(1):78–90.

14. Gillespie B, Polit D, Hamlin L, Chaboyer W. The influence of personal characteristics on perioperative nurses' perceived competence: implications for workforce planning. Aust J Adv Nurs. 2013;30:14–25.

15. Gillespie B, Polit D, Hamlin L, Chaboyer W. Developing a model of competence in the OR: psychometric validation of the perceived perioperative competence scale-revised. Int J Nurs Stud. 2012;49(1):90–101.

16. Gillespie B, Hamlin L. Synthesis of the literature on "competence" as it applies to perioperative nursing. AORN J. 2009;90(2):245–58.

17. Gillespie B, Chaboyer W, Wallis M, Chang A, Werder H. Operating theatre nurses' perceptions of competence: a focus group study. J Adv Nurs. 2009;65(5):1019–28.

18. Gillespie B, Chaboyer W, Wallis M, Chang A, Werder H. Managing the list: OR nurses' dual role of coordinator and negotiator. Acorn Journal. 2009;22(1):5–12.

19. Gillespie B, Pearson E. Perceptions of self-competence in theatre nurses and operating department practitioners. AORN J. 2013;24(1):78–90.

20. Jaensson M, Falk-Brynhildsen K, Gillespie B, Wallentin F, Nilsson U. Psychometric validation of the perceived perioperative competence scale-revised in the Swedish context. J Perianesth Nurs. 2017;

21. Cohen J: Statistical power analyses for Behavioural sciences: Lawrence Erlbaum associates, NY; 1988.

22. Tzeng H. Nurses' self-assessment of their nursing competencies, job demands and job performance in the Taiwan hospital system. Int J Nurs Stud. 2004;41:487–96.

23. Meretoja R, Leino-Kilpi H, Kaira A-M. Comparison of nurse competence in different hospital work environments. J Nurs Manag. 2004;12(5):329–36.

24. Hamlin L, Gillespie B. Beam me up Scotty, but not just yet: understanding generational diversity in the perioperative milieu. Acorn Journal. 2011;24(4):36–43.

25. What is Lagom?. https://somethingswedish.wordpress.com/lagom/. Accessed 23 Oct 2017.

26. Lofmark A, Smide B, Wikblad K. Competence of newly-graduated nurses – a comparison of the perceptions of qualified nurses and students. J Adv Nurs. 2006;53:721–8.

27. Grönroos E, Perälä M-L. Self-reported competence of home nursing staff in Finland. J Adv Nurs. 2008;64(1):27–37.

28. Clark S, Aiken L. Failure to rescue: needless deaths are prime examples of the need for more nurses at the bedside. Am J Nurs. 2003;103(1):42–7.

29. Chang Z-X, Yang G-H, Yuan W. Competency-based management effects on satisfaction of nurses and patients. Int J Nurs Stud Sci. 2014;1:121 e125.

30. Scholz U, Doña B, Sud S, Schwarzer RI. Is general self-efficacy a universal construct? Psychometric findings from 25 countries. Eur J Psychol Assess. 2005;18(3):242–51.

31. Owen SV, Froman RD. Why carve up your continuous data? Research in Nursing & Health. 2005;28(6):496–503.

8

Effects of interprofessional education for medical and nursing students: enablers, barriers and expectations for optimizing future interprofessional collaboration

Sabine Homeyer[1], Wolfgang Hoffmann[1], Peter Hingst[2], Roman F. Oppermann[3] and Adina Dreier-Wolfgramm[1*]

Abstract

Background: To ensure high quality patient care an effective interprofessional collaboration between healthcare professionals is required. Interprofessional education (IPE) has a positive impact on team work in daily health care practice. Nevertheless, there are various challenges for sustainable implementation of IPE. To identify enablers and barriers of IPE for medical and nursing students as well as to specify impacts of IPE for both professions, the 'Cooperative academical regional evidence-based Nursing Study in Mecklenburg-Western Pomerania' (Care-N Study M-V) was conducted. The aim is to explore, how IPE has to be designed and implemented in medical and nursing training programs to optimize students' impact for IPC.

Methods: A qualitative study was conducted using the Delphi method and included 25 experts. Experts were selected by following inclusion criteria: (a) ability to answer every research question, one question particularly competent, (b) interdisciplinarity, (c) sustainability and (d) status. They were purposely sampled. Recruitment was based on existing collaborations and a web based search.

Results: The experts find more enablers than barriers for IPE between medical and nursing students. Four primary arguments for IPE were mentioned: (1) development and promotion of interprofessional thinking and acting, (2) acquirement of shared knowledge, (3) promotion of beneficial information and knowledge exchange, and (4) promotion of mutual understanding. Major barriers of IPE are the coordination and harmonization of the curricula of the two professions. With respect to the effects of IPE for IPC, experts mentioned possible improvements on (a) patient level and (b) professional level. Experts expect an improved patient-centered care based on better mutual understanding and coordinated cooperation in interprofessional health care teams. To sustainably implement IPE for medical and nursing students, IPE needs endorsement by both, medical and nursing faculties.

Conclusion: In conclusion, IPE promotes interprofessional cooperation between the medical and the nursing profession. Skills in interprofessional communication and roles understanding will be primary preconditions to improve collaborative patient-centered care. The impact of IPE for patients and caregivers as well as for both professions now needs to be more specifically analysed in prospective intervention studies.

Keywords: Interprofessional education, Education research, Education, medical, graduate, Education, nursing, Qualitative research

* Correspondence: adina.dreier@uni-greifswald.de
[1]Institute for Community Medicine, Department Epidemiology of Health Care and Community Health, University Medicine Greifswald, Ellernholzstr. 1-2, 17487 Greifswald, Germany
Full list of author information is available at the end of the article

Background

A changing health care system with increasingly complex health needs of patients require innovative and efficient concepts of patient care. These concepts require key competencies, such as effective communication, teamwork and interprofessional collaboration between healthcare professionals [1, 2]. Interprofessional education (IPE), whereby students from several healthcare professions learn and work together [3, 4], has shown a positive impact on team work in daily health care practice [5] and is recommended for training programs of healthcare professionals [6–8]. Several advantages of IPE have been reported: (a) increased mutual respect and trust [9, 10], (b) improved understanding of professional roles and responsibilities [10–13], (c) effective communication [1, 7], (d) increased job satisfaction [11, 13, 14], and (e) positive impact on patient outcomes (e.g. decreased patient's length of hospital stay and a reduced number of medical errors) [8, 15, 16]. Previous studies have proven that students trained in an IPE approach have better interprofessional collaborative practice competencies compared to students without an IPE-training [8, 15, 17]. This can be attributed to students' more positive attitudes towards each other, a better understanding about each other's competencies, the ability to share knowledge and skills, and improved team identity [10, 13, 17]. Nevertheless, there are various challenges for sustainable implementation of IPE including (a) non-coordinated and strictly separate curricula of different health care professions, (b) an insufficient number of specifically qualified teaching staff and (c) limited financial resources of the institutions [9, 12, 18, 19]. As a result, most existing IPE courses are optional and only a few of them are sustainably implemented in the curricula of the health care professionals involved.

In Germany, IPE and research on the impact for interprofessional collaboration (IPC) in routine care is still in its iunfancy. First IPE activities concerned interprofessional communication in hospitals [20], interprofessional seminars in ethics [21], and interprofessional emergency management [22]. To support a sustainable implementation of IPE the GMA Committee - 'Interprofessional Education for the Health Care Professions' was founded in 2011. In its position statement, the committee developed recommendations to integrate interprofessional approaches into education for health professions and required continuous evaluation regarding outcomes of IPE [23]. In addition, the Advisory Council on the Assessment of Developments in the Health Care System emphasize in its report "Cooperation and Responsibility" in 2007 positive effects of IPE for IPC including a better mutual understanding and the acquisition of cooperative skills for all professions involved [24]. A better interaction between the different health care professions is a further positive effect that the GMA Committee stated [23].

To specify the impacts of IPE for medical and nursing students and to identify enablers and barriers of IPE, the Cooperative academical regional evidence-based Nursing Study in Mecklenburg-Western Pomerania (Care-N Study M-V) was conducted. A starting point of the study was the development of an academic nursing program [25]. The study evaluated (1) IPE acceptance between medical and nursing students, and four further research dimensions: (2) further development of academic nursing training, (3) identification of the task fields for graduates with bachelor degrees or master degrees in nursing, (4) specification of learning contents for academic bachelor and master training programs and (5) implications for health politics. The research dimensions comprised 25 research questions. A detailed study design and selected preliminary results were published elsewhere [25, 26].

Research dimension (1) IPE between medical and nursing students addressed the following research questions: (a) what are the enablers and barriers of IPE for nursing and medical students? (b) what are the expectations for the future impact of IPC between both professions?. The aim of the investigation is to explore, how IPE should be designed and implemented in medical and nursing training programs to optimize students' impact for IPC in routine care.

Methods

Design

The present analyses are based on data derived from the Care-N Study M-V, which was a qualitative study using the Delphi method (type: aggregation of ideas) and consisted of two qualitative semi-structured mailed questionnaires, and a group discussion. The details of the study have been described elsewhere [25].

Participants

To guide recruitment of experts for the study, inclusion criteria based on Häder 2009 were defined: (a) each expert is able to answer every research question, one question particularly competent, (b) interdisciplinarity, (c) sustainability and (d) status [27]. To be able to cover a wide range of ideas several disciplines were involved (interdisciplinarity). The sustainable implementation of the study results was supported by experts from different stakeholders associations and politics (sustainability) [28]. It was expected that expert answers will depend on their hierarchy level. Thereby, it could not readily assume that experts in higher positions have all the necessary expertise [29]. Therefore, experts representing various hierarchy levels were included (status of the person).

Participants were purposely sampled. Recruitment was based on existing collaborations and a web based search.

A fixed order for enquiry of experts was defined. When a 'first' requested expert declined to participate, the 'second' expert from the respective list was contacted. This process was repeated until for every research question an adequate expert could be recruited. The first contact was made by telephone: the study was described and the interest for participation was solicited. When the feedback was positive, experts received written study information detailing study aims, methods, data management and a written informed consent. When the written informed consent was completed, signed, and returned to the study center, experts were enrolled in the Care-N Study M-V [25].

Nine experts rejected their participation. Reasons for non-participation provided included: (a) lack of time, (b) stay abroad during the data collection phase of the study, and too short-term request. Over the course of the study none of the experts dropped out.

Overall, 25 experts were enrolled in the Care-N Study M-V. Each expert was categorized to one of following six professional areas: (1) Science, (2) Practitioner from the Professional Fields of Nursing and Medicine, (3) Education and Training, (4) Health Care Provision, (5) Politicians, Associations, Organizations and (6) Health Insurance (see Fig. 1).

Experts were invited to participated in all data collection rounds and to answer all questions. They decide by themselves, in which data collection round they want to participate and which questions they answer. The distribution was: (a) first qualitative mailed questionnaire $n = 13$, (b) second qualitative mailed questionnaire $n = 14$ and (c) group discussion $n = 9$. At least, each expert was involved in one of the three data collection rounds. Most of them participate in two of the three data collection rounds. Detailed description can be found by Dreier et al. 2016, doi: https://doi.org/10.1016/j.zefq.2016.03.003.

The majority of experts were female ($n = 16$). Of them, 13 experts (52%) participated in the first mailed questionnaire, 14 (56%) in the second and nine (36%) in the focus group discussion. All 25 respondents participated at least in one of the three data collections [25].

Data collection

The three data collection rounds were conducted in intervals of 3 months between June 2013 and April 2014.

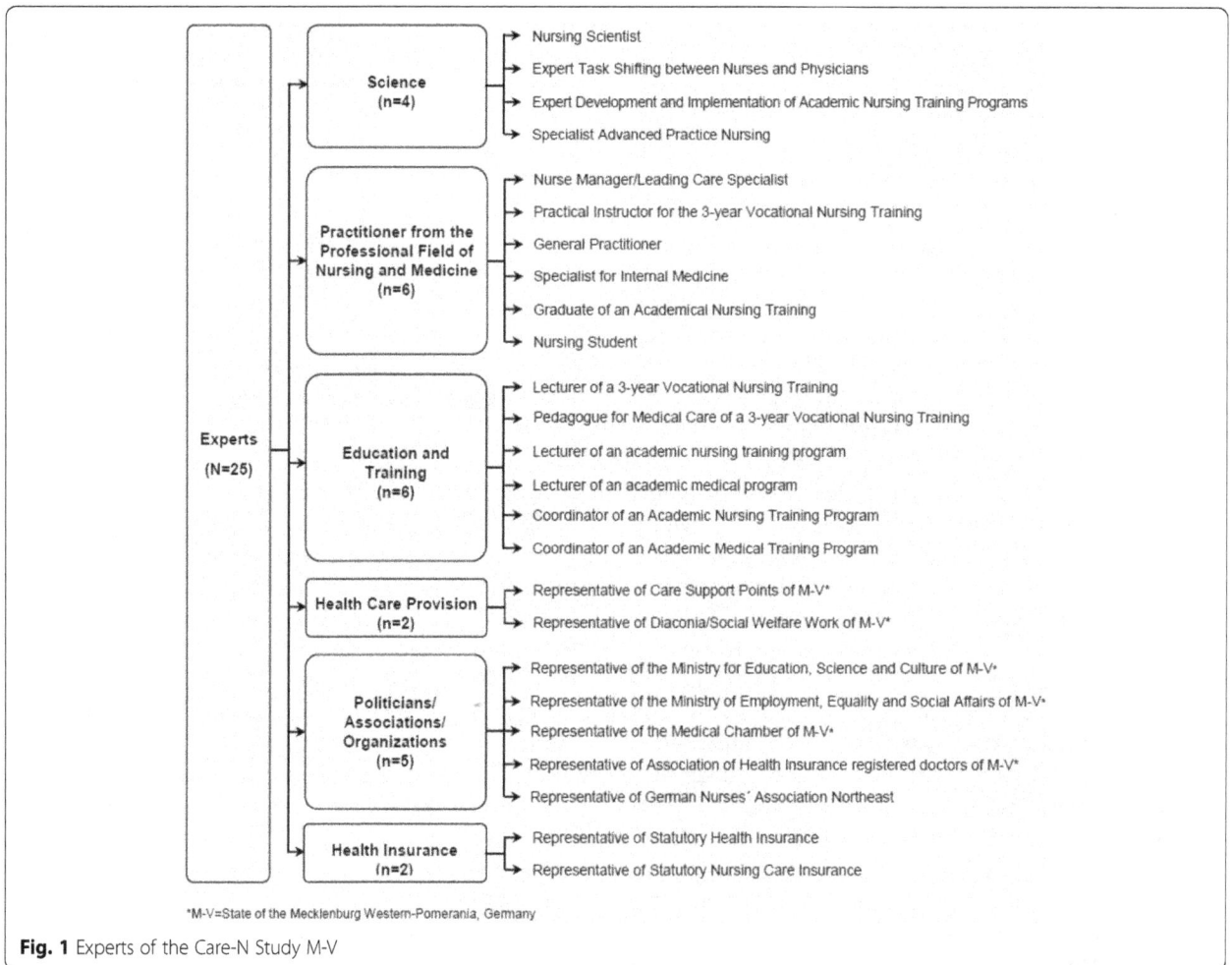

Fig. 1 Experts of the Care-N Study M-V

The first qualitative mailed questionnaire consisted of 25 semi-structured research questions. Its completion took 30–50 min. Of this, five research questions addressed IPE. Results of the first qualitative semi-structured interviews with 13 experts were sent to all experts as a written summary. This summary is a key feature of a Delphi method [27]. And was the basis for the second mailed questionnaire with 14 experts, which consisted of 17 semi-structured research questions (two of those specifically addressing IPE) of the overall 25 research questions. Experts completed and specified their answers based on the results of the first semi-structured mailed questionnaire. The completion took 20–35 min. A written summary with the results were sent to all experts by mail. Results were the basis for the group discussion to clarify specific aspects of both semi-structured questionnaires.

The focus group discussion was conducted with nine experts and comprised five semi-structured research questions. It took approximately 3 h. One team member was the interviewer. The focus group discussion took place in the study center of the Institute for Community Medicine, University Medicine Greifswald, Mecklenburg-Western Pomerania, Germany. All experts received the results as a written summary by mail. Data saturation was evident in the way that no new information was forthcoming during the focus group interviews for the 20 of overall 25 research questions.

The survey instrument for the two semi-structured questionnaires was digitized using TeleForm® (Electric Paper Information Systems GmbH Lüneburg Germany, version 10.2). The completed questionnaires were scanned and verified in TeleForm®. For analysis, the data were documented in a word-data base and transferred to the software MAXQDA, Version 10 (VERBI GmbH, Berlin). The focus group discussion was audio recorded and transcribed with the f4transkript software (dr. dresing & pehl GmbH, Marburg).

Data analysis

To analyze both qualitative semi-structured interviews and the group discussion, a qualitative content analysis as suggested by Kuckartz et al. [30, 31] using the software MAXQDA was conducted. Analysis steps were: (1) Initiating textual work (highlight important text passages, writing memos), (2) development of thematic major categories, (3) coding of the questionnaires and group discussion transcripts by the thematic major categories, (4) assort text passage with the same thematic major categories, (5) inductive development of sub-categories based on the questionnaires and group discussion, (6) coding of the complete text material by the differentiated category system (with thematic major categories and sub-categories) and (7) category based

analysis and result presentation. This analysis structures qualitative data into an order and by frequencies [30].

Two study team members (SH, ADW) coded the interviews and the group discussion according to the consensual coding approach [30]. First, both team members coded separately. Subsequently, both resulting category systems were compared for similarities and differences. In case of differences, the codes were discussed and modified if both coders agreed. This process caused an extension of the category system. Finally, a system with categories, sub-categories and codes based on the code systems of both coders was developed [25].

Results

Enablers and barriers for IPE

Experts stated more enablers then barriers for IPE for medical and nursing students (see Table 1). Overall, four primary arguments for IPE in medical and nursing training programs were mentioned: (1) development and promotion of interprofessional thinking and acting (2) acquirement of shared knowledge, (3) promotion of beneficial information and knowledge exchange, and (4) promotion of mutual understanding.

'Interprofessional education for medicine and nursing students promotes the recognition and understanding

Table 1 Enablers and barriers of IPE for medical and nursing students

Enablers
Development and promotion of interprofessional thinking and acting
patient centered care
Acquisition of shared knowledge
Promotion of information and knowledge exchange
Promotion of mutual understanding
mutual acceptance
respect for each other
reduction of hierarchies
Prerequisites for successful IPC
specific skills and knowledge
communication
specific roles and tasks of medical and nursing profession
ability to put oneself in the other profession's perspective

Barriers
Standardization of learning content levels
Different levels of knowledge
Chronological harmonization of medical and nursing curricula
Organization of IPE lectures
personal resources
time resources
financial resources
Low mutual respect between medical and nursing students and resulting limited willingness for IPE
Low appreciation of medical students towards nursing students
Capacity-legal issues[a]

[a] In Germany, the number of medical students, that a University hast to accept, is determined by a formula that contains the faculty's total teaching hours and class sizes. As a consequence, any engagement of faculty members in additional teaching formats provides an argument for additional medical students to enforce their acceptance legally

of interdisciplinary correlations, the competence for interprofessional acting [...] and the clinical expertise.' (FB_1114: 137–137).

One argument for IPE *'[...] is the mutual benefit to investigate themes from medical's and nursing's perspectives.'* (FB_1119: 88–88).

According to experts' opinions a mutual understanding particularly supports the acceptance and respect for each other in caring for patients in daily work. The reduction of hierarchies is an additional positive side effect.

IPE *'[...] improves the acceptance and thus the mutual understanding of both professions.'* (FB_1113: 59–59).

'Interprofessional education can dismantle hierarchies between both professions.' (FB_1115: 92–92).

To further develop IPC, experts mentioned three main skills or competences, which need to be taught by IPE for medical and nursing students: (1) interprofessional communication, (2) profession specific roles and tasks as well as (3) put oneself in the other profession's perspective. In consequence, experts concluded that these are the main preconditions for improving IPC in the long run to address the overall aim of optimization of needs-oriented and patient centered care.

'IPE promotes skills and competences to work effectively in an interprofessional team. Improved communication enhances coordinated interprofessional collaborative practice.' (FB_1115: 92–92).

'The recognition and understanding of interdisciplinary relation help to identify threatening or current health problems.' (FB_1114: 137–137).

Hence, for any broader rollout of IPE, various barriers must be overcome (see Table 1).

The experts emphasized (1) standardization of learning content levels, (2) different levels of knowledge and (3) the chronological harmonization of medical and nursing curricula as the major challenges of IPE.

'The different levels of knowledge should be noted, training programs have to be synchronized.' (FB_1115: 95).

'Width and depth of the medical knowledge differ from the nursing knowledge.' (FB_1112: 66).

Furthermore, implementing IPE for all students in medical and nursing curricula may cause capacity-legal challenges.

IPE *'[...] leads to capacity-legal problems, because of the restricted acceptance of medical students at medical faculties.'* (FB_1115: 95–95).

This also includes the organization of IPE lectures, which requires personnel, time and financial resources. To overcome existing challenges of IPE for medical and nursing students, experts stated, that the willingness of both students groups and the mutual respect are the most important prerequisites for successful implementation.

'The feasibility of IPE is associated with a high effort which needs essential personal, time and financial resources.' (FB_2114: 51).

Expectations for future IPC in routine care

Judging the effects of IPE for medical and nursing students for future IPC to experts differentiated the (a) patient level and (b) professional level (see Fig. 2).

On the patients' level, experts mentioned possible improvements in following areas: (a) collaborative treatment planning (b) coordinated treatment and implementing individualized health care interventions, (c) collaborative development of innovative treatment measures, (d) improved communication and enhanced cooperation during the care process, and (d) continuous interprofessional information and knowledge exchange to be able to adapt a care plan quickly when necessary.

'I expect an improved collaborative treatment planning as well as an enhanced integrated care of patients.' (FB_1111: 73–73)

'[...] the shared development and implementation of new concepts of patient care.' (FB_1101: 122)

'[...] an improved competence to work as a team in the daily health care practice in consideration of patients' interest.' (FB_1119: 107–107)

Based on this further development of IPC, experts expect changes on the professional level including (a) reduction of stereotypes, (b) improvement of mutual attitude toward the medical and the nursing profession and, (c) mutual appreciation by understanding of roles (see Fig. 2).

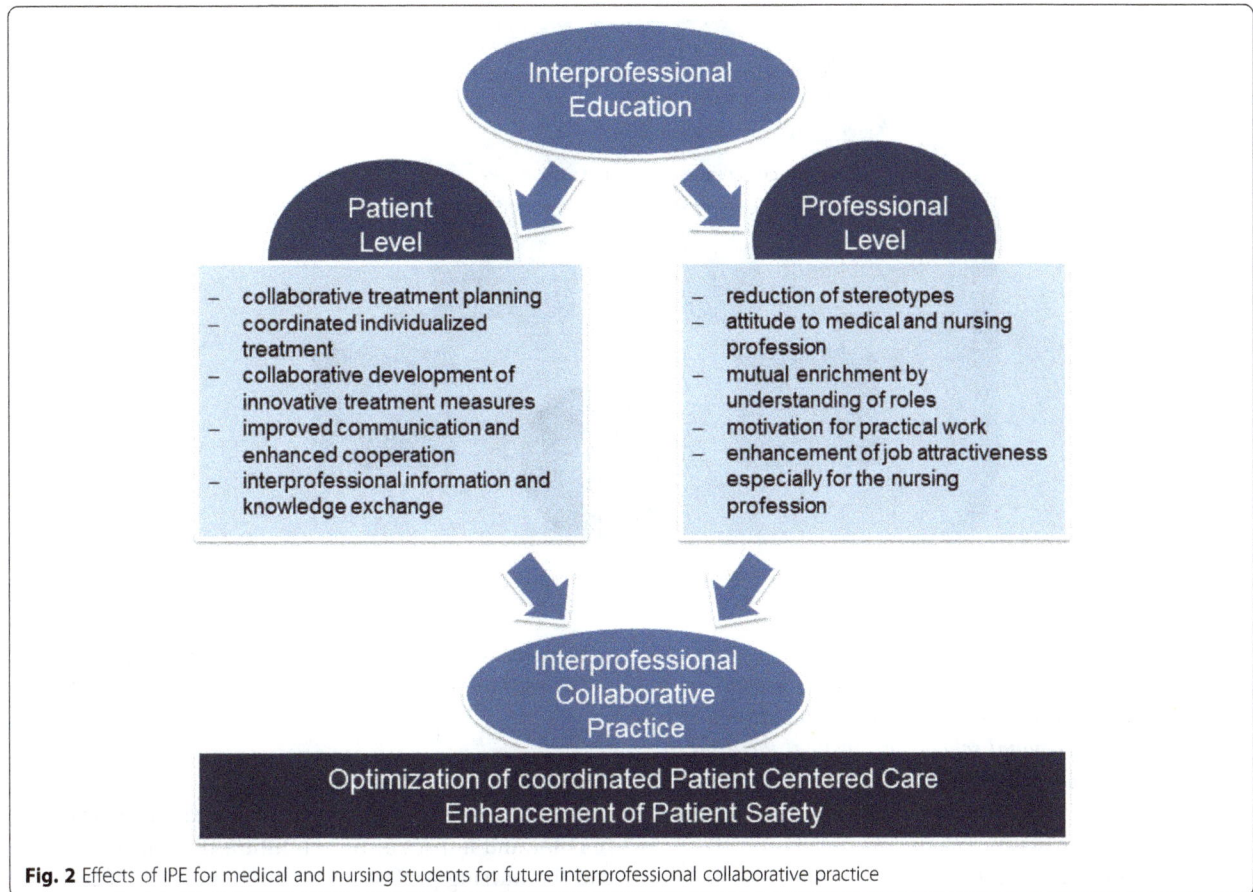

Fig. 2 Effects of IPE for medical and nursing students for future interprofessional collaborative practice

'I expect a reduction of stereotyped behaviors' as well as improved confidence and understanding in working with the other professional group.' (FB_1103: 89–89)

'Everybody has an improved understanding of professional responsibilities of all team members.' (FB_1101: 121)

This might also enhance motivation for practical work in both professions as well as increase job attractiveness especially for the nursing profession (see Fig. 2).

'[...] increase of motivation for the practical work.' (FB_1103: 89)

'[...] improvement of job attractiveness for the nursing profession.' (FB_1115: 115)

In consequence, experts assume an optimization of patient centered care by coordinated collaboration, which results in an enhancement to patient safety (see Fig. 2).

'I expect a coordinated procedure of both professions in patient care as well as the development of new cooperation models.' (FB_1114: 165–165)

'[...] patient safety will be improved' (FB_1101: 120–122)

Implications for sustainable implementation of IPE in medical and nursing curricula

To achieve possible positive effects on IPC, a sustainable implementation of IPE in the education of medical and nursing students is required. Experts stated four primary influencing factors, which need to be considered: (a) the commitment of medical and nursing faculties for IPE, (b) the necessity to synchronize currently existing medical and nursing curricula with respect to comparable learning content deepness and learning aims, (c) the qualification of lecturers to adequately prepare them for teaching in an IPE approach and, (d) prioritize IPE learning contents with regard to the added value for patients and their caregivers of interprofessional collaborative practice (see Fig. 3).

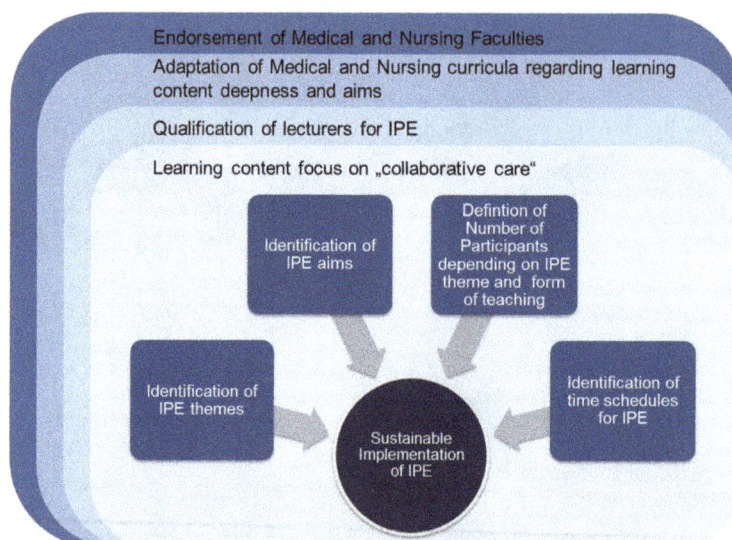

Fig. 3 Influencing factors for sustainable implementation of IPE in medical and nursing curricula

'The implementation of IPE depends on overcome of different structural factors of the both educational institutions (vocational schools vs. medical faculties of universities).' (Fragebögen\FB_2103: 45 - 46)

'Different designs of both training programs - with different depths and scopes of individual fields - are taken into account.' (FB_2115: 40–40)

'It could be critical if lectures are not adequately prepared for interprofessional teaching.' (FB_2103: 49–49)

The experts point out, that it is necessary to comprehensively define IPE themes for both professions followed by the identification of learning aims, the determination of the optimum number of participants depending on IPE theme and teaching format as well as to define the optimal time schedule to implement IPE lectures into both training programs (Fig. 3).

'A possible disadvantage arises when curricular decisions and reforms include needs and targets for only one (and not for both) professional group(s).' (FB_1104: 100–100)

It should be asked at which interfaces the mutual understanding and the collaborative practice will provide the best possible health benefit to patients. Here interprofessional education should take place. It

is important to learn in competence-focused (not fact-focused) useful learning settings. (FB_2119: 29–29)

Discussion

The Care-N study M-V aimed to identify enablers, barriers for and impact of IPE on future IPC for the medical and the nursing profession. Overall, the experts surveyed mentioned more enablers then barriers for IPE. Expected impacts for future IPC were stated on patient and professional level to make a contribution toward optimizing coordinated patient centered care and to enhance patient safety in the future.

The results showed that IPE for medical and nursing students can encourage positive mutual attitudes, better understanding of professional roles in caring for patients and their caregivers as well as improved information and knowledge exchange to cooperate during their daily practical work. Previous studies reported similar results and emphasized that students' improved attitude towards teamwork increased mutual respect and understanding between different groups of health care professionals [10, 32]. Furthermore, IPE provides opportunities to develop interprofessional communication skills [33, 34], and to exercise how to cooperate in an interprofessional team [7]. The acquirement of profession-specific roles during patient treatment is one of the primary enablers of IPE in the Care-N Study. This result agrees with findings of previous studies showing that IPE prepares students to better understand their own professional identity as well as their roles and perspectives on patients and their caregivers [19, 35, 36].

Furthermore, IPE enables students to learn and exercise interprofessional communication. By improving knowledge about their own roles and responsibilities as well as the roles of the other profession an improvement for interprofessional team working can be expected [36, 37]. Finch stated that students can also be better prepared for performing roles traditionally taken over by the other profession [38]. Due to the fact, that tasks and roles of medical and nursing professionals increasingly overlap [39], and both healthcare professions have expanded their roles and responsibilities [40]. IPE might provide the opportunity to better prepare students to taking over the future extended roles and responsibilities already during their training programs.

The Care-N Study M-V experts identify several barriers against a sustainable implementation of IPE in the medical and nursing curricula. These include difficulties in coordinating the two programs. This finding is consistent with previous studies, which showed that program structures and timetables of both curricula are quite different. This has been reinforced by different regulations for professional training programs and the fact that the programs are offered by different providers (university, university of applied science, vocational school, public and private sector etc.) [8, 12, 18, 23].

Nevertheless, from the experts' points of view there are various positive impacts for IPC on patient level in the future including an improved patient-centered care and improved coordinated cooperation in interprofessional health care teams. Previous studies showing that an effective cooperation between nursing and medical professionals improves efficiency and quality of patient care as well as patient safety and patient satisfaction. The University of Colorado integrated patient safety into medical and nursing school curricula and tested models for interprofessional student involvement in clinical improvement [41]. As a result medical and nursing students improved the efficiency of discharge processes, safety of patient transfers from intensive care, and care for bedsores [41]. In their evaluation of an interprofessional student clinical program, Lawrence et al. could show that patients reported high levels of satisfaction with the patient care team and the facility quality [42]. In particular results of the items students 'listen to you', 'take enough time with you', 'explain what you want to know', 'answer your questions' described high levels of patient satisfaction [42].

To achieve these positive impacts for IPC, IPE must be widely implemented in both professions' curricula. One important precondition is, that existing curricula need to be opened and revised for this learning approach. Experts of the Care-N Study stated that IPE should focus on collaborative care to maximize the value for both patients and caregivers. Liang et al. examined outcomes of Neighborhood Health Screening (NHS), an in-home service provided by medical and nursing undergraduate students

for 355 patients in a low-income neighborhood [43]. Overall, 240 medical and 34 nursing students were involved in management of chronic diseases, particularly hypertension. NHS had a positive impact on hypertension management. Demonstrably the rates of treatment for blood pressure (63 to 93%) and control of blood pressure (27 to 73%) could be improved already over 1 year [43].

The Care-N Study M-V has several limitations. First, the use of purposive sampling can be highly prone to selection bias. The definition of clear inclusion criteria should antagonize this potential bias. Second, the purposive sampling focuses on particular characteristics of an expert population enabling them to best answer the research questions. Thus, generalization to the whole population is limited.

Conclusion

The Care-N Study M-V describes enablers, barriers and impact of IPE for medical and nursing students. IPE promotes interprofessional cooperation between both professions and enhance mutual respect and understanding. For future IPC in routine care it can be expected that skills in interprofessional communication and roles understanding will be primary preconditions to improve collaborative patient-centered care. A sustainable implementation of IPE programs faces various barriers, including the coordination of IPE with the medical and nursing core curricula. In consequence, it is necessary to specify overlapping tasks fields to comprehensively identify IPE themes for both professions. Furthermore, the actual impact on patients health and on caregiver burden as well as on the development of both professions need to be studied in controlled prospective designs in the future.

Abbrevations
Care-N Study M-V: Cooperative academical regional evidence-based Nursing Study in Mecklenburg-Western Pomerania; GMA: Society for Medical Education (Gesellschaft für Medizinische Ausbildung); IPC: Interprofessional collaboration; IPE: Interprofessional education; NHS: Neighborhood health screening; WHO: World Health Organization

Acknowledgements
The authors acknowledge the support of the nursing board of the University Medicine Greifswald, who enabled the Care-N Study M-V. Furthermore special thanks to the participating experts who have provided the grounds to the success of the study.

Funding
This study was funded by the nursing board of the University Medicine Greifswald (Director: P. Hingst). PH was involved in data interpretation and critical review of the manuscript. SH received full financial support for her time as a Research Assistant from nursing board.

Authors' contributions
SH made substantial contributions to the data collection, data management, data analysis, data interpretation and drafting the manuscript. WH developed

the study design, made substantial contribution in data interpretation and critically reviewed the manuscript. RFO and PH were involved in data interpretation and critical review of the manuscript. ADW as the PI of the study developed the study design and made substantial contributions to recruitment of experts, data collection, data analysis, data interpretation and critical review of the manuscript. All authors read and approved the final manuscript.

Competing interests

The authors declare that they have no competing interests.

Author details

[1]Institute for Community Medicine, Department Epidemiology of Health Care and Community Health, University Medicine Greifswald, Ellernholzstr. 1-2, 17487 Greifswald, Germany. [2]Nursing Board, University Medicine Greifswald, Fleischmannstraße 8, 17475 Greifswald, Germany. [3]Department Nursing, Health and Administration, University of Applied Science Neubrandenburg, Brodaerstr. 2, 17033 Neubrandenburg, Germany.

References

1. Liaw SY, Zhou WT, Lau TC, Siau C, Chan SW. An interprofessional communication training using simulation to enhance safe care for a deteriorating patient. Nurse Educ Today. 2014;34:259–64.
2. Herrmann G, Woermann U, Schlegel C. Interprofessional education in anatomy: learning together in medical and nursing training. Anat Sci Educ. 2015;8:324–30.
3. World Health Organization. Framework for action on interprofessional education & collaborative practice, vol. 64. Switzerland; 2010. p. 64.
4. Thistlethwaite J, Moran M. Learning outcomes for interprofessional education (IPE): literature review and synthesis. J Interprof Care. 2010;24:503–13.
5. Speakman E, Sicks S. Nursing in the 21st century: find opportunities to practice in Interprofessional healthcare teams. Imprint. 2015;63:35–7.
6. Wagner J, Liston B, Miller J. Developing interprofessional communication skills. Teach Learn Nurs. 2011;6:97–101.
7. Institute of Medicine Committee on the Health Professions Education Summit: Health professions education: a bridge to quality. In Health professions education: a bridge to quality. Edited by Greiner AC, Knebel E. Washington (DC): National Academies Press (US); 2003: 192.
8. Buring SM, Bhushan A, Broeseker A, Conway S, Duncan-Hewitt W, Hansen L, Westberg S. Interprofessional education: definitions, student competencies, and guidelines for implementation. Am J Pharm Educ. 2009;73:59.
9. Interprofessional Education Collaborative Expert Panel. Core competencies for interprofessional collaborative practice: report of an expert panel, vol. 56. Washington, D.C: Interprofessional Education Collaborative; 2011. p. 56.
10. Karim R, Ross C. Interprofessional education (IPE) and chiropractic. J Can Chiropr Assoc. 2008;52:76–8.
11. Angelini DJ. Interdisciplinary and interprofessional education: what are the key issues and considerations for the future? J Perinat Neonatal Nurs. 2011;25:175–9.
12. Sottas B. Learning outcomes for health professions: the concept of the swiss competencies framework. GMS Z Med Ausbild. 2011;28:Doc11.
13. Ebert L, Hoffman K, Levett-Jones T, Gilligan C. "They have no idea of what we do or what we know": Australian graduates' perceptions of working in a health care team. Nurse Educ Pract. 2014;14:544–50.
14. Lindeke LL, Sieckert AM. Nurse-physician workplace collaboration. Online J Issues Nurs. 2005;10:5.
15. Barr H, Koppel I, Reeves S, Hammick M, Freeth D. Effective interprofessional education: argument, assumption and evidence. London: Blackwell Publishing; 2005.
16. Freeth D, Hammick M, Reeves S, Koppel I, Barr H. Effective Interprofessional education: development, delivery, and evaluation. UK: Wiley-Blackwell; 2005.
17. Reeves S, Zwarenstein M, Goldman J, Barr H, Freeth D, Koppel I, Hammick M. The effectiveness of interprofessional education: key findings from a new systematic review. J Interprof Care. 2010;24:230–41.
18. Nisbet G, Lee A, Kumar K, Thistlethwaite J, Dunston R: Interprofessional health education - a literature review: overview of international and Australian developments in interprofessional health education (IPE). pp. 43. San Francisco: Centre for Research in Learning and Change, University of Technology, Sydney; 2011:43.
19. Hou J, Michaud C, Li Z, Dong Z, Sun B, Zhang J, Cao D, Wan X, Zeng C, Wei B, et al. Transformation of the education of health professionals in China: progress and challenges. Lancet. 2014;384:819–27.
20. Klapper B, Lecher S, Schaeffer D, Koch U. Patient records: supporting interprofessional communication in hospital. Pflege. 2001;14:387–93.
21. Neitzke G. Interprofessional education in clinical ethics. GMS Z Med Ausbild. 2005;22(2):Doc24.
22. Quandt M, Schmidt A, Segarra L, Beetz-Leipold C, Degirmenci Ü, Kornhuber J, Weih M. Teamwork elective: results of a German pilot project on interprofessional and interdisciplinary education with formative team OSCE. GMS Z Med Ausbild. 2010;27(4):Doc60.
23. Walkenhorst U, Mahler C, Aistleithner R, Hahn EG, Kaap-Frohlich S, Karstens S, Reiber K, Stock-Schroer B, Sottas B. Position statement GMA committee—"Interprofessional education for the health care professions". GMS Z Med Ausbild. 2015;32:Doc22.
24. Advisoray Council on the Assessment of Developments in the Health Care System Cooperation. Cooperation and responsibility. Prerequisites for target-oriented health care. Report for 2007 (abridged version). Bonn: Advisory Council on the Assessment of Development in the Health Care System Cooperation; 2007. p. 102.
25. Dreier A, Homeyer S, Oppermann RF, Hingst P, Hoffmann W. Academic training of nursing professionals in Germany: further development of nursing expertise - results of the care-N study M-V. Z Evid Fortbild Qual Gesundhwes. 2016;115-116:63–70.
26. Dreier A, Rogalski H, Homeyer S, Oppermann RF, Hingst P, Hoffmann W. Expectations, requirements and limitations of future task sharing between the nursing profession and the medical profession: results from the care-N study M-V. Pflege. 2015;28:287–96.
27. Häder M. Delphi-interviews. An exercise book. Wiesbaden: VS Publisher for Social Science; 2009.
28. Duffield C. The Delphi technique: a comparison of results obtained using two expert panels. Int J Nurs Stud. 1993;30:227–37.
29. Meuser M, Nagel U. Expert interviews - tested many times, but poorly conceived: an article on qualitative method discussion. In: Garz D, Kraimer K, editors. Qualitative empirical social research - concepts, methods, analysis. Opladen: West-German Publisher; 1991. p. 441–71.
30. Kuckartz U. Qualitative content analysis. Methods, practice, computer support. Weinheim: Beltz Juventa; 2012.
31. Kuckartz U, Dresing T, Rädiker S, Stefer C. Qualitative evaluation. Entry into practice. Wiesbaden: VS Publisher for Social Science; 2008.
32. Reeves S, Zwarenstein M, Goldman J, Barr H, Freeth D, Hammick M, Koppel I. Interprofessional education: effects on professional practice and health care outcomes. Cochrane Database Syst Rev. 2008;23(1):Cd002213.
33. Robson W. Eliminating avoidable harm: time for patient safety to play a bigger part in professional education and practice. Nurse Educ Today. 2014;34:e1–2.
34. Edwards S, Siassakos D. Training teams and leaders to reduce resuscitation errors and improve patient outcome. Resuscitation. 2012;83:13–5.
35. Frenk J, Chen L, Bhutta ZA, Cohen J, Crisp N, Evans T, Fineberg H, Garcia P, Ke Y, Kelley P, et al. Health professionals for a new century: transforming education to strengthen health systems in an interdependent world. Lancet. 2010;376:1923–58.
36. Wilhelmsson M, Pelling S, Uhlin L, Owe Dahlgren L, Faresjo T, Forslund K. How to think about interprofessional competence: a metacognitive model. J Interprof Care. 2012;26:85–91.
37. Inuwa IM. Interprofessional education (IPE) activity amongst health sciences students at Sultan Qaboos University: the time is now! Sultan Qaboos Univ Med J. 2012;12:435–41.
38. Finch J. Interprofessional education and teamworking: a view from the education providers. BMJ. 2000;321:1138–40.
39. Parsell G, Bligh J. The development of a questionnaire to assess the readiness of health care students for interprofessional learning (RIPLS). Med Educ. 1999;33:95–100.

40. Currie J, Crouch R. How far is too far? Exploring the perceptions of the professions on their current and future roles in emergency care. Emerg Med J. 2008;25:335–9.

41. Headrick LA, Barton AJ, Ogrinc G, Strang C, Aboumatar HJ, Aud MA, Haidet P, Lindell D, Madigosky WS, Patterson JE. Results of an effort to integrate quality and safety into medical and nursing school curricula and foster joint learning. Health Aff. 2012;31:2669–80.

42. Lawrence D, Bryant TK, Nobel TB, Dolansky MA, Singh MK. A comparative evaluation of patient satisfaction outcomes in an interprofessional student-run free clinic. J Interprof Care. 2015;29:445–50.

43. Liang En W, Koh GC, Lim VK. Caring for underserved patients through neighborhood health screening: outcomes of a longitudinal, interprofessional, student-run home visit program in Singapore. Acad Med. 2011;86:829–39.

9

Nursing staffs self-perceived outcome from a rehabilitation 24/7 educational programme – a mixed-methods study in stroke care

M. I. Loft[1,2*], B. A. Esbensen[3,4], K. Kirk[5], L. Pedersen[5], B. Martinsen[2], H. Iversen[1,4], L. L. Mathiesen[1] and I. Poulsen[2,6]

Abstract

Background: During the past two decades, attempts have been made to describe nurses' contributions to the rehabilitation of inpatients following stroke. There is currently a lack of interventions that integrate the diversity of nurses' role and functions in stroke rehabilitation and explore their effect on patient outcomes. Using a systematic evidence- and theory-based design, we developed an educational programme, Rehabilitation 24/7, for nursing staff working in stroke rehabilitation aiming at two target behaviours; working systematically with a rehabilitative approach in all aspects of patient care and working deliberately and systematically with patients' goals. The aim of this study was to assess nursing staff members' self-perceived outcome related to their capability, opportunity and motivation to work with a rehabilitative approach after participating in the stroke Rehabilitation 24/7 educational programme.

Methods: A convergent mixed-method design was applied consisting of a survey and semi-structured interviews. Data collection was undertaken between February and June 2016. Data from the questionnaires ($N = 33$) distributed before and after the intervention were analysed using descriptive statistics and Wilcoxon sign rank test. The interviews ($N = 10$) were analysed using deductive content analysis. After analysing questionnaires and interviews separately, the results were merged in a side by side comparison presented in the discussion.

Results: The results from both the quantitative and qualitative analyses indicate that the educational programme shaped the target behaviours that we aimed to change by addressing the nursing staff's capability, opportunity and motivation and hence could strengthen the nursing staff's contribution to inpatient stroke rehabilitation. A number of behaviours changed significantly, and the qualitative results indicated that the staff experienced increased focus on their role and functions in rehabilitation practice.

Conclusion: Our study provides an understanding of the outcome of the Rehabilitation 24/7 educational programme on nursing staff's behaviours. A mixed-methods approach provided extended knowledge of the changes in the nursing staff members' self-percived behaviours after the intervention. These changes suggest that educating the nursing staff on rehabilitation using the Rehabilitation 24/7 programme strengthened their knowledge and beliefs about rehabilitation, goal-setting as well as their role and functions.

Keywords: Behaviour change, Complex intervention, Feasibility, Stroke, Rehabilitation

* Correspondence: belle.mia.ingerslev.loft@regionh.dk
[1]Department of Neurology, Rigshospitalet, Nordre Ringvej 57, 2600 Glostrup, Denmark
[2]Institute of Public Health, Department of Nursing Science, Aarhus University, Aarhus, Denmark
Full list of author information is available at the end of the article

Background

Every year, 15 million people worldwide are affected by stroke. Stroke has physical, mental and social consequences for patients, with many patients subsequently needing rehabilitation. We know that both early initiation and the intensity of patients' rehabilitation affect functional outcomes [1–3]. However, patients experience time wastage during inpatient rehabilitation that could profitably have been used for active rehabilitation [4, 5].

The term 'rehabilitation' refers to a targeted and time-delimited process that involves collaboration between different professionals, the patient and the relatives. This process should be undertaken with defined, meaningful goals that are formulated together with the patient [6, 7]. In this understanding of rehabilitation, a holistic approach to disease is adopted, where physical, psychological and social consequences are taken into account. The goals for rehabilitation are thus not merely the absence of disease and symptoms, but relate to the patient getting to live independently and participate in meaningful social activities with the highest possible self-perceived quality of life. Patients affected by stroke require specialized skills from staff as they often have motor, cognitive, speech and behavioural sequelae that complicate their involvement in the rehabilitation process [6].

Nurses play an important role in stroke rehabilitation and are a natural member of the interdisciplinary rehabilitation team [8, 9]. However, their role and functions appear to be therapeutically unclear and the nursing staff in a stroke rehabilitation unit often fail to fully incorporate rehabilitation practices into their daily routines[RW.ERROR - Unable to find reference:562]. Previous, mainly descriptive, research on nurses' role and functions in stroke rehabilitation gave rise to a call for interventions that focused on strengthening their contributions [8–10].

Research indicates that nursing interventions are often underdeveloped, and this likely explains why they have difficulties showing effect [11, 12]. Furthermore, research findings are poorly integrated in practice [11, 13]. It is therefore important to develop theory- and evidence-based interventions where also the implementation strategy is incorporated from the beginning [13–15]. An intervention for stroke rehabilitation that could strengthen the nursing staff's contributions is a complex intervention that largely centres on behavioural change. We therefore chose to develop an evidence- and theory-based intervention guided by the British Medical Research Council's (MRC) framework for complex interventions [15] to ensure a systematic and evidence based development and Michie's Behaviour Change Wheel (BCW) [14] as the intervention would address behaviour change [16]. Furthermore, we addressed implementation from the outset by developing a strategy following the steps recommended by Grol and Wensing [13]. Trials of complex interventions are by nature complex in their design and overall process; thus, feasibility studies are valuable for informing trials that relate to clinical, procedural or methodological issues before setting up an effect study [11]. We have previously investigated the educational programme for its feasibility and acceptability (under review). As a next step, we in this study investigate if there is any self-perceived changes in the nursing staff members' behaviours related to capability, opportunity and motivation (COM-B factors) [14]. To our knowledge, this is the first study to investigate whether an intervention obtained on the basis of BCW benefits the COM-B factors or whether something should be changed before a larger effect study is carried out.

Aim

The aim of this convergent mixed-methods study was to asses nursing staff members' self-perceived outcome on their capability, opportunity and motivation to work with a rehabilitative approach after participating in the stroke Rehabilitation 24/7 educational programme.

Methods

Design

A convergent mixed-method design was applied that included a questionnaire to obtain quantitative data and semi-structured interviews to obtain qualitative data. The rationale for choosing a mixed-methods design was the recognition of a need for different methods that, in combination, can give a better understanding of the complex contextual environment of healthcare [11, 17, 18]. For a study overview, see Fig. 1.

Setting and intervention

The educational programme named "Rehabilitation 24/7" was designed to strengthen the nursing staff's rehabilitative practices. The intervention addressed key barriers identified within the COM-B model with the purpose of achieving behavioural change in the nursing staff [16]. The specific goals of the intervention for the nursing staff were as follows:

- To work systematically with a rehabilitative approach in all aspects of patient care
- To work deliberately and systematically with patients' goals.

The intervention was designed as an educational programme that comprised three workshops lasting 3 h each, interspersed with work-in-practice. Over the course of a 3-month period in the spring of 2016, all registered nurses (RNs) ($n = 19$) and all nurse assistants (NAs) ($n = 18$) in a 15-bed acute stroke unit were enrolled in the educational programme. Participation was mandatory, except for substitute staff. Together with the first and last author of this paper, the two charge nurses of the unit and three

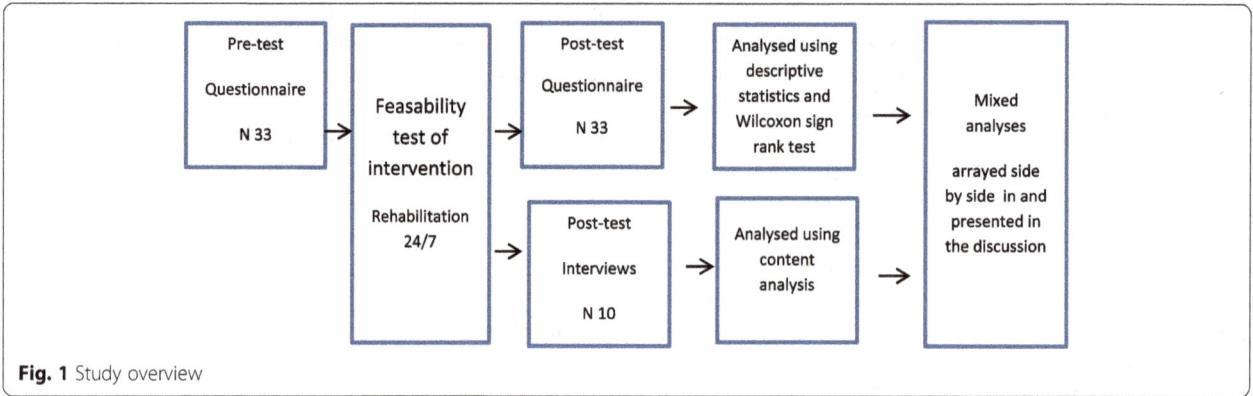

Fig. 1 Study overview

nursing staff members were involved in designing and planning the intervention and took an active role in training. In developing and modelling the intervention, two professional advisers were also involved, a Master of Science (MSc) in Economics and a Master in Organisational Psychology. These two professional advisers contributed with knowledge of and experience in patient involvement, process improvement and change management. Moreover, they had insider perspectives as a former patient and as a relative, respectively. The intervention was developed based on existing relevant research and empirical research undertaken by the developers of the intervention (interviews and field observations in the chosen stroke unit) [16, 19, 20]. In the early development stages, field observations were also conducted in another rehabilitation in-patient setting to broaden perspectives and later to validate the findings. Each component in the intervention was furthermore based on theory and evidence hence for instance the didactic considerations were drawing on educational theory [21].

The main elements of the educational programme outlined in Fig. 2 were as follows:

1. Improving the participants' theoretical understanding of how nursing contributes to patients' rehabilitation. Every workshop comprised theoretical input, including rehabilitation theory and history, theory related to nursing role and functions, patient narratives, and evidence related to goal-setting.
2. Presenting and providing training on tools for improving rehabilitation tasks. In workshop 1, the focus was on learning to give peer-to-peer feedback and performing patient-centred observations, which should be performed 2 to 3 h in the participants' own practice. Guidelines were handed out for both of these elements. In workshop 2, the participants' own experiences that derived from the observations were used to reflect on theoretical aspects of the nursing role.

3. Effecting change in practice. Each participant identified own areas for further development and was asked to formulate individual goals on which to work. The charge nurses were involved in developing the educational programme, and participated as well. This was done to increase 'ownership' of the changes at all levels, as well as ensure that the programme was designed to fit the particular needs of the stroke rehabilitation unit.

Participants

All RNs and NAs participating in the educational programme were asked to answer the questionnaire immediately before and after the 7-week educational programme was completed.

For the semi-structured interviews, RNs and NAs were selected to obtain a purposive sample to ensure breadth

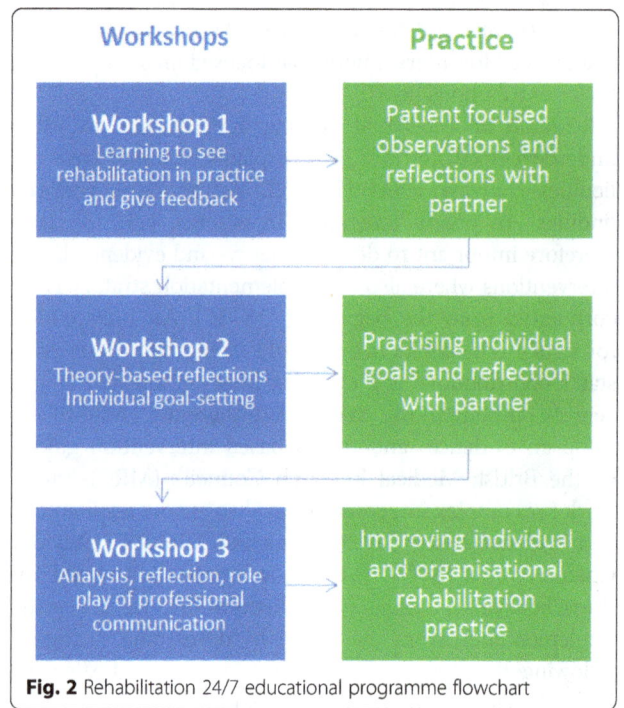

Fig. 2 Rehabilitation 24/7 educational programme flowchart

and variety in perspectives [22]. Thus, RNs and NAs with differing degrees of seniority and ages were selected. The principle of data saturation, defined as the point at which no additional new information was obtained, guided sampling. After 10 interviews, the interviewer (BAE) and the first author (MIL) agreed that saturation had been reached, and data collection ceased.

For characteristics of the sample for the questionnaire and interviews, see Table 1.

Data collection
Questionnaire
The questionnaire was inspired by the COM-B Self-Evaluation Questionnaire and the COM-B Behavioural Diagnosis Form [14]. It was intended to examine self-perceived outcomes before and after the educational programme that related to the COM-B factors (capability [C], opportunity [O] and motivation [M]) [14] and patient involvement. The questionnaire was completed electronically before and after the educational programme. After the programme, the questionnaire was expanded with an additional 11 questions (see Table 3) addressing how the participants assessed their professional knowledge and skills after participating in the intervention. The questionnaire was reviewed for its comprehensibility and face validity with a convenience sample ($n = 5$) prior to being administered. The questionnaire used a 4-point Likert scale ranging from very bad to very good and totally disagree to totally agree (Table 4).

Table 1 Sample characteristics for questionnaire and semi-structured interviews

Characteristics	N Questionnaire	Percentage (%) Questionnaire	N Interviews
Professional group			
Registered nurse	17	51.5	6
Nurse assistant	16	48.5	4
Sex			
Male	2	6	1
Female	31	94	9
Education (years since graduation)			
< 2 years	7	21	2
2–5 years	1	3	0
> 5 years	25	76	8
Supplementary education			
Yes	12	36	3
No	21	64	7
Current employment			
< 2 years	13	40	3
2–5 years	6	18	1
> 5 years	14	42	6

Numbers answering questionnaire: 33 out of 37 participants

Interviews
The interviews were conducted using a semi-structured interview guide [22] that explored participants' perceptions of the relevance of the educational programme and its learning outcomes. The interviews were also aimed at uncovering areas that related to RNs' and NAs' daily practice, indicating possible changes in the identified COM-B factors. All interviews were conducted in an outlying office at the hospital and lasted between 37 and 50 min (mean duration 45 min). The interviewer was unknown to the participants and had not been directly involved in the development or delivery of the educational programme. The interviews were digitally recorded and transcribed verbatim.

Analyses
The questionnaires were analysed using descriptive statistics and Wilcoxon sign rank test using IBM SPSS Statistics [23].

The qualitative interview data were analysed using deductive content analysis as described by Elo and Kyngäs [24] as we aimed at investigating already predefined categories. COM-B factors were employed to develop a structured categorisation matrix [24]. This matrix was used as a lens for the analysis. The theme of the interviews was chosen to facilitate answering the research questions about the nursing staff members' capability, opportunity and motivation in relation to their daily work in the stroke unit. Changes in the nursing staff members' perceptions of their competence were analysed, coded and compared with the COM-B factors. The development of the intervention also involved identifying barriers which suggested the need to make changes to the COM-B factors, and this information constituted the basis for what we looked for in relation to each COM-B factor (Table 2). The material was transcribed verbatim and NVivo® software (QSR International Pty Ltd., Victoria, Australia) was used to provide an overview and facilitate a systematic approach to analysing the material. Three members of the research team (first, second and last author) independently read the transcripts multiple times to become familiar with the data and acquire an overview of the text. Then, the transcripts were reviewed for content. Text corresponding to the matrix categories was coded and transferred to these categories. Any coding inconsistencies among the researchers were discussed until consensus was reached. A description of each category was then developed.

In the mixed analysis, results from the two individual analyses were brought together in a discussion where they are arrayed side by side this is in accordance with the methods as presented by Creswell [17, 18].

Results
Quantitative results
Self-perceived outcome
The nursing staff assessed the overall outcome of Rehabilitation 24/7 as having had a positive influence on both

Table 2 COM-B factors to look for in the analysis

COM-B factors:	Identified as:
Physical Capability	Having the physical skills to work towards the patient's goals; having the physical skills to work systematically with a rehabilitative approach
Psychological Capability	Understanding nursing roles and functions in the rehabilitation process; understanding the concept of rehabilitation; knowing and understanding the reason for working with goals in rehabilitation; knowing how to collaborate with the patient; knowing how to collaborate with the interdisciplinary collaborators.
Physical Opportunity	Having the opportunity to document goal-setting, progress, etc.; having time, resources and the physical space to work systematically with a rehabilitative approach
Social Opportunity	Fostering a culture in which the nursing staff can work effectively and take co-responsibility for achieving the patient's goals; observing senior nurses working deliberately and systematically with the patient's goals in mind; having social and cultural norms that strengthen respect for nursing roles and functions; appreciating the value of a rehabilitative approach
Automatic Motivation	Following established routines and habits for working deliberately and systematically towards the patient's goals and with a rehabilitative approach
Reflective Motivation	Having a strong professional identity; believing that it is possible to integrate rehabilitation principles into daily care; believing that a rehabilitative approach is important; believing that a systematic rehabilitative approach will improve the patient's outcome

their professional identity and competencies (Table 3). Regarding the two target behaviours, 71% answered that they agreed or totally agreed feeling stronger in relation to working deliberately with the patient's goals as part of their daily care; and 74.2% answered that they felt stronger working with a rehabilitative approach. This was also reflected in the result that 74.2% agreed or totally agreed about becoming aware of the possibilities of affecting rehabilitation within the profession (Table 3). When asked about the effect of the feedback element of the educational programme, 80.6% and 87.1% agreed or totally agreed, respectively, that they had improved as a result of giving feedback to or receiving feedback from their colleagues.

Among the participants 80.8% agreed or totally agreed that they had become more competent in relation to communicate their professional contribution to the interdisciplinary team, patients and relatives (Table 3).

Assessing own skills
When looking at the COM-B factors assessed before and after the educational programme, we found that the nursing staff assessed their skills in collaborating with doctors as having increased after the intervention ($p = 0.038$). There were no changes in skills involved in collaborating with colleagues within the nursing staff group. However, descriptive statistics showed a statistically near significant ($p = 0.059$) positive change in monodisciplinary collaboration. There were no reported changes in relation to skills used to involve patients in daily work. Skills that related to giving feedback increased significantly ($p = 0.017$), but no change was found with respect to receiving feedback (Table 4).

Competencies in relation to care and rehabilitation
The nursing staff assessed their knowledge of working with a rehabilitative approach ($p = 0.013$), knowing what

Table 3 Nursing staffs assessment of self-perceived outcome after participating in the educational programme

%	Totally agree	Agree	Disagree	Totally disagree
I feel more secure in my professional role and function	22.6	61.3	16.1	0.0
I feel more competent involving the patient in my work	16.1	67.8	16.1	0.0
I feel stronger about working deliberately with patients' goals in daily care	12.9	58.1	29.0	0.0
I feel stronger working with a rehabilitative approach	25.8	48.4	25.8	0.0
I become aware of the possibilities within my profession to affect the patient's rehabilitation	12.9	61.3	25.8	0.0
I improved at giving feedback to my colleagues	16.1	64.5	19.4	0.0
I improved at receiving feedback from my colleagues	22.6	64.5	12.9	0.0
I feel more competent at collaborating with the interdisciplinary team	19.4	67.7	12.9	0.0
I feel more competent at communicating my professional contribution to the interdisciplinary team	9.8	71.0	19.4	0.0
I feel more competent at communicating my professional contribution to the patient	16.1	64.5	19.4	0.0
I feel more competent at communicating my professional contribution to patients' relatives	16.1	64.5	19.4	0.0

Table 4 Nursing staffs self-perceived outcome before and after participating in the educational programme

Question		Before %				After %				Wilcoxon signed rank test	P-value
How do you assess your skills?		Very good	Good	Bad	Very bad	Very good	Good	Bad	Very bad	z	P
1	To work patient involving	36	64	–	–	39	61	–	–	0.000	1.0
2	To work with the patients goals in daily care	15	79	–	–	23	74	3	–	−0.966	0.334
3	Focusing on rehabilitative principles in daily care	15	85	–	–	26	74	–	–	−1.732	0.083
4	Collaborating with mono professional colleagues	30	70	–	–	45	55	–	–	−1.890	0.059
5	Collaborating with nursing staff colleagues	39	61	–	–	35	61	–	–	−0.832	0.405
6	Collaborating overall in the rehabilitation team	21	70	9	–	39	55	6	–	−1.371	0.170
7	Collaborating with therapists	18	70	12	–	39	55	6	–	−1.529	0.126
8	**Collaborating with the doctor**	18	70	12	–	23	74	3	–	− 2.070	**0.038**
9	Learning from colleagues on the interdisciplinary team	18	76	6	–	23	77	–	–	−1.613	0.107
10	**Giving feedback on colleagues' work**	6	67	27	–	26	61	13	–	−2.379	**0.017**
11	Receiving feedback from colleagues	6	76	18	–	13	77	10	–	−1.333	0.182
	Rate your level of agreement or disagreement with the following statements regarding your competencies in the care and rehabilitation of patients admitted for rehabilitation after a stroke.	Totally agree	agree	dis -agree	Totally dis-agree	Totally agree	agree	dis -agree	Totally disagree	z	P
12	**I know how to work with a rehabilitative approach**	25	72	3	–	52	48	0	–	−2.496	**0.013**
13	**I know what patient involvement in rehabilitation means**	34	63	3	–	55	45	0	–	−2.111	**0.035**
14	I know how to motivate the patient to participate in their rehabilitation	31	66	3	–	45	55	0	–	−1.155	0.248
15	**I am sure of how to work with patients towards their goals for rehabilitation**	22	69	9	–	48	52	–	–	−2.653	**0.008**
16	**I am competent in performing the tasks I think are expected of me as a nurse/nurse assistant in a stroke rehabilitation unit**	31	63	6	–	52	48	–	–	−2.179	**0.029**
	Indicate your level of agreement or disagreement with the following statements regarding your role and function as a nurse/ nurse assistant in the care and rehabilitation of patients admitted for rehabilitation after a stroke.										
17	**I know what is expected of me as an RN/NA in a rehabilitation unit**	19	71	10	–	47	53	–	–	−2.486	**0.013**
18	I know what patients expect of me	23	65	13	–	23	63	13	–	−0.543	0.587
19	I know what patients' relatives expect of me	23	55	23	–	17	60	20	3	−1.273	0.203
20	I know what my colleagues in the care group expect of me	23	65	13	–	27	73	–	–	−1.473	0.141
21	I know what the doctor expects of me	16	65	19	–	17	77	7	–	−0.812	0.,417
22	I know what the therapist expects of me	16	68	16	–	17	77	7	–	−0.933	0.351
23	I estimate that I am so strong in my professional function that I can clearly communicate it to patients	29	52	16	3	33	63	3	–	−1.789	0.074
24	**I am so strong in my professional function that I can communicate it clearly to my interdisciplinary colleagues**	29	48	23	–	37	60	3	–	−1.979	**0.048**

Table 4 Nursing staffs self-perceived outcome before and after participating in the educational programme *(Continued)*

Question		Before %				After %				Wilcoxon signed rank test	P-value
How do you assess your skills?		Very good	Good	Bad	Very bad	Very good	Good	Bad	Very bad	z	P
25	I am competent to work with the other staff in the patient's rehabilitation	35	58	6	–	47	50	3	–	−0.237	0.083
26	I know where my professional function differs from others in the interdisciplinary team	32	55	13	–	43	53	3	–	−0.722	0.470
27	I am happy with my work	42	48	10	–	47	43	–	–	−0.690	0.490
28	I am proud of my professional group's contribution to patients' rehabilitation	35	58	6	–	50	47	–	–	−1.732	0.083
29	I asses that my professional group has an untapped potential to contribute to the rehabilitation of patients admitted after a stroke	32	61	7	–	40	50	10	–	−0.087	0.931
	Indicate your level of agreement or disagreement with the following statements regarding how you work in the unit in terms of patient involvement.										
30	Within my professional group, we always know who is responsible for a patient	16	49	32	3	20	53	23	3	−0.549	0.583
31	It is in our department's culture to involve patients throughout their rehabilitation	36	55	10	–	27	67	6	–	−0.749	0.454
32	We are good at translating the individual's experiences/wishes into solutions that suit the patient	7	74	19	–	23	60	17	–	−1.027	0.305
33	Our division of labour between professional groups allows the patients to be involved	10	71	19	–	17	67	16	–	−0.104	0.917
34	In the department we are continuously discussing what is actually meant by involving patients	6	52	32	10	17	37	46	–	−0.514	0.607
35	The way we work together in the interdisciplinary team gives the patient a coherent experience of the rehabilitation course/pathway	13	74	10	3	17	70	13	–	−0.426	0.670
36	We have the resources to be able to involve the patients as a permanent practice	10	36	48	6	10	50	40	–	−1.079	0.281
37	The way the stroke unit works as an organisation supports patient involvement in the rehabilitation	13	64	23	–	17	60	23	–	−0.484	0.628
38	**We have organised the work so that the patients' views and resources come into play**	23	64	13	–	10	70	20	–	−2.271	**0.023**
39	The way our work is organised enables us to have a holistic view of the patient	13	52	35	–	10	60	30	–	−0.302	0.763
40	In our department, we prioritise the contact person system	6	42	42	10	10	33	47	10	0.000	1.0
41	In our department, we prioritise the patient to experience continuity in contact with the nursing staff	19	52	23	6	7	63	30	–	−0.179	0.858
	Rate your level of agreement or disagreement with the following statements related to what you think you need in order to be even better at working with a rehabilitative approach.										

Table 4 Nursing staffs self-perceived outcome before and after participating in the educational programme *(Continued)*

Question		Before %				After %				Wilcoxon signed rank test	P-value
How do you assess your skills?		Very good	Good	Bad	Very bad	Very good	Good	Bad	Very bad	z	P
42	**I need to know more about why it is important to work using a rehabilitative approach**	10	45	42	3	3	20	57	20	−2.216	**0.027**
43	**I need education to know more about how to work with a rehabilitative approach**	13	58	29	–	3	27	60	10	−3.063	**0.002**
44	**I need more practical skills**	6	52	39	3	6	27	57	10	−2.166	**0.030**
45	I need more mental skills	6	58	36	–	3	50	40	7	−1.054	0.292
46	I need more time	42	39	19	–	43	37	20	–	−0.302	0.763
47	I need a different structure in the unit	6	62	29	3	13	57	27	3	−0.091	0.927
48	I need more colleagues in the nursing staff group	39	45	16	–	30	47	20	3	−1.127	0.260
49	I need support from management	42	42	16	–	23	60	17	–	−0.401	0.689
50	I need support from my colleagues in the nursing staff group	39	55	6	–	27	60	13	–	−1.384	0.166
51	I need support from my colleagues in the interdisciplinary team	39	51	10	–	30	60	10	–	−0.540	0.589
52	I need to believe that it has a positive effect on the patients	32	61	3	3	23	60	7	10	−1.611	0.107
53	I need to believe that it has a positive effect on me	16	74	7	3	13	60	17	10	−1.755	0.079
54	**I need to develop habits for working with a rehabilitative approach, which means incorporating it into my everyday life**	29	58	10	3	17	50	33	–	−2.170	**0.030**
55	**I need to develop plans for how to practically adopt a rehabilitative approach in my everyday work**	35	52	13	–	13	50	34	3	−2.977	**0.003**

Bold text indicates a statistically significant difference with a p-value less than 0.05

patient involvement in rehabilitation means ($p = 0.035$), being sure about how to work with patients towards their goals for rehabilitation ($p = 0.008$) and their competence in performing tasks expected of an RN or NA in stroke rehabilitation to increase ($p = 0.029$). There were no changes in self-perceived competencies in respect to motivating patients to participate ($p = 0.248$) (Table 4).

Role and functions
We found an increase in knowledge of what was expected of them ($p = 0.013$). Before the educational programme10% stated that they did not know what was expected of them, whereas none stated this after. Furthermore, after the intervention, participants either agreed or totally agreed that they were so clear about their professional functions that they could communicate them to colleagues in the interdisciplinary team ($p = 0.048$).

Working with patient involvement
After the educational programme, the nursing staff stated that they totally agreed (10%), agreed (70%) or disagreed (20%) that the work in the unit was organised so that patients' views and resources came into play, which contrasted with the responses before the educational programme ($p = 0.023$) (Table 4). The other 11 questions had no statistically significant changes.

Needs in order to get better
After the educational programme the nursing staff needed to a lesser degree than before to know more about why it was important to adopt a rehabilitative approach ($p = 0.027$) and expressed les need for education to know how to do so ($p = 0.002$). Furthermore, they professed less need for more practical skills ($p = 0.030$) after the educational programme (Table 4). Before the educational programme, they highlighted the need to

develop the habit of working towards rehabilitation and planning for how this could be done practically; this result showed a statistically significant change in terms of a diminished need after the intervention ($P = 0.003$) (Table 4).

Qualitative results
Physical capability
Participants articulated how working with patients in rehabilitation required experience, special abilities and skills. Physical capability was described as being related to basic and general nursing skills, but complex patients could require more than that:

> It may be that patients cannot move their extremities at all. It can be complex because they cannot speak or because they do not understand and cannot remember, or because they need complete help with all that is called ADL. (NA1)

The nurse experienced physical capability as being linked to knowledge as a prerequisite physical skill. This includes knowledge of how, as a RN or NA, one is affected if they do not come to deploy one's skills properly and how this could affect the patient. However, there was no direct expression of any effect on physical capability after participating in the educational programme.

Psychological capability
Nursing staff increased their knowledge and awareness of the importance of setting goals for patients. Goal-setting was described as a daily part of clinical practice. However, before the educational programme this was often not prioritised in a busy work day. The nursing staff became more aware of the need to establish rehabilitation goals after completing the programme. They also perceived a greater number of challenges associated with goal-setting, such as lack of documentation and continuity, and there was greater awareness of the benefits and relevance of goal-setting for patients: We are working with the goals. I have greater insight into this now than I had previously (NA1).

The nursing staff described having greater empathy for patients as well as greater understanding of their experiences of inpatient rehabilitation. This new knowledge inspired individual RNs or NAs to adjust their behaviour and actions in their daily practice:

> I was just wondering how much it really meant, how you [nursing staff] enter and are present. We often just act and think we have asked and involved the patient, but we may, in fact, only have mentioned it [what we are going to do] and then done it. (NA2)

The observation exercise (Table 1) was described as increasing participants' knowledge. It gave the observer

insights into the patient's perspective; what it meant to be under rehabilitation after suffering a stroke. The observation exercise was an eye opener to seeing the importance of nursing staff taking their time to involve the patients in activities of daily living (ADLs).

For some participants, it was surprising that their role and functions were described as therapeutically unspecific in the literature, but it helped to put things that they had been wondering about into perspective. Their understanding of their nursing role and functions increased after the intervention. They perceived the value of their contribution to patients' physical training; for example, they recognised that they influenced patients' rehabilitation as much as therapists did: Well, I had the opinion (before) that training ... was something that therapists did. It was an eye opener (NA3).

The theory that was presented regarding their role and functions was new for most of the nursing staff, and they described not having experienced their role and functions in this light before, but that it made sense to them and provided the basis for increased capability.

> Well, now it is obvious after the project that we are a rehabilitation department. It became evident in the process that many of us, especially nurses and nursing assistants, are not [as] good at explaining or describing our professionalism and our role in rehabilitation as [those in] the other professional groups. (RN1)

Greater awareness of one's own role and functions was linked to increased motivation and ability to verbalise the contribution of the nursing staff to both the patients and the interdisciplinary team.

Participants described interdisciplinary collaboration as challenging; but increasing their knowledge of their own role and functions seemed to relieve some of these difficulties. They described having achieved a better understanding of a shared vision for the interdisciplinary team:

> I have come to understand the importance of working jointly to achieve goals that are set across disciplines. [...] I think that I have got better at arguing for my own nursing versus their [the therapists'] training. Also, the things I can contribute with ... are just as relevant as what they provide, because it is important for the patient. (RN2)

In line with an increased understanding of their own role and functions, participants described gaining greater understanding of the concept of rehabilitation.

> The difference is that, for me, it has provided greater understanding and more knowledge of the specialism of stroke rehabilitation. For the patient, this means, of

course, that there is now continuity in the way we work. I think all the things we've talked about – using each other and using everyone on the interdisciplinary team – that the physiotherapist and occupational therapist also use the same goals as us and work on them... and give time to the patients and train with patients – all those things help us to work using a rehabilitative approach. (NA 1)

The nursing staff described that they were much more aware after the programme that little things they did with patients every day could be therapeutic in several ways, such as getting patients in and out of bed, helping them walk to the dining room, helping them get dressed etc.

Physical opportunities

The nursing staff described a lack of resources, especially relating to time and staffing levels. However, their participation in the educational programme and physical changes such as the new way of documenting the patients goals, emphasised by the programme, altered their understanding:

Besides directly influencing patient care, participants described lack of time and resources as affecting opportunities for professional advancement, as professional and mono- and interdisciplinary learning were not prioritised. Participation in the educational programme challenged their perceptions of professional advancement. Hence, the nursing staff came to view it not only as a personal professional gain, but also as having a direct impact on patient rehabilitation.

Social opportunity

The nursing staff lacked the mono- and interdisciplinary culture required to support the rehabilitative approach and the culture of goal-setting and systematic liaison with patients to work towards achieving their goals. A part of this culture could be documenting explicitly how and whether they worked rehabilitative or with goal-setting and what they expected more from their colleagues: *Personally, I think my colleagues document very little. There are some who do not write as much as I would like them to (RN 3).*

The nursing staff thought it was likely that a new common language and their enhanced professional role and functions would influence the work culture both internally among the nursing staff and in the interdisciplinary team.

Automatic motivation

The nursing staff expressed the wish to establish new work routines and habits, a process that some of them had already initiated:

It's not that I go around thinking about it for 8 hours, but there are times where there is a click in my head, and I think of it and try to do things differently.[...]. You have to repeat it over and over until it becomes automatic. But I'm getting better at it. (RN4)

The newly acquired focus and knowledge from the educational programme were perceived to constitute the first step in establishing new behaviours. However, there were concerns that it would be difficult to continue to progress because of time pressure and lack of possibilities for ongoing development. The importance of management offering guidance and prioritising change was emphasised in that respect.

Reflective motivation

The value of having a stronger professional identity was expressed both implicitly and explicitly. Such a belief was also expressed as having the possibility of growing in their current circumstances: *I think it has been a really good offer in relation to strengthening professionalism and becoming aware of what is, in fact, necessary to care for these patients, doing straightforward things that we can easily benefit from like making changes within our existing framework* (RN5).

The nursing staff members had achieved a stronger professional identity and enhanced awareness of the possibilities of working with a rehabilitative approach:

Because we are here 24 hours... and occupational and physiotherapists [are] not. We work [all] day, evening and night. There is actually training at night, because when patients need to get up from their bed and out into the hallway and go to the toilet. (RN6)

This reflective motivation also related to making a difference for the patients; there was awareness that using a rehabilitative approach and working on goal-setting and patient involvement meant that nurses' contributions could lead to important improvements in patients' outcomes and experiences.

Discussion

The results from both the qualitative and quantitative analyses, which in this discussion is merged, indicate that the educational programme shaped the target behaviours that we aimed to change by addressing the nursing staff's capability, opportunity and motivation through an educational intervention, and hence had the potential to strengthen the nursing staff's contribution to inpatient stroke rehabilitation.

The workshops mainly addressed cognitive functions. This was reflected in the interviews, where physical capability was considered not to have been directly changed after the intervention. However, in the quantitative data, the participants after the programme expressed less need for more practical skills to be able to work using a rehabilitative approach. This could be explained by the fact that the nursing staff in this study expressed the opinion that knowledge formed the basis of their clinical skills. A part of the Rehabilitation 24/7 educational programme included a role play exercise where the participants practiced communicating their professional functions to interdisciplinary collaborators (practiced skills). Appling this element as a practical skill exercise may be the reason why knowledge of how to collaborate and communicate with members of the interdisciplinary team stood out from the rest of the results, and it could indicate that this rehearsal positively influence the nursing staff's learning. The fact that practical exercises had a positive influence on the learning is supported by the findings from an earlier study on nursing staff members' beliefs, attitudes and actions in inpatient stroke rehabilitation. Here the participants stated that bedside training and peer-to-peer training was the best sources of learning [19]. This indicates the importance of integrating different approaches to learning.

Psychological capability seemed to increase overall in relation to the target behaviours. The quantitative results indicate a significant positive change from before to after the intervention with respect to working with patients towards achieving their goals. The qualitative results complemented this findings by illuminating how increased knowledge of the evidence behind goal-setting and why it is important in rehabilitation caused the nursing staff to prioritise goal-setting in their busy everyday practice. The quantitative and qualitative data also show that having a stronger professional identity is based on deeper insight into one's own role and functions as well as increased understanding of the concept of rehabilitation. Mauk et al. [25] also found that education increased the nursing staff's knowledge of nursing competencies in rehabilitation. Mauk et al. [25] argue that the specialism of rehabilitation requires rehabilitation-specific education both before and after graduation from nursing school. This was also suggested by Clark [9], who argues that stroke-specific education needs to be enhanced if nurses are to perceive more fully their rehabilitative role and enhance their rehabilitation skills. In previous research, nursing staff education is shown to have a positive effect on nurses' self-perceived competence and job satisfaction and to increase quality in patient care [25]. However, only a few previous studies have addressed the issue of strengthening nurses' contributions to inpatient stoke rehabilitation. Differences in content and duration of such educational initiatives make it difficult to compare our study to these prior studies [26–29]. Our previous study showed a high level of feasibility and acceptability of the educational programme

among nursing staff [30]. According to Sidani [31], the acceptability of an intervention depends on the participants' perception of the intervention. Hence, the high levels of acceptability and feasibility of the educational programme may have had a positive influence on the participants' self-perceived outcome. However, recognizing that self-perceived effect has some degree of limitation when looking at effect, is important. First, a self-perceived effect does not necessarily report on the actual effect or change, but rather on the participants' beliefs [13]. However, using a self-perceived outcome in a feasibility study can be a good indicator of the expected behaviour change. In an intervention aimed at professional behaviour change, intention, defined as the individual motivation concerning the performance of a given behaviour, is a good predictor for change [32]. According to Nielsen et al. [32], effect can only be expected if healthcare professionals have positive attitudes and good intentions.

Changes with respect to physical and social opportunities were seen at different levels. The quantitative results revealed no significant change regarding whether more time is needed to be better at working using a rehabilitative approach. However, the qualitative results are at variance with this as they offered descriptions of immediate changes in the structure of the unit after running the educational programme. Hence, increased understanding of the possibilities of integrating rehabilitation into basic daily care, thereby illustrating some differences in the perception of time. In a Q-methodology study whereby the participants sort a set of statements about nursing practice in inpatient stroke rehabilitation, Clarke and Holt [10] found that despite very real time and workload pressures, routinely integrated rehabilitation principles in care could be followed without extra time pressure. With respect to social opportunity, specifically having a supportive culture and norms for working with a rehabilitative approach, it was interesting from our study that more was expected from collaboration mono professional and among RNs and NAs and in the qualitative results were highlighted for fostering a good rehabilitative culture.

Overall, it appears that changes occurred in relation to all COM-B factors in our study. However the quantitative results relating to patient involvement did not show statistical significant changes in 11 out of 12 questions. This might reflect that the participant in the main part of these questions assess them self with a high level of agreement before the intervention. However the participants also stated that 83.9% felt stronger in working patient involving after participating which also was revealed in the qualitative analysis. This inconsistence in the results therefor calls for further investigation in order to strengthen the intervention.

While developing the educational programme, which was guided by the MRC framework and the BCW, we developed an implementation strategy by conducting a need assessment and following the steps proposed by Grol and Wensing for implementing change in health care [13]. This meant incorporating a multifaceted strategy for implementation during the testing period to support the educational programme, which allowed us to address several potential barriers. This strategy pointed to include, besides an educational intervention, other elements, such as feedback, reminders, etc. An educational intervention has been proven as effectual for increasing the knowledge of nursing staffs and is often a necessary step in implementing changes in practice [13]. However, the evidence for educational intervention is neither strong nor one-sided. When guided towards education as an element to achieve the desired behaviour change, considerations should be given to how. The Cochrane Effective and Organisation of Care Group (EPOC) distinguishe between different educational strategies, from e-learning to large-scale educational meetings [33]. In the current study, small-scale educational meetings were chosen. This decision was based on stronger evidence for effect [33] and didactic considerations and was deemed the most pragmatic in relation to the clinical practice. As such, we believe that it provided a strong foundation for a clinically relevant educational programme.

Limitations

This study has several limitations. First, the tailoring of the intervention and the implementation strategy raise questions about the transferability of our results. We tried to address this issue by also conducting field observations in another context during the development phase to broaden both perspectives and context. Second, the questionnaire was only pre-tested on a small sample; therefore, its face validity could be questioned. Third, the study reports on results from a small sample; it is therefore important to interpret the statistical analyses cautiously. However, given the mixed-methods design, we interpreted the results in the light of both qualitative and quantitative data. Using a deductive approach in the qualitative analysis could mean a more narrowed insight into the perceived strengths and weaknesses of the program than an inductive approach might have been open for. However, applying a deductive approach using the COM-B factors as categories enhanced the possibility to draw clear lines back to the theoretical and empirical foundations of the intervention and thereby evaluate on these in line with the aim of the study. Fourth, a limitation of the study could be that the first author developed, delivered and evaluated the intervention. However, precautions were taken to limit any confounders; the interviews, for example, were performed by the second author, who were not directly involved in the

development and delivery of the intervention, and analysis was performed collaboratively by the research team.

Conclusions

The results of our study provide an understanding of the of the self-perceived outcome of the Rehabilitation 24/7 educational programme on nursing staff members' behaviour. A mixed-methods approach provided us with in-depth knowledge of the changes in the nursing staff members' behaviours following the intervention. These changes suggest that the different aspects of the Rehabilitation 24/7 programme strengthened the nursing staff's knowledge and beliefs about rehabilitation as well as heightened their awareness of their own role and functions. Using a structured theory- and evidence-based approach guided by the BCW to address the COM-B factors and using a multifaceted implementation strategy appeared to enhance the effectiveness of the intervention.

In this study we created an educational intervention for nursing staff in practice. The intervention cost staffing hours during the test but was feasible and acceptable. The intervention was developed within thefra-mework of an already existing context, which means it is possible to make behavioural changes for acollective staffing group within an already existing context. Hence this intervention should be considered as a way to enhance neuro-nursing.

The feasibility study of the rehabilitation educational programme seemed promising. Testing theintervention on a larger population in a controlled trial would be the natural next step. It could bebeneficial to do this as a multicentre study to increase the external generalisability. The present studywill contribute important knowledge about the process, content and structure. Before further investigation, future research should gain further understanding and testing of relevant outcome measurements both related to the nursing staff and patient outcomes.

Abbreviations
ADL: Activities of daily living; COM-B: Capability Opportunity Motivation Behaviour; MRC: Medical Research Council; NA : Nurse Assistants; RN: Registered Nurse

Acknowledgements
We would like to express our gratitude to the participants for supporting this study by their unevaluable participation.

Funding
The study was supported by grants from the Novo Nordic Foundation, Tømmerhandler Johannes Fogs Fond, the Research Council at Glostrup Hospital and Department of Neurology, Rigshospitalet, Glostrup, Denmark. The funders had no role in the design of the study, the collection, analysis and interpretation of the data or the writing of the manuscript.

Authors' contributions
Study design: MIL, IP, KK, LP, HKI, LLM and BAE and BM; data collection MIL, BAE; data analysis: MIL, IP and BAE; manuscript preparation: MIL, KK, LP, HKI, LLM, BAE, BM and IP. All authors read and approved the final manuscript.

Competing interests
The authors declare that they have no competing interests.

Author details
[1]Department of Neurology, Rigshospitalet, Nordre Ringvej 57, 2600 Glostrup, Denmark. [2]Institute of Public Health, Department of Nursing Science, Aarhus University, Aarhus, Denmark. [3]Copenhagen Centre for Arthritis Research (COPECARE), Centre for Rheumatology and Spine Diseases VRR, Head and Orthopaedics Centre, Rigshospitalet, Glostrup, Denmark. [4]Falcuty of Health and Medical Sciences, Department of Clinical Medicine, University of Copenhagen, Copenhagen, Denmark. [5]Partner PAR3(consulting firm), Copenhagen, Denmark. [6]Research Unit on Brain Injury Rehabilitation Copenhagen (RuBRIC), Clinic of Neurorehabilitaion, TBI unit Rigshospitalet, Glostrup, Denmark.

References
1. Bernhardt J, Godecke E, Johnson L, et al. Early rehabilitation after stroke. Curr Opin Neurol. 2017;30:48–54. https://doi.org/10.1097/WCO. 0000000000000404.
2. Langhorne P, Bernhardt J, Kwakkel G. Stroke rehabilitation. Lancet. 2011;377: 1693–702. https://doi.org/10.1016/S0140-6736(11)60325-5.
3. Bernhardt J, Indredavik B, Langhorne P. When should rehabilitation begin after stroke? Int J Stroke. 2013;8:5–7. https://doi.org/10.1111/ijs.12020.
4. West T, Bernhardt J. Physical activity in hospitalised stroke patients. Stroke Res Treat. 2012; https://doi.org/10.1155/2012/813765.
5. Bernhardt J, Dewey H, Thrift A, et al. Inactive and alone: physical activity within the first 14 days of acute stroke unit care. Stroke. 2004;35:1005–9.
6. Hjerneskaderehabilitering – en medicinsk teknologivurdering. Hovedrapport. Available at: http://sundhedsstyrelsen. dk/publ/publ2011/MTV/ Hjerneskaderehabilitering/ Hjerneskaderehabilitering.pdf., 2016.
7. Marselisborgcentret, Rehabiliteringsforum Danmark. Rehabilitering i Danmark: hvidbog om rehabiliteringsbegrebet. Århus: Marselisborgcentret 2004:71 sider.
8. Kirkevold M. The role of nursing in the rehabilitation of stroke survivors: an extended theoretical account. ANS 2010;33:E27–E40 doi:https://doi.org/10. 1097/ANS.0b013e3181cd837f.
9. Clarke DJ. Nursing practice in stroke rehabilitation: systematic review and meta-ethnography. J Clin Nurs. 2014;23:1201–26. https://doi.org/10.1111/ jocn.12334.
10. Clarke DJ, Holt J. Understanding nursing practice in stroke units: a Q-methodological study. Disabil Rehabil. 2015;37:1870–80. https://doi.org/10. 3109/09638288.2014.986588.
11. Richards DA, Hallberg IR. Complex interventions in health : an overview of research methods. London, England; New York, New York: Routledge 2015:1 online resource (409 pages).
12. Richards DA, Coulthard V, Borglin G. The state of european nursing research: dead, alive, or chronically diseased? A systematic literature review. Worldviews Evid-Based Nurs. 2014;11:147–55. https://doi.org/10. 1111/wvn.12039.
13. Grol R, Wensing M, Eccles M, et al. Improving patient care : the implementation of change in health care. Chichester, West Sussex: Wiley-Blackwell/BMJ Books; 2013. p. 374.
14. Michie S, Atkins L, West R. The behaviour change wheel. A guide to designing interventions

: Silverback 2014.
15. Craig P, Dieppe P, Macintyre S, et al. Developing and evaluating complex interventions: the new Medical Research Council guidance. BMJ. 2008;337
16. Loft MI, Martinsen B, Esbensen BA, et al. Strengthening the role and functions of nursing staff in inpatient stroke rehabilitation: developing a complex intervention using the behaviour change wheel. International Journal of Qualitative Studies on Health and Well-being. 2017;12:1392218. https://doi.org/10.1080/17482631.2017.1392218.
17. Creswell JW. Research design : qualitative, quantitative, and mixed methods approaches. Thousand Oaks, CA.: SAGE Publications 2014:xxix, 273 s., illustreret.
18. Creswell JW. A concise introduction to mixed methods research. Thousand Oaks, California: SAGE 2015:xiv, 132 pages, illustrations.
19. Loft MI, Poulsen I, Esbensen BA, Iversen HK, Mathiesen LL, Martinsen B. Nurses' and nurse assistants' beliefs, attitudes and actions related to role and function in an inpatient stroke rehabilitation unit-A qualitative study. J Clin Nurs. 2017;26(23/24):4905-14. https://doi.org/10.1111/jocn.13972.
20. Loft MI, Martinsen Woythal B, Esbensen BA, et al. Call for human contact and support: an interview study exploring patients' experiences with inpatient stroke rehabilitation and their perception of nurses' and nurse assistants' roles and functions. Disabil Rehabil. 2017:1–9. https://doi.org/10. 1080/09638288.2017.1393698.
21. Entwistle N. Teaching for understanding at university: deep approaches and distinctive ways of thinking. Basingstoke: Palgrave Macmillan; 2009.
22. Kvale S, Brinkmann S. Interviews : learning the craft of qualitative research interviewing. Thousand Oaks, Calif.: Sage Publications 2014:xviii, 405 sider.
23. IBM SPSS Version 22.0. IBM Corp. Released 2013. IBM SPSS statistics for windows, version 22.0. Armonk, NY: IBM Corp.
24. Elo S, Kyngäs H. The qualitative content analysis process. J Adv Nurs. 2008; 62:107–15.
25. Mauk KL. The effect of advanced practice nurse-modulated education on rehabilitation nursing staff knowledge. Rehabil Nurs. 2013;38:99–111. https://doi.org/10.1002/rnj.70.
26. Forster A, Dowswell G, Young J, et al. Effect of a physiotherapist-led training programme on attitudes of nurses caring for patients after stroke. Clin Rehabil. 1999;13:113–22.
27. Jones A, Carr EK, Newham DJ, et al. Positioning of stroke patients: evaluation of a teaching intervention with nurses. Stroke. 1998;29:1612–7.
28. Gibbon B. A reassessment of nurses' attitudes towards stroke patients in general medical wards. J Adv Nurs. 1991;16:1336–42. https://doi.org/10. 1111/j.1365-2648.1991.tb01562.x.
29. Burton C, Gibbon B. Expanding the role of the stroke nurse: a pragmatic clinical trial. J Adv Nurs. 2005;52:640–50. https://doi.org/10.1111/j.1365-2648. 2005.03639.x.
30. Loft IM, Poulsen I, Woythal Martinsen B, et al. Strengthening nursing role and functions in stroke rehabilitation 24/7: a mixed methods study assessing the feasibility and acceptability of an educational intervention programme. In: Unpublished article; 2017.
31. Sidani S. Braden CJ,1944-. Design, evaluation, and translation of nursing interventions. Chichester, west Sussex. Ames, Iowa: Wiley-Blackwell; 2011.
32. Nilsen P, Roback K, Broström A, et al. Creatures of habit: accounting for the role of habit in implementation research on clinical behaviour change. Implement Sci. 2012;7 https://doi.org/10.1186/1748-5908-7-53.
33. Cochrane effective practice and organisation of care group, 2017-last update, EPOC 2013 EPOC: Cochrane Effective Practice and Organisation of Care Group. Available:http://epoc.cochrane.org/our-reviews.

10

Impact of the introduction of an endotracheal tube attachment device on the incidence and severity of oral pressure injuries in the intensive care unit

Jaye Hampson[1], Cameron Green[1*], Joanne Stewart[1], Lauren Armitstead[1], Gemma Degan[1], Andrea Aubrey[1], Eldho Paul[2,3] and Ravindranath Tiruvoipati[1,2]

Abstract

Background: Endotracheal tube (ETT) fasteners such as the AnchorFast™ claim to assist with the prevention of oral pressure injuries in intubated patients, however evidence to support their clinical efficacy is limited. This retrospective observational study aimed to investigate the impact of the introduction of the AnchorFast™ device on the incidence of oral pressure injuries in mechanically ventilated patients.

Methods: Data was collected from patient case notes and clinical incident reports for October 2010 to June 2013 (*pre-AnchorFast*) and July 2013 to March 2016 (*post-AnchorFast*). Incidence and location of oral pressure injuries associated with securing device, and compliance with institutional policies related to reducing oral pressure injuries were recorded.

Results: Incidence of oral pressure injuries increased from 1.53/100 intubated patients in the pre-AnchorFast period to 3.73/100 intubated patients in the post-AnchorFast period (IRR = 2.43, 95%CI = 1.35–4.38; p = 0.003). Across both study periods, patients with an ETT secured using AnchorFast™ had significantly increased risk of oral pressure injuries (IRR = 2.03, 95%CI = 1.17–3.51; p = 0.02). There was also a significant difference in location of pressure injuries sustained with ETTs secured using cloth tapes (53.6% in corner of the mouth) vs. AnchorFast™ (75% on the lips) (p = 0.008). Among patients with oral pressure injuries, compliance with institutional policies relating to the prevention of pressure injuries was significantly greater after the introduction of the AnchorFast™ (9.1% vs 64.5%, p = 0.004).

Conclusions: The incidence of oral pressure injuries increased significantly following the introduction of the AnchorFast™ device. Further research is required to establish the reasons for this observed increase to and identify ways to reduce the risk of pressure injuries with ETT securement devices.

Keywords: Pressure injury, Pressure wound, AnchorFast, Endotracheal intubation, Critical care

* Correspondence: CGreen@phcn.vic.gov.au
[1]Department of Intensive Care Medicine, Peninsula Health, Frankston Hospital, 2 Hastings road, Frankston, VIC 3199, Australia
Full list of author information is available at the end of the article

Background

Pressure injuries are a leading cause of preventable harm to hospitalised patients worldwide, affecting between 1 and 11% of patients in acute-care settings [1]. Among all hospitalised patients the prevalence rate of pressure injury is highest for patients in Intensive Care Units (ICU) [2]. Globally, the incidence of pressure injuries among patients admitted to ICU ranges from 5 to 20%, with a prevalence of between 14 and 47% [3–5]. Patients in ICU have many unique factors that make them vulnerable to the development of pressure injuries. Risk factors for pressure injury development in critically ill patients may include impaired sensation, altered level of consciousness, reduced mobility, sedation, decreased tissue perfusion, nutritional compromise, and vasoactive medications [3, 6–8].

Medical devices are often an essential component in delivering necessary care to critically ill patients, yet are also increasingly being recognised as a potential cause of pressure injury. Medical device-related pressure injuries (MDRIs) are defined as a localised injury to the skin or underlying tissue as a result of sustained pressure from a device [9]. The majority of MDRIs occur on the head, neck and face [10], and may be caused by poor device fit, improper securement, or poor visualisation of the skin under the device making it difficult to perform skin assessment [9, 11]. A lack of practice guidelines and staffing workload and experience may also impact on the risk of a medical device related pressure injury [12]. The proportion of pressure injuries that are device-related varies in the literature from 10% to 40% [2, 6, 13]. Black et al. [9] reported that patients with a medical device were 2.4 times more likely to develop a pressure injury.

Although there is an increasing awareness of the risk of MDRIs, there are few studies that have addressed specific devices and their impact on the development of pressure injury. Two recent studies have found endotracheal tubes (ETT) and nasogastric tubes to be leading causes of MDRIs [13, 14], with intubated patients at risk of developing pressure injuries from the ETT and/or the methods or devices used to secure it [15]. ETTs are secured to prevent tube migration, and to avoid unplanned extubation. There are several methods for securing ETTs, including adhesive or cloth tapes, and endotracheal tube attachment devices (ETADs). These devices are designed specifically to hold the ETT securely in a way that facilitates regular repositioning of the ETT to prevent the development of pressure injuries caused by the tube resting on the inside of the mouth or lips for prolonged periods. These devices are therefore marketed as having the potential to reduce rates of oral pressure injuries [16]; however evidence to support these claims is limited [15, 17–20]. Two studies have found reduced skin breakdown with commercial ETT holders when compared to adhesive tape [19, 20]. Furthermore

ETT holders were shown to significantly reduce internal and external movement of endotracheal tubes [20]. A systematic review and meta-analysis found significant reduction in lip excoriation with commercial devices ($p <$ 0.001; OR = 0.2, 95%CI = 0.1–0.5), but no significant reduction in facial trauma (p = 0.11; OR = 0.4, 95%CI = 0.1–1.2) [17]. The degree of ETT displacement was found to be less with commercial devices than with adhesive tape in the setting of significant heterogeneity of the studies included [17]. A recent study comparing sixteen ETT securement methods using anatomically correct intubation models with embedded pressure sensors found that commercial devices exerted more pressure on the face than non-commercial devices and commercial ETT holders allowed for rapid and secure movement of ETT from one side of the mouth to the other. [15].

A commercially available ETAD, the AnchorFast™ (Hollister), was introduced into clinical practice in our department in mid-2013.

This study aimed to retrospectively evaluate the impact of the introduction of the AnchorFast™ device on the incidence of oral pressure injuries in our ICU.

Methods

Study setting

The study hospital ICU is a 15-bed university-affiliated non-tertiary Metropolitan medical and surgical ICU located in Victoria, Australia. Approximately 1100 patients are treated in this ICU each year, with about 40% requiring invasive mechanical ventilation (IMV).

AnchorFast™ devices were introduced into clinical practice in this unit from the start of July 2013. Prior to, and following the introduction of the AnchorFast™ into this department, nurses have received ongoing education in the proper use and placement of this device. Prior to the introduction of AnchorFast™, ETTs were secured using cloth tapes; after its introduction, both methods of ETT securement (AnchorFast and cloth tapes) were available for use. The choice of ETT securement method used in the post-AnchorFast period was at the discretion of the bedside nurse, with the exception of specific contraindications listed below.

Institutional pressure injury prevention guidelines state that cloth tapes should be changed and ETT repositioned every 6 h, or when the cloth is soiled; while the ETTs should be repositioned every 2 h for patients with an AnchorFast™ in situ. AnchorFast™ devices should be replaced every 3–5 days as per manufacturers' instructions or clinical need. Repositioning of the ETT and replacement of tapes or AnchorFast™ devices should also be clearly documented on the patient's ICU flow chart. Pressure injuries are reported using the Victorian Health Incident Management System, a database for the collection of clinical incidents and adverse events.

Severity of pressure injuries is graded by the nurse generating the report, according to the current National Pressure Ulcer Advisory Panel (NPUAP) staging system [21].

Study design

This was a retrospective observational study, investigating the incidence of reported pressure injuries to the mouth and lips of patients, prior-to and following the introduction of the AnchorFast™ device into clinical practice The time period from 01/10/2010–31/06/2013 was defined as the 'pre-AnchorFast' period; while 01/07/2013–31/03/2016 was defined as the 'post-AnchorFast' period.

AnchorFast™ Endotracheal tube attachment device

The AnchorFast™ device is produced by Hollister (Hollister Incorporated, Libertyville, IL USA). AnchorFast™ (Fig. 1) includes a number of features aimed at reducing the occurrence of pressure injuries to the mouth and lips, such as a 'gliding tube shuttle' which enables the ETT to be easily repositioned while being held securely in place, and a 'lip stabiliser' that prevents the ETT from resting on the patient's upper lip.

AnchorFast™ devices are contraindicated for patients without teeth, with facial oedema, or with protruding teeth, facial hair, profuse diaphoresis, or allergic reaction to the device's skin barrier pads.

Data collection

The total number of admissions to the study ICU, number of patients receiving mechanical ventilation, and the total hours of mechanical ventilation required by patients during each study period was retrieved from ICU patient databases. The medical records of all patients receiving invasive mechanical ventilation in the study ICU during the post-AnchorFast period were reviewed to identify whether patients ever had their ETT secured using an AnchorFast™ device.

All pressure injuries reported during the study period were retrieved from Victorian health incident management system (VHIMS). These reports were reviewed by one of the investigator (JH), and pressure injuries to the mouth or lips were identified. The date and time of pressure injury documentation, and severity and location of the pressure injury was retrieved from VHIMS reports. Location of pressure injuries was classified as 'corner of mouth', 'lip' (for injuries on the outer surface of the lip), or 'mouth' (for injuries on the inner surface of the mouth).

The case notes for patients with reported oral pressure injuries were reviewed. The following variables were collected: length of ICU and hospital stay; length of mechanical ventilation; location of intubation (e.g. ambulance, emergency department, ICU); method of ETT securement at intubation; ICU admission diagnosis; comorbidities; use of long term steroids, Adult Physiology and Chronic Health Evaluation (APACHE-III) illness severity score; Waterlow pressure injury risk score at ICU admission and prior to pressure injury documentation; and whether there was documentation of compliance with institutional pressure injury prevention guidelines in the 48 h prior to pressure injury documentation.

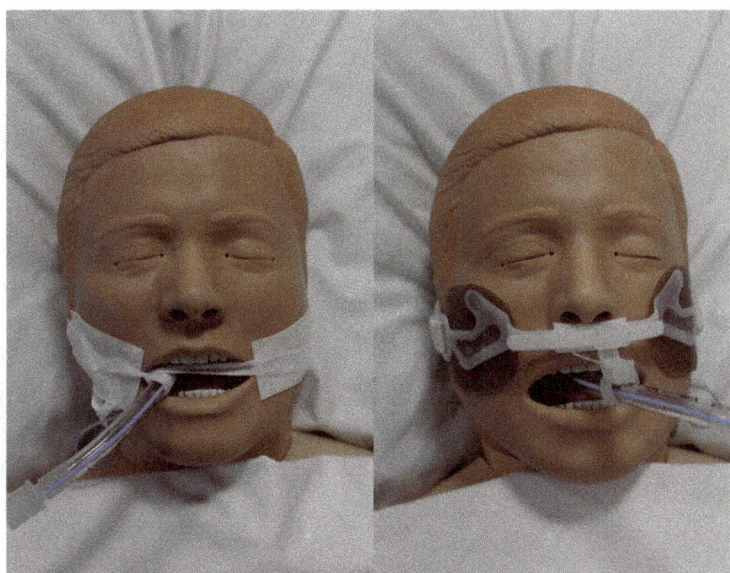

Fig. 1 Two methods of endotracheal tube (ETT) securement used in the study hospital. Cloth tapes (left) are looped around the ETT and tied around the patient's head, passing under their ears. A foam dressing is placed between the cloth tape and the patient's skin, and an adhesive tape is used to secure it in place. The AnchorFast™ device is shown on the right

Ethical considerations

This study was reviewed and approved as an audit by Research Governance of Peninsula Health (ref.: QA/16/PH/8). As this was a retrospective study requiring no patient contact, no informed consent was required.

Statistical analysis

Continuous variables were assessed for normality and expressed as mean (standard deviation) or median (inter-quartile range) depending on the distribution of data. Categorical variables were summarised using frequencies, presenting the subject counts and percentages. Comparisons between groups were made using Wilcoxon rank-sum test for continuous variables and chi-square or Fisher's exact test as appropriate for categorical variables. The incidence of pressure injuries were compared using Poisson regression with results reported as incidence rate ratios (IRR) and 95% confidence intervals. All calculated p values were two-tailed and $p < 0.05$ indicated statistical significance. Analyses were performed with Stata software version 14 (StataCorp, College Station, Texas, USA).

Results

Incidence of oral pressure injuries

Throughout the study period 2008 patients received invasive mechanical ventilation in ICU (1043 pre-

AnchorFast, 965 post-AnchorFast). There were a total 230 pressure injury incident reports, of which 22.6% (n = 52) were oral pressure injuries to the mouth or lips (16 pre-AnchorFast, 36 post-AnchorFast). During the post-AnchorFast period, 61.8% (n = 596) of mechanically ventilated patients had their ETT secured with an AnchorFast™.

Throughout both study periods, there were 42 patients with 52 reported oral pressure injuries.

There was no significant difference between the pre- and post-AnchorFast periods in patient age, gender distribution, ICU or hospital length of stay, Waterlow score on ICU admission, risk factors for pressure injury development, and length of mechanical ventilation (Table 1). There was a significant difference in compliance with institutional policies aimed at preventing pressure injuries between the two periods. There was greater documented compliance with pressure injury prevention protocols in the 24 h prior to pressure injury documentation for patients in the post-AnchorFast period compared to those in the pre-AnchorFast period (64.5% vs. 9.1%; p = 0.004).

Similarly, there was no difference in patient demographics between patients that developed pressure injuries with AnchorFast devices or cloth tape in situ across study periods (Table 2). Those with AnchorFast™ devices in–situ at the time of the pressure injury report were significantly more likely to have documented compliance

Table 1 Comparison of characteristics of patients with pressure injuries between pre- and post-AnchorFast periods

Variable	All patients (N = 42)	Pre-AnchorFast (n = 11)	Post-AnchorFast (n = 31)	p-value
Age (median, IQR)	56 (47.7–72.6)	52.2 (37.7–63.0)	56.7 (47.8–73.6)	0.43
Male Sex (%, n)	66.7% (28)	81.8% (9)	61.3% (19)	0.28
Malnourished at ICU admission (%, n)	19.0% (8)	36.4% (4)	12.9% (4)	0.17
Peripheral vascular disease (%, n)	2.4% (1)	9.1% (1)	0% (0)	0.26
Diabetes (%, n)	14.3% (6)	27.3% (3)	9.7% (3)	0.31
Current Smoker (%, n)	26.2% (11)	27.3% (3)	25.8% (8)	1.00
Long-term steroid therapy (%, n)	16.7% (7)	9.1% (1)	19.4% (6)	0.65
Serum albumin	34.5 (27.8–39.0)	30.0 (26.0–39.0)	35.0 (29.0–39.0)	0.45
Restricted mobility (%, n)	26.2% (11)	27.3% (3)	25.8% (8)	1.00
Waterlow score at ICU admission (median, IQR)	24 (17–28)	23.5 (14–24.5)	24 (17–28)	0.28
Length of mechanical ventilation, days (median, IQR)	7.6 (3.8–15.2)	8.7 (6.7–16.9)	6.9 (3.0–14.0)	0.10
ICU length of stay, days (median, IQR)	9.9 (4.6–21.2)	9.4 (7.8–23.1)	10.1 (4.2–20.9)	0.13
Hospital length of stay, days (median, IQR)	27.0 (11.6–36.3)	31.6 (14.9–38.3)	20.9 (10.6–36.3)	0.35
APACHE-III Score (median, IQR)	92.5 (72.8–111.3)	86.0 (73.0–121.0)	96.0 (69.0–107.0)	0.71
Time from intubation to PI reporting, days (median, IQR)	3 (1.9–6)	5 (2–6)	3 (1–7)	0.50
ICU Mortality (%, n)	14.3% (6)	18.2% (2)	12.9% (4)	0.64
Hospital Mortality (%, n)	28.6% (12)	27.3% (3)	29.0% (9)	1.00
Pressure injury severity				
1	21.4% (9)	18.2% (2)	22.6% (7)	1.00
2	78.6% (33)	81.8% (9)	77.4% (24)	

Table 2 Comparison of characteristics of patients with pressure injuries based on ETT securement method

Variable	All patients (N = 42)	Tape (n = 21) *	AnchorFast (n = 21)	p-value
Age (median, IQR)	56 (47.7–72.6)	53.2 (39.2–67.1)	58.6 (49.3–73.6)	0.22
Male Sex (%, n)	66.7% (28)	81.0% (17)	52.4% (11)	0.10
Malnourished at ICU admission (%, n)	19.0% (8)	28.6% (6)	9.5% (2)	0.24
Peripheral vascular disease (%, n)	2.4% (1)	4.8% (1)	0% (0)	1.00
Diabetes (%, n)	14.3% (6)	23.8% (5)	4.8% (1)	0.18
Current Smoker (%, n)	26.2% (11)	19.0% (4)	33.3% (7)	0.48
Long-term steroid therapy (%, n)	16.7% (7)	9.5% (2)	23.8% (5)	0.41
Serum albumin	34.5 (27.8–39.0)	36.0 (27.0–39.5)	32.0 (27.5–36.0)	0.26
Restricted mobility (%, n)	26.2% (11)	28.6% (6)	23.8% (5)	1.00
Waterlow score at ICU admission (median, IQR)	24 (17–28)	23.5 (15.3–26.0)	25.0 (17.5–28.0)	0.20
Length of mechanical ventilation, days (median, IQR)	7.6 (3.8–15.2)	7.1 (3.8–16.7)	7.9 (3.6–13.9)	0.10
ICU length of stay, days (median, IQR)	9.9 (4.6–21.2)	8.31 (4.1–21.8)	10.7 (4.9–20.8)	0.51
Hospital length of stay, days (median, IQR)	27.0 (11.6–36.3)	26.0 (8.6–33.7)	28.0 (13.8–60.8)	0.36
APACHE-III Score (median, IQR)	92.5 (72.8–111.3)	93.0 (72.5–119.5)	92.0 (71.5–101.5)	0.41
Time from intubation to PI reporting, days (median, IQR)	3 (1.9–6)	3 (1–5.5)	4 (2–9)	0.12
ICU Mortality (%, n)	14.3% (6)	19.0% (4)	9.5% (2)	0.66
Hospital Mortality (%, n)	28.6% (12)	19.0% (6)	28.6% (6)	1.00
Pressure injury severity				
1	21.4% (9)	23.8% (5)	19.0% (4)	1.00
2	78.6% (33)	76.2% (16)	81.0% (17)	

with pressure injury prevention protocols within the previous 24 h of pressure injury development, compared to those with cloth tapes in-situ at the time of pressure injury documentation (81.0% vs 19.0%; $p < 0.001$).

The incidence of reported oral pressure injuries was 1.53 per 100 mechanically ventilated patients during the pre-AnchorFast period, compared to 3.73 oral pressure injuries per 100 mechanically ventilated patients in the post-AnchorFast period (IRR: 2.43, 95% CI: 1.35–4.38; $p = 0.003$). Across both study periods, the incidence of oral pressure injuries among those with ETTs secured with tape was 1.98 per 100 ventilated patients, compared to 4.03 per 100 ventilated patients with an AnchorFast™ (IRR: 2.03, 95% CI: 1.17–3.51; $p = 0.02$). The incidence

of oral pressure injuries by time period and method of ETT securement is shown in Table 3.

Across both study periods, there was a statistically significant difference in the location of oral pressure injuries between those sustained with an AnchorFast™ device or cloth tape in-situ ($p = 0.008$). Those with an ETT secured using AnchorFast™ devices were most likely to sustain injuries to their lip (75%); while patients with their ETT secured using cloth tape were most likely to sustain injuries to the corner of their mouths (53.6%) (Table 4).

There was no significant difference in the time from intubation to pressure injury development between patients with tape and AnchorFast™ ETT securement

Table 3 Incidence of oral pressure injuries by study period (pre- vs. post- introduction of the AnchorFast™ device), and by method of ETT securement (cloth tapes vs. AnchorFast™ device) across both study periods

	All patients	Pre-AnchorFast period	Post-AnchorFast Period	Tape ETT securement	AnchorFast ETT securement
Number of Mechanically ventilated patients	2008	1043	965	1412	596
Total Ventilation Hours	201,152	93,602	107,550	109,711	91,441
Number of Oral Pressure Injuries reported	52	16	36	28	24
Oral Pressure Injuries per 100 ventilated patients	2.59	1.53	3.73*	1.98	4.03#
Oral pressure Injuries per 10,000 ventilation hours	2.59	1.71	3.35^	2.55	2.63‡

* p = 0.003; # p = 0.02; ^ p = 0.03; ‡ p = 0.92

Table 4 Location of oral pressure injuries across study period, by method of ETT securement (cloth tapes vs. AnchorFast™ device) at the time of pressure injury report

	ETT secured using cloth tape	ETT secured with AnchorFast device	p-value
Number of pressure Injuries reported	28	24	
Location of Pressure Injury (%, n)			
Corner of mouth	53.6% (15)	20.8% (5)	**0.008**
Lip	32.1% (9)	75% (18)	
Inside of lip or mouth	14.3% (4)	4.2% (1)	

(median 3 vs 4 days respectively; $p = 0.12$). There was also no significant difference in the severity of pressure injuries sustained with tapes (median = 2, range = 1–2) vs Anchor-Fast™ devices (median = 2, range = 1–2; $p = 0.71$). A majority of injuries in both groups were assessed as being stage 2 (tape = 76.2%, AnchorFast = 81.0%).

Discussion

Medical devices are a leading cause of pressure injuries in critically ill patients [2, 6], with ETTs and nasogastric tubes accounting for the majority of these [13, 14]. Oral pressure injuries related to endotracheal intubation accounted for 22.6% of all documented pressure injuries over a 6.5-year period in our ICU.

The incidence of reported oral pressure injuries appears to have increased significantly following the introduction of the AnchorFast™ device in our unit. Overall, patients with an AnchorFast™ in place were approximately twice as likely to develop oral pressure injuries. To our knowledge, only one previous study has investigated the impact of the introduction of the AnchorFast™ device on the incidence of oral pressure injuries. This retrospective 20-month study found a decrease in incidence of oral pressure injuries following the introduction of the AnchorFast™ device, from an incidence of 1.25 injuries per 100 ventilated patients to 0.06/100 ventilated patients [22]. These findings are at odds with those of the present study. It is unclear where this discrepancy may arise from, however variations in staffing and patient mix may contribute. In particular, Zaratkiewicz and colleagues reported an average of over 300 patients per month receiving IMV [22], compared to an average of 26 patients per month in our unit during the study period. This is likely to influence staffing experience and workload, as well as the length of mechanical ventilation that patients received. No information regarding patient acuity, length of mechanical ventilation, or staffing was provided in this article to enable comparisons with the present study.

Compliance with institutional policies aimed at reducing oral pressure injuries improved significantly following the introduction of the AnchorFast™ device. Similarly, compliance was significantly better among patients that developed oral pressure injuries with their ETT secured using an AnchorFast™ device compared to patients with cloth tape during the post-AnchorFast period.

According to promotional materials, the design of the AnchorFast™ device allows nursing staff to more easily reposition the ETT. This is likely to have contributed to the improved compliance with pressure injury prevention policies observed in this study; however, this does not appear to relate to a decrease in pressure injury incidence when implemented in routine practice. The reasons for this warrant further investigation.

The location of pressure injuries to the mouth and lips varied significantly between those sustained with AnchorFast™ devices and cloth tapes in place. The locations of pressure injuries reported with each method reflect areas of pressure exerted by these devices on the underlying skin (see Fig. 1), and these findings therefore have implications for the prevention of pressure injuries using these devices. This may include adjusting the way that cloth tapes are secured to reduce pressure across the corners of the mouth, and potential modifications to the AnchorFast™ device.

The severity of oral pressure injuries did not differ between those sustained with tapes and AnchorFast™ devices, with the majority of injuries reported as being stage 2 or "partial thickness skin loss with exposed dermis" [21]. The appropriateness of using standard pressure wound staging systems for the assessment of oral pressure wounds has previously been questioned [23].

Limitations

This study has a number of limitations that must be acknowledged. As it was conducted at a single centre the findings may have been influenced by a number of aspects of clinical practice that vary between centres, including staffing and patient characteristics.

The incidence of oral pressure injuries over the study period was relatively low, at 2.59 injuries per 100 invasively-ventilated patients. This limited the sample size available to compare the characteristics of patients who developed oral pressure injuries on the basis of their method of ETT securement.

As this is a retrospective observational study causality cannot be clearly established for the increased incidence in oral pressure injuries observed following the introduction of the AnchorFast™ device. It is possible that this finding also reflects an increased awareness and reporting of pressure injuries following the introduction of this device; however within the post-AnchorFast period, where both securement methods were used, two-thirds of oral pressure injuries occurred with AnchorFast™ devices in situ. In addition, after adjusting for the proportion of all mechanically ventilated patients who received each method of ETT securement, those with AnchorFast™ devices were found to be at significantly increased risk of oral pressure injuries. This is despite no significant differences in risk factors for pressure injuries between those that developed oral pressure injuries with cloth tapes or AnchorFast™ devices.

The retrospective nature of this study limits discussion to those pressure injuries that were documented. Clinical practice guidelines state that all pressure injuries must be reported appropriately, and all nursing staff in this unit received regular training in the identification and reporting of pressure injuries. Despite this, it is possible that some pressure injuries were never documented. In addition, assessment of nursing compliance with pressure injury prevention guidelines relied upon existing documentation.

Finally, despite being highly statistically significant, effect size confidence intervals were relatively large for comparisons of oral pressure injuries between the pre- and post-AnchorFast periods (IRR = 2.43; 95% CI = 1.35–4.38), and between patients with AnchorFast devices and cloth tapes (IRR = 2.13; 95% CI = 1.17–3.51).

Despite these limitations, this study represents a significant contribution to the existing body of literature regarding the utility of the AnchorFast™ device (and ETADs more broadly) to prevent oral pressure injuries associated with endotracheal intubation.

Recommendations

These findings highlight the importance of continually evaluating the efficacy of medical devices, particularly where there is limited empirical evidence to support their use. Given the present findings, the lack of available evidence, and the limitations of retrospective observational studies, a prospective randomised controlled trial may be warranted to investigate whether ETADs demonstrate any benefit for the prevention of oral pressure injuries when compared to cloth tape. A cost-benefit analysis may also be of relevance, given the increased financial costs associated with such devices.

Conclusion

Incidence of oral pressure injuries increased significantly following the introduction of the AnchorFast™ ETT securement device. Patients with an ETT secured using an AnchorFast™ device were found to be at a significantly increased risk of developing oral pressure injuries.

Abbreviations

95% CI: 95% Confidence Interval; APACHE-III: Adult Physiology and Chronic Health Evaluation illness severity score, version three; ETAD: Endotracheal tube attachment device; ETT: Endotracheal tube; ICU: Intensive Care Unit; IMV: Invasive mechanical ventilation; IRR: Incidence rate ratio; MDRI: Medical device-related injury; NPUAP: National Pressure Ulcer Advisory Panel; VHIMS: Victorian health incident management system

Acknowledgements

The authors would like to acknowledge the input of Angela Clinkaberry, Christine Clemence, Laurel Walker, and Kate Jones for their assistance with this study.

Funding

This study received no funding.

Authors' contributions

JH and RT were responsible for the conceptualisation of this study; CG and RT were responsible for study design. JH, JS, LA, GD, and AA were responsible for data acquisition and for reviewing the manuscript and revising it for important intellectual content. CG and EP were responsible for data analysis. CG, JH, and RT were responsible for manuscript preparation. All authors have reviewed the final manuscript and agree to be accountable for all aspects of the work in ensuring that questions related to the accuracy or integrity of any part of the work are appropriately investigated and resolved.

Competing interests

The authors declare that they have no competing interests to declare. The authors have received no financial or material support from Hollister.

Author details

[1]Department of Intensive Care Medicine, Peninsula Health, Frankston Hospital, 2 Hastings road, Frankston, VIC 3199, Australia. [2]Department of Epidemiology and Preventive Medicine, School of Public health and Preventive Medicine, Faculty of Medicine, Nursing and Health Sciences, Monash University, Clayton, VIC, Australia. [3]Clinical Haematology Department, The Alfred Hospital, Melbourne, Victoria 3181, Australia.

References

1. Keller BP, Wille J, van Ramshorst B, van der Werken C. Pressure ulcers in intensive care patients: a review of risks and prevention. Intensive Care Med. 2002;28:1379–88.
2. VanGilder C, Amlung S, Harrison P, Meyer S. Results of the 2008-2009 international pressure ulcer prevalence survey and a 3-year, acute care, unit-specific analysis. Ostomy Wound Manage. 2009;55:39–45.

3.   Elliott R, McKinley S, Fox V. Quality improvement program to reduce the prevalence of pressure ulcers in an intensive care unit. Am J Crit Care. 2008; 17:328–34. quiz 335; discussion 336-327

4.   Manzano F, Navarro MJ, Roldan D, Moral MA, Leyva I, Guerrero C, Sanchez MA, Colmenero M, Fernandez-Mondejar E, Granada UPPG. Pressure ulcer incidence and risk factors in ventilated intensive care patients. J Crit Care. 2010;25:469–76.

5.   de Laat EH, Schoonhoven L, Pickkers P, Verbeek AL, van Achterberg T. Epidemiology, risk and prevention of pressure ulcers in critically ill patients: a literature review. J Wound Care. 2006;15:269–75.

6.   Cooper KL. Evidence-based prevention of pressure ulcers in the intensive care unit. Crit Care Nurse. 2013;33:57–66.

7.   Cox J, Roche S. Vasopressors and development of pressure ulcers in adult critical care patients. Am J Crit Care. 2015;24:501–10.

8.   Krupp AE, Monfre J. Pressure ulcers in the ICU patient: an update on prevention and treatment. Curr Infect Dis Rep. 2015;17:468.

9.   Black JM, Cuddigan JE, Walko MA, Didier LA, Lander MJ, Kelpe MR. Medical device related pressure ulcers in hospitalized patients. Int Wound J. 2010;7:358–65.

10. Black J, Alves P, Brindle CT, Dealey C, Santamaria N, Call E, Clark M. Use of wound dressings to enhance prevention of pressure ulcers caused by medical devices. Int Wound J. 2015;12:322–7.

11. Apold J, Rydrych D. Preventing device-related pressure ulcers: using data to guide statewide change. J Nurs Care Qual. 2012;27:28–34.

12. Dyer A. Ten top tips: preventing device-related pressure ulcers. Wounds International. 2015;6:9–13.

13. Hanonu S, Karadag A. A prospective, descriptive study to determine the rate and characteristics of and risk factors for the development of medical device-related pressure ulcers in intensive care units. Ostomy Wound Manage. 2016;62:12–22.

14. Coyer FM, Stotts NA, Blackman VS. A prospective window into medical device-related pressure ulcers in intensive care. Int Wound J. 2014;11:656–64.

15. Fisher DF, Chenelle CT, Marchese AD, Kratohvil JP, Kacmarek RM. Comparison of commercial and noncommercial endotracheal tube-securing devices. Respir Care. 2014;59:1315–23.

16. Clinical Benefits of the AnchorFast and AnchorFast Guard. http://www. anchorfast1.com/clinical-benefits.html. Accessed 31 Jan 2018.

17. Gardner A, Hughes D, Cook R, Henson R, Osborne S, Gardner G. Best practice in stabilisation of oral endotracheal tubes: a systematic review. Aust Crit Care. 2005;18(158):160–55.

18. Kaplow R, Bookbinder M. A comparison of four endotracheal tube holders. Heart Lung. 1994;23:59–66.

19. Levy H, Griego L. A comparative study of oral endotracheal tube securing methods. Chest. 1993;104:1537–40.

20. Tasota FJ, Hoffman LA, Zullo TG, Jamison G. Evaluation of two methods used to stabilize oral endotracheal tubes. Heart Lung. 1987;16:140–6.

21. Prevention and treatment of pressure ulcers: quick reference guide. http://www.npuap.org/wp-content/uploads/2014/08/Updated-10-16-14-Quick-Reference-Guide-DIGITAL-NPUAP-EPUAP-PPPIA-16Oct2014.pdf. Accessed 31 Jan 2018.

22. Zaratkiewicz S, Teegardin C, Whitney JD. Retrospective review of the reduction of oral pressure ulcers in mechanically ventilated patients: a change in practice. Crit Care Nurs Q. 2012;35:247–54.

23. Reaper S, Green C, Gupta S, Tiruvoipati R. Inter-rater reliability of the reaper oral mucosa pressure injury scale (ROMPIS): a novel scale for the assessment of the severity of pressure injuries to the mouth and oral mucosa. Aust Crit Care. 2017;30(3):167–71.

11

When east meets west: a qualitative study of barriers and facilitators to evidence-based practice in Hunan China

Wendy Gifford[1,2]* , Qing Zhang[3], Shaolin Chen[3], Barbara Davies[1,2], Rihua Xie[4,5], Shi-Wu Wen[6,7] and Gillian Harvey[8,9]

Abstract

Background: Research into evidence-based practice has been extensively explored in nursing and there is strong recognition that the organizational context influences implementation. A range of barriers has been identified; however, the research has predominantly taken place in Western cultures, and there is little information about factors that influence evidence-based practice in China. The purpose of this study was to explore barriers and facilitators to evidence-based practice in Hunan province, a less developed region in China.

Methods: A descriptive qualitative methodology was employed. Semi-structured interviews were conducted with staff nurses, head nurses and directors ($n = 13$). Interviews were translated into English and verified for accuracy by two bilingual researchers. Both Chinese and English data were simultaneously analyzed for themes related to factors related to the evidence to be implemented (Innovation), nurses' attitudes and beliefs (Potential Adopters), and the organizational setting (Practice Environment).

Results: Barriers included lack of available evidence in Chinese, nurses' lack of understanding of what evidence-based practice means, and fear that patients will be angry about receiving care that is perceived as non-traditional. Nurses believed evidence-based practice was to be used when clinical problems arose, and not as a routine way to practice. Facilitators included leadership support and the pervasiveness of web based social network services such as Baidu (百度) for easy access to information.

Conclusion: While several parallels to previous research were found, our study adds to the knowledge base about factors related to evidence-based practice in different contextual settings. Findings are important for international comparisons to develop strategies for nurses to provide evidence-based care.

Keywords: Qualitative study, Evidence-based practice, Barriers, Facilitators, China

Background

As the largest group of healthcare professionals, nurses play an essential role in delivering evidence-based practice (EBP) for positive patient outcomes [1]. However, gaps exist between recommendations for EBP and the actual care nurses provide in practice [2, 3]. A range of barriers has been identified, however, and while factors that influence EBP have been extensively explored by researchers in many countries, this has predominantly taken place in Western cultures; little information exists about EBP in China [4, 5]. As a relatively new concept, a recent scoping review ($n = 95$ articles) found barriers not commonly documented in western countries [6]. For example, the values embedded in traditional Chinese culture continue to have a strong influence on the ways in which Chinese people think and behave, which in turn affects the ways healthcare is delivered. Reverence for authority and obedience to superiors typically influences Chinese nurses' motivation to change their practice independently, particularly as they are perceived to have little decision-making autonomy and low professional status [5, 7]. Order and

* Correspondence: wgifford@uottawa.ca
[1]School of Nursing, Faculty of Health Sciences, University of Ottawa, 451 Smyth Road, Ottawa, ON K1H 8M5, Canada
[2]Nursing Best Practice Research Center, 451 Smyth Road, Ottawa, ON K1H 8M5, Canada
Full list of author information is available at the end of the article

harmony are expected social behaviours in China, and many people expect healthcare to be rooted in traditional Chinese practices that may not have a strong evidence base [8, 9]. Such reverence for authority and expectation for tradition impedes nurses from implementing EBP or considering it a routine way of practice [8, 9].

Large health and healthcare inequities exist between China's more developed urban provinces that are largely coastal and generate a large proportion of the country's wealth [10], and its less developed rural provinces that lack resources and infrastructure to meet healthcare needs [11, 12]. Across different provinces, inconsistencies also exist in nurses' understanding and acceptance of EBP [13]. Research has indicated that nurses in some provinces of China are more advanced in understanding, accepting and implementing EBP when compared to other provinces where healthcare systems are less developed [13].

Effecting change across healthcare settings and organizations can be challenging. With recognition that the contextual factors influence EBP, there has been recent interest in factors that influence the successful implementation of EBP in mainland China. The majority of research has been quantitative in design and few studies have explored nurses' experiences of the EBP implementation process [6]. Strategies for implementing EBP have a higher chance of success if they are tailored to known contextual barriers and facilitators both internal and external to the practice settings [14].

The Ottawa Model of Research Use (OMRU) is an implementation framework based on planned change theories that outline the interrelationships and complex organizational dimensions of translating research or new knowledge into practice [15]. The OMRU describes factors that influence the process of implementing research evidence into practice, classifying barriers and facilitators at the levels of the: 1) innovation or evidence to be implemented, 2) potential adopters or healthcare practitioners who will use the evidence and 3) practice environment in which the evidence will be used [15]. However, limited knowledge exists about nurses' perceptions of factors that hinder or facilitate EBP in China, particularly in less developed regions where healthcare is less developed and resources are scarce.

Qualitatively understanding Chinese nurses' perceptions of factors that influence the implementation processes of EBP is important to develop strategies for organizational leaders and decision-makers to improve the effectiveness of patient care for positive patient outcomes. To this end, we undertook a qualitative study to understand nurses' perceptions of the factors that influence nurses' implementation of EBP in Hunan province, a less developed region in China [16]. The following research questions were addressed:

1. What sources of the knowledge do nurses use to make decisions in their clinical practice?
2. What are the barriers and supports for clinical nurses to use research evidence in their daily practice?

Methods

Drawing on principles of naturalistic inquiry, a qualitative descriptive study was conducted [17]. Descriptive qualitative research is valuable to explore the experiences of a phenomenon when a comprehensive summary is desired [17]. The aim of qualitative descriptive studies is a descriptive summary of the information in the data desired. Descriptive qualitative analysis is considered the method of choice when straight descriptions of phenomena are desired [17].

Participants

Convenience sampling was first initiated at a two day "China-Canada" colloquium on best practices in nursing education and practice held in Hunan province where academic researchers in nursing, epidemiology and medicine from Canada and China were featured. Over 400 nurses and healthcare leaders from Hunan province, a mountainous province in south central China, attended. Hunan is a largely agricultural with approximately 60% of the 68.2 million residents living rural lives [18]. Confucianism values are prominent, with the virtues of loyalty, etiquette, ritual and customs strongly influencing the behaviours and social structures of Hunan society [19].

Information about the study was distributed, and interested participants identified themselves to the bilingual research assistants who were present. Snowball sampling was used to further recruit participants after the colloquium ended.

Data collection

Data were collected through individual, face-to-face semi-structured interviews between November and December 2015 in Hunan province. All interviews were conducted in Mandarin by two bilingual researchers. The principal investigator (WG) did not speak Mandarin but was present for the first five interviews with a bilingual researcher who translated participant responses as the interview progressed, allowing for probes and clarification of meanings and context.

Interviews were conducted with staff nurses, head nurses and senior nursing directors. The interview guide consisted of open-ended questions regarding participants' views about the type of knowledge they used to make practice decisions, and their experiences of using research evidence to inform practice. Examples of interview questions included: What are the main sources of knowledge that you use to make clinical decisions? From your experience, what would you say are the barriers or challenges for nurses to use research evidence in their clinical decisions? What are some of the facilitators or supports? The full interview schedule can be found in Additional file 1.

Interviews averaged between 40 and 60 min, were audio-recorded, transcribed verbatim into Chinese and translated into English by two bilingual researchers from Hunan province (QZ, SC). The same two researchers independently crosschecked the translation and came to consensus on contextual meanings. Different bilingual investigators (XR, SWW) provided confirmation of the translation and back-translation; any discrepancies were discussed with the research study team until consensus was reached. Both Chinese and English transcriptions were imported together into QSR NVIVO© 10 qualitative software.

Ethical considerations
Ethical approval was obtained from University of Ottawa Research Ethics Board, and recognized by the Hunan University of Medicine in China. Ethical principles of informed consent, anonymity and right to withdraw were maintained throughout the study. Written information about the study was reviewed with each participant by a Chinese research assistant and verbal consent to participate was received from all participants prior to recording the interviews.

Data analysis
Analysis proceeded as a group process with the principal investigator (WG) and the two bilingual researchers from China (QZ, SC), hereafter referred to as the 'analysis team.' Transcripts were reviewed numerous times to ensure familiarization with the data. The analysis team reviewed the English and Chinese data together and discussed the explicit and implicit meanings in response to the interview questions. If agreement could not be reached about meaning, a fourth party was consulted until consensus was reached.

Qualitative content analysis was informed by procedures described by Graneheim and Lundman [20]. Data were initially coded by the analysis team into meaning units and codes using relevant words and phrases of participants in both English and Chinese. Next, English codes for each of the research questions were collapsed into inductive sub-categories. Barriers and facilitators to EBP were then classified into three broad deductive categories based on the OMRU: 1) Innovations, 2) Potential Adopters and 3) Practice Environment [15].

The analysis process was iterative, with ongoing and simultaneous examination of the Chinese and English data and codes to ensure the analysis team captured appropriate meanings. Larger meetings with the research team were held throughout the analysis to confirm interpretations and findings.

Results
Description of participants
Thirteen nurses from tertiary and community hospitals participated in the study (see Table 1). All participants were female with more than five years' work experience.

Sources of knowledge
To inform their clinical practice decisions-making, nurses described using multiple sources of knowledge that included colleagues (peers, head nurses and doctors), educational seminars and conferences, original nursing education, social media applications (apps) and the internet web service "Baidu." WeChat, a mobile text and voice messaging service developed in China, was consistently detailed as a primary source for accessing information to make practice decisions, as described by a head nurse in a community hospital:

Baidu Search or website of Nursing Association, and the public channel "nurses learning notes" in WeChat, where there are some new views about nursing practice or research. (Source 9 Community)

Participant believed the information they found through their social media apps and on Baidu was accurate, trustworthy and reliable.

Awareness of EBP
Less than half of the sample ($n = 6/13$; 46%) was aware of the concept of EBP, and only two of the six participants from community had heard of it. Directors and head nurses were more aware than clinical staff.

We have not started to implement evidence-based nursing practice yet. I heard the concept of EBP a few years ago when I worked in [a tertiary hospital]. I know that the concept has been around for many years, however, implementing EBP has not been long, even in tertiary hospitals. I know little about EBP and there are less complex nursing problems in community that need it. (Source 7 Community)

Table 1 Participant positions and previous awareness of EBP

	Community hospital ($n = 6$)	Tertiary hospital ($n = 7$)	Total ($n = 13$)
Position			
Director	1	1	2
Head Nurse	2	4	6
Staff nurse	3	2	5
Previous awareness of EBP	2 (33%)	4 (57%)	6 (46%)

For participants who had heard of EBP, it was not perceived to be a routine way of providing care. Rather, EBP was believed to be a way of practice for addressing individualized clinical problems when they could not be dealt with through established routines and traditional ways. This perception did not vary between community and tertiary settings. Respondents believed medical practice was more research-based than nursing, and that tertiary hospitals provided more evidence-based care than community hospitals.

> *Nursing is less important than medical science in China. Our hospital leaders do not support us to do research... We just want to do the things required by the superior leaders, and make sure no medical errors happen. (Source 6 Urban)*

Barriers to EBP

Barriers to applying research evidence in everyday practice were expressed as they related to the innovation, potential adopters and practice settings. A summary of barriers are presented in Table 2.

Innovation

Respondents reported that the majority of nursing research journals and guidelines were published in English, and therefore a barrier to EBP was the lack of readable and understandable research evidence in Chinese. When guidelines were available, some felt they did not have enough details about how to apply it in practice.

Table 2 Barriers to evidence-based practice

Innovation
- Lack of evidence written in Chinese language
- Not enough details in guidelines

Potential Adopters

Nurse-related
- Fear of patients' and families' reacting to something new or non-traditional
- Lack of awareness, knowledge and skills
- Negative attitudes and beliefs toward EBP

Patient-related
- Lack of money
- Lack of trust

Practice Environment
- Lack of leadership support
- Little/no opportunities for EBP education and training
- Limited resources (physical and human)

Potential adopters
Nurse-related barriers

Many respondents reported fearing patients and families if they did something that was considered new or non-traditional to what was expected, such as a new practice based on research evidence. Nurses described fear of being blamed or assaulted both physically and verbally if patients had a bad outcome, and this fear discouraged nurses from considering doing something that could be perceived as different to or outside the traditional practices. All nurses interviewed described some level of fear of patients and families, as one participant related:

> *We tend to be conservative here; we will not use some new medicine or new nursing practices until the practices are generally accepted by everyone, because if there is a bad outcome, the patient will be angry and blame us. (Source 9 Community)*

Participants spoke about a lack of knowledge and skills of clinical nurses about finding, accessing and understanding research evidence, exemplified as follows:

> *Nurses' scientific research knowledge base is very low; therefore, they do not know how to find or appraise evidence or use. (Source 4 Community)*

> *But I guess the ordinary clinical nurses may not know what to do, just know the assignments which head-nurse asked them to do. The head-nurses told them if there are some problems, they should use EBP approach to solve them. They feel it is difficult to understand and accept. The reason for this phenomenon may be nurses' training has not been done well. The Nursing Department of the hospital carried out some training lectures, but most of nurses who attended were head-nurses, most ordinary nurses were busy in clinical care; they could not attend. (Source 1 Urban)*

Holding negative attitudes and beliefs towards research in general was another barrier described by participants. Most respondents reported that they and their nursing colleagues preferred to practice in ways they had learnt in nursing school or that were consistent with routines in their practice settings. EBP was described as being difficult to understand, and participants did not believable that the evidence was always applicable in China:

> *... it is much easier to use the traditional method. ... The [research] evidence may work for some patients, but may not work for patients in China. (Source 2 Urban)*

Patient-related barriers

Participants identified costs to patients and their inability to afford the best care as a barrier to EBP:

Patients and their families worry about the expense. For example, according to the evidence, we may use a better material to help patients' recovery, but they cannot afford it. (Source 3 Urban)

Nurses spoke about patients' lack of trust when doing things that were considered different or unfamiliar to traditional care. This was emphasized when caring for the elderly patients, where communication difficulties were present:

Most of our patients are elderly, so it's hard to communicate with them.... Sometimes, because of generational culture gap, old patients do not trust us, and they do not want to see a change in routine based on something new. (Source 10 Community)

Practice setting

Lack of leadership support from head nurses and hospital administrators was a barrier to EBP and included an absence of leaders with EBP knowledge to promote, encourage and facilitate EBP:

Another main barrier is the way of management. If there was someone to take the responsibility of EBP and educating nurses for EBP, implementation would be much better in clinical practice. (Source 4 Community)

Even some nursing leaders do not know what EBP means or how to appraise and implement the evidence. If EBP is needed in clinical practice, nurses will have to learn it by themselves. (Source 7 Community)

Participants also expressed senior leaders' lack of understanding and commitment to the implementation of EBP:

...if the senior leaders of the hospital do not stress on the issues [EBP], why do the clinical nurses do it? Some senior leaders of the hospital do not pay attention to this issue. Evidence-based practice has not been fully carried out at present... some of them [nursing managers] do not even understand the inner meaning of evidence-based practice, they just say it. They know it is priority, but they don't know how to do it in practice. (Source 3 Urban)

Participants indicated there were little or no opportunities for EBP education and training, and limited resources for nurses to implement new evidence-based practices, as emphasized:

Our hospital's condition is not good enough, and the equipment are not advanced, so evidence-based practice cannot be implemented. (Source 10 Community)

Limited resources included an insufficient number of nursing staff, resulting in heavy workloads. Participants felt that they had limited time during their scheduled working hours to provide patient care and EBP was seen as extra work:

Chinese nursing conditions are different from other countries. Chinese nurses' basic workload is very heavy; we do not have enough time to practice based on new evidence. (Source 4 Community)

Facilitators of EBP

Facilitators to EBP in nursing were seldom discussed, however, respondents identified two facilitators related to the potential adopters (i.e. nurses), and four related to the practice setting (Table 3).

Potential adopter

Participants emphasized that EBP would increase the credibility of the nursing profession, and bring recognition to the importance of nursing practice for positive patients outcomes.

I believe evidence-based practice is a very effective way to improve nursing... I believe EBP working method will avoid many medical disputes or contradictions with medical staff...and the evidences will direct our nursing work in future. For example, a patient suffers from pressure ulcer, if we find out some evidences and accumulate these evidences...when we come across another similar patient, we can find out the best nursing method quickly. If we can work this way, I believe it is helpful for our clinical nursing. (Source 4 Community)

Table 3 Facilitators to evidence-based practice

Potential Adopter
• Understanding that EBP improves patient care
• Belief that EBP improves credibility of nursing

Practice Setting
• Education and training
• Leadership promotion and support of EBP
• Presence of EBP team
• Mechanism to access evidence

Now, we head-nurses believe it [EBP] is a wonderful scientific method. If we encounter some problems in clinical, we will search literatures and find evidence, apply these evidence to address problems, then evaluate outcomes or effects. I feel this kind of work method is perfect for nursing (Source 3 Urban)

Practice setting

Participants described nursing leadership at many levels as an important EBP facilitator. The role of the government was emphasized in both urban and community hospitals to set the stage for conducting and using research in practice:

The Ministry of Health can develop some rules about doing research in community hospitals, so the leaders of our hospital will support using research; from the patient's point of view, it is beneficial to them, and nurses will get pleasure and fulfillment from this and increase our professional self-identity. Everybody likes a good work environment, so that we can work in a good mood and work more efficiently. (Source 9 Community)

Leadership to develop international collaborations has assisted with raising awareness of the importance of EBP and the resources required to provide quality nursing care:

The collaborations, which are not just among personnel but increasingly with nursing associates and governments with other countries, improves the Chinese government to change their decisions so they know the importance of giving more human resources and more support for the nurses - hire more nurses - so the nurses can do the right job and feel good and strong. Secondly, now our country is advocating for medical reform and high-quality nursing care programs. (Source 3 Urban)

Senior nursing leaders played a significant role in bringing awareness to organizational leaders regarding the importance of EBP in nursing:

Nursing care is paid more attention to than before in our country now, and so does our hospital leadership. The nursing group plays a great role in influencing the decisions of hospital leadership... to improve the awareness of EBP in nursing... and there is someone to lead us to improve. ...the facilitators mainly include two aspects: hospital leadership's attention and improvement of nurse education level. (Source 2 Urban)

Hospital leadership is important as well; they should pay attention to the hospital future planning and medical safety management. (Source 10 Community)

The presence of clinical nursing leaders was discussed as a necessary direction to increase awareness and engage staff in research activities that included conducting and using research in practice, as discussed by a head nurse in a large urban hospital.

The government set up a "Clinical Nursing Key Specialty Program," which is similar with doctors,' and they give some funding. Our hospital gained about 3 million RMB from this program for supporting nursing research, training nurses, sending nurses to go abroad for studying and communicating with Taiwan and Hong Kong... The aim of the research is to direct the practice, implement into practice. (Source 3 Urban)

Education was further described as necessary to facilitate EBP in China. In addition, social media and electronic platforms, which are integral to people's daily lives, were consistently detailed as a primary resources for accessing information to make practice decisions, as described by a head nurse in a community hospital:

Baidu Search or website of Nursing Association, and the public channel "nurses learning notes" in WeChat (a mobile text and voice messaging communication service developed by Tencent in China), where there are some new views about nursing practice or research. (Source 9 Community)

Discussion

In this study, nurses in a less-developed province in mainland China discussed the knowledge they used to make practice decisions, and the barriers and facilitators to EBP. While several parallels to previous research were found, our study revealed new and important findings that have not been previously reported. Our findings are discussed as they relate to the innovation, the individual and the organization.

The innovation

One unique finding was the use of mobile social media apps by nurses and other healthcare professionals as a source of knowledge to inform patient care. Fast-paced technological developments that link mobile apps to smartphones and tablet computers are integral to everyday life in China [21]. Previous research has shown that medical professionals' use of mobile technology was beneficial to making evidence-based decisions and lowering error rates [22, 23]. However, despite all participants in this study regularly using electronic mobile technology at work, they infrequently used it to inform practice decisions, nor did they question the accuracy or reliability of the information they found on popular social media sites.

In 2016, a 21-year-old college student in China died after receiving an experimental cancer treatment that was promoted on a hospital website through the Chinese search engine Baidu [24]. The student's death drew widespread international attention when the family accused Baidu of promoting false medical information that was supported by staff at the hospital. The ubiquitous use of electronic mobile technology underscores the need for nurses to have critical appraisal knowledge and skills to safely use information from electronic sources to inform their practice decisions. This is particularly relevant today where information from electronic technology is increasingly part of people's everyday lives. Incorporating evidence-based decision-making tools from trustworthy sources into electronic mobile devices is a promising strategy for increasing EBP nursing in China.

The individual

Our study found that, in general, bedside nurses had a limited awareness and understanding of EBP and how it could improve care and outcomes. Using research evidence to routinely inform practice decisions was not considered standard practice as traditional ways were deemed the most desirable, and many nursing leaders considered EBP as a way to manage problems when traditional practice failed. This finding provides further insights into previous survey research that showed Chinese nurses do not use research findings in their daily practice decisions [25, 26] and lacked understanding of EBP [27].

To use research evidence routinely in practice, nurses must first be aware of EBP and then have the knowledge and skills to access, appraise, and integrate evidence with patient preferences and clinical experience [27]. Results of our study showed that participants lacked awareness and knowledge of EBP, particularly in community settings. While nurses from tertiary hospitals had greater awareness of EBP, they lacked the knowledge of how to find, appraise and judicially apply the evidence. With nursing research poorly developed in China [28–30], many nurses lack knowledge of the research process and do not understand how research could improve nursing care and outcomes [30–32].

The need to increase awareness and knowledge of EBP in China is an important first step to attenuate barriers and enable evidence-based nursing. This is consistent with an updated systematic review (n = 45 articles) that indicated that beliefs and attitudes, information seeking and education influenced nurses' use of research [33]. In our study, respondents had negative beliefs and attitudes

about EBP, and preferred to practice the way they had learned or according to the expected tradition. These findings are similar to cross-sectional survey studies conducted in other non-western countries. Farokhzadian et al. [34] found that nurses in Iran (n = 182) had unfavorable attitudes towards EBP, and Lai, Teng, & Lee [35] had similar findings in Malaysia. In our study, nurses stated they did not believe that research evidence was applicable to their settings because the research was not conducted in China, and they would not adopt EBP as routine practice unless they could see positive results on patient care and outcomes.

EBP was seen as a useful way to increase the credibility of the nursing profession and recognize nursing's contributions to quality patient care. Using research evidence to inform practice was emphasized as a way to recognize nursing as a science-based profession, improving nursing's credibility, particularly with physicians. These results concur with findings from studies in Iran [36] and Germany [37] that highlight EBP as a way of strengthening understanding of nurses' contributions to patient care. Aiken et al. [38] showed nursing care was significantly associated with patient mortality and length of stay in nine European countries, emphasizing the role nurses have in influencing patient care and outcomes.

Lack of research studies and evidence-based guidelines in Chinese was identified as a barrier to EBP, and this finding has been similarly reported in other non-English-speaking countries [27, 39–41]. With English being the international language of science [42], the majority of nursing research is published in English; however, less than 1 % of people in China are able to fluently understand it [43]. Translating evidence-based guidelines into Chinese could help overcome language obstacles to accessing research evidence in China [4, 44]. In Canada, the Registered Nurses' Association of Ontario (RNAO) has produced evidence-based guidelines for nursing care that are freely available on their website (http://rnao.ca/bpg/language), and a number are being translated into Chinese. Interestingly, participants in our study felt that guidelines did not have enough details related to the evidence, which is inconsistent with a survey of almost 1500 nurses in Hong Kong that found guidelines and research reports had too much information [45].

A unique finding in our study was the fear of patients and families that nurses had when doing something new or different from what is expected. This fear is arguably accentuated by the perceived lack of organizational support nurses received when patients and families were unsatisfied with their care or outcomes [5]. Nurses in China face increasingly heavy workloads and stressful work environments that affect the quality of patient care [46]. The lack of leadership support they perceived in our study may partially explain why they are hesitant to implement new or non-traditional practices.

Our findings provide contextual data on work environment barriers within the Chinese healthcare context that may contribute to nurses' use of evidence in practice.

Patient involvement is an integral part of EBP; however, participants described difficulties getting patients involved in care because of factors such as cultural traditions with aging patients. Reports indicate that the Chinese medical system is not fully prepared to manage the aging trend in China and fails to meet healthcare demands due to lack of resources and expertise [12]. This includes the costs patients assume because of lack of socially funded healthcare, particularly in rural areas where inequalities exist in healthcare services [47].

In our study, the cost of care was identified as problematic for patients; health reforms are providing wider coverage of costs to alleviate financial burdens caused by illness [48, 49], and government policies have been developed for rural farmers to have access to basic health services [12]. However, lax governance regulatory and enforcement systems are an obstacle to reducing out-of-pocket spending for healthcare, as healthcare delivery often concentrates on services that generate the most profit rather than the evidence base [50]. The influence of government health reforms to facilitate EBP and improve health outcomes for people in China warrants further investigation.

The organizational setting

Using research evidence for decision-making in practice is a complex process and factors related to the organizational setting consistently explain a large amount of the variance in EBP [5]. Lack of leadership support, heavy workload, no opportunities for continuing education and lack of specialized staff were organizational factors found to be barriers in this study.

Previous studies indicate that leadership support is related to successful implementation of EBP [2, 51–53]. In our study, staff nurses reported the need for support from head nurses and, in turn, head nurses needed support from their superiors, which were often hospital directors. Leadership and the management of healthcare in China have been built on traditional hierarchical structures in which hospital administrators and medical doctors have higher status and authority over nurses [5].

Confucian principles of loyalty, obedience and respect for the social order, where everyone knows the behaviours expected in relation to others, have strongly influenced the norms and behaviours of Chinese people [54, 55]. Full support from superiors like head nurses, directors and physicians is required for nurses to deviate from the status quo and make changes to routine practices, such as EBP. In light of the hierarchies embedded in Chinese cultural values, nurses lack the authority to initiate change; therefore, leadership support is essential

to facilitate EBP in China [5]. As healthcare reform continues in China [56], leadership is required to promote EBP as a routine part of nursing practice. Leadership commitment and support are positively related to the implementation of EBP in western countries [2, 51, 57].

The leadership of bedside nurses, as champions for EBP, has also been shown to facilitate implementation [58]. Establishing key personnel to promote and share research findings with staff can support nurses' understanding and implementing of EBP. An organizational intervention that included having designated champions to facilitate staff accessing and understanding of research evidence influenced nurses to use research findings in their practice [59].

Prior studies have indicated that a lack of education is a barrier to EBP [34, 60]. Most participants in our study stated that they had not had any professional education about EBP, and felt that educational opportunities would enhance their inquiry and appraisal skills to practice EBP. With little focus on research in nursing school, the majority of nurses in China have not received education about research or using research findings in their basic nursing education, nor have they had continuing education on EBP in the workplace [5]. Education and training were described as necessary to facilitate EBP in our study; however, research has shown that implementation is complex and education alone will not ensure research findings are used in practice [61, 62], particularly where respect for social order is a strong influence on how people act.

Organizational characteristics such as location, size, infrastructure and resources, have been associated with knowledge and attitudes towards EBP in China [5]. Healthcare inequities between more-developed urban provinces and less-developed rural provinces contribute to differences in organizational characteristics [11, 12]. Consistent with our study, survey research has revealed nurses in rural hospitals are less knowledgeable about EBP than nurses in tertiary hospitals [5, 36].

Evidence based practice is a complex process that requires multidimensional change at the individual, organizational and cultural levels. This study brings us closer to understanding some of the changes that could support nurses to use rigorous research evidence to guide their clinical practice in China. With the ubiquitous use of electronic internet devices, nurses require critical appraisal skills to safely and judiciously use evidence that is readily available on the internet. Evidence-based guidelines in Chinese are needed to provide nurses access to research knowledge for making practice decisions. Further research is required into the process of translating and adapting clinical practice guidelines and other knowledge translation tools into Chinese language and context to support nurses use evidence based knowledge in practice.

Our study acknowledged the importance of nursing leadership in creating a work environment that supports EBP. However it also demonstrates the complexity of the leadership process to influence change. Further research is required to understand leadership in China and how to effectively develop nursing leaders to facilitate and support the implementation of evidence based practices.

Study strengths and limitations

We used a small sample in order to perform in-depth qualitative interviews with bilingual translation during the interviews, allowing for rich data collection and interpretations of meanings. Nurses from multiple levels of the organizations were interviewed providing insights into the structures and processes that impact direct patient care. While translation and back-translation processes were conducted, other semantic meanings and cultural norms may have been present and not captured.

Conclusions

Our findings from Hunan province provide an important understanding of the barriers and facilitators of EBP in nursing from the narratives of three stakeholder groups: staff nurses, head nurses and nursing directors. While several parallels to previous research were found, this study adds to the knowledge base about factors related to EBP in different geographic and contextual settings. To realize a successful implementation of EBP in mainland China, it is important that strategies consider nurses' perspectives from multiple levels within an organization. Findings are important for international comparisons so that strategies can be developed for nurses to deliver evidence-based practice and improve the quality of patient care.

Abbreviations
Apps: Social media applications; EBP: Evidence-based practices

Acknowledgements
The authors would like to thank Nursing Best Practice Research Center (NBPRC), a joint partnership between the University of Ottawa and the Registered Nurses' Association of Ontario, for their continued support of visiting scholars from the Hunan University of Medicine. We would also like to acknowledge the investigator team of the international FLAME study, the parent study in which this work was conceptualized, namely Paul Wilson and Roman Kislov at the University of Manchester, UK; Lars Wallin and Anna Ehrenberg at Dalarna University, Sweden; Greta Cummings at University of Alberta, Canada; and Alison Kitson at University of Adelaide, Australia. We recognize the contributions of Jinfeng Ding (丁金锋), Central South University, Changsha, China, and Liquaa Waazni, University of Ottawa, for their work as research assistants on this study.

Funding
This study was partially supported by funding from the Hunan Province Ministry of Education China (received by Dr. Davies and Dr. Gifford), and Canadian Institute of Health Research (CIHR) Foundation grant (received by Dr. Wen; FDN-148438) to support project related activities including international travel, supplies and services.

Authors' contributions
WG and QZ are co-first authors and were major contributors to writing the manuscript. WG, GH and BD each made substantial contributions to the conception and design of the study. QZ, SC, RX and SWW provided continuous forward and back-translation of data during analysis, and contributed substantially to interpretation and analysis of the data. All authors (WG, QZ, SC, RX, SWW, BD, GH) contributed substantially to the interpretation of results and implications of findings. All authors critically reviewed drafts of the manuscript and gave final approval before submission.

Competing interests
The authors declare that they have no competing interests.

Author details
[1]School of Nursing, Faculty of Health Sciences, University of Ottawa, 451 Smyth Road, Ottawa, ON K1H 8M5, Canada. [2]Nursing Best Practice Research Center, 451 Smyth Road, Ottawa, ON K1H 8M5, Canada. [3]School of Nursing, Hunan University of Medicine, 492 Jinxinan Road, Huaihua, Hunan, China. [4]Nanhai Hospital, Southern Medical University, 45 ZhenXing Road, Lishui Town, Nanhai District, Foshan 528244, Guangdong, China. [5]OMNI Research Group, Department of Obstetrics, Gynecology and Newborn Care, Faculty of Medicine University of Ottawa, Ottawa, Canada. [6]Clinical Epidemiology Program, Ottawa Hospital Research Institute, Ottawa, Canada. [7]Department of Epidemiology and Community Medicine, University of Ottawa, 501 Smyth Box 51, Ottawa, ON K1H 8L6, Canada. [8]Adelaide Nursing School, The University of Adelaide, Adelaide, Australia. [9]Alliance Manchester Business School, University of Manchester, Manchester, UK.

References
1. Melnyk BM, Fineout-Overholt E, Stetler C, Allan J. Outcomes and implementation strategies from the first U.S. evidence-based practice leadership summit. Worldviews Evid-Based Nurs. 2005;2(3):113–21.
2. Gifford WA, Davies BL, Graham ID, Tourangeau A, Woodend AK, Lefebre N. Developing leadership capacity for guideline use: a pilot cluster randomized control trial. Worldviews Evid Based Nurs. 2013;10(1):51–65.
3. Squires JE, Hutchinson AM, Bostrom AM, O'Rourke HM, Cobban SJ, Estabrooks CA. To what extent do nurses use research in clinical practice? A systematic review. Implement Sci. 2011;6:21.
4. He M, Hu Y. Integrating the online nursing evidence-based information resources for evidence-based nursing study in China. Int J Nurs Pract. 2012;18(5):429–36.
5. Wang LP, Jiang XL, Wang L, Wang GR, Bai YJ. Barriers to and facilitators of research utilization: a survey of registered nurses in China. PLoS One. 2013;8(11):e81908.
6. Cheng L, Feng S, Hu Y. Evidence-based nursing implementation in mainland China: a scoping review. Nurs Outlook. 2017;65(1):27–35.

7.   Chien WT, Bai Q, Wong WK, Wang H, Lu X. Nurses' perceived barriers to and facilitators of research utilization in mainland China: a cross-sectional survey. Open Nurs J. 2013;7:96–106.

8.   Y-c C. Chinese values, health and nursing. J Adv Nurs. 2001;36(2):270–3.

9.   Dodgson JE. The cocreating environment: a nexus between classical Chinese and current nursing philosophies. ANS Adv Nurs Sci. 2008;31(4):356–64.

10. Kanbur R, Zhang X. Fifty years of regional inequality in China: a journey through central planning, reform, and openness. Rev Dev Econ. 2005;9(1):87–106.

11. Dai B. The old age health security in rural China: where to go? Int J Equity Health. 2015;14:119.

12. Liang Y, Lu P. Medical insurance policy organized by Chinese government and the health inequity of the elderly: longitudinal comparison based on effect of new cooperative medical scheme on health of rural elderly in 22 provinces and cities. Int J Equity Health. 2014;13:37.

13. Chang J, Guan Z, Chi I, Yang KH, Bai ZG. Evidence-based practice in the health and social services in China: developments, strategies, and challenges. Int J Evid Based Healthc. 2014;12(1):17–24.

14. Brown CE, Wickline MA, Ecoff L, Glaser D. Nursing practice, knowledge, attitudes and perceived barriers to evidence-based practice at an academic medical center. J Adv Nurs. 2009;65(2):371–81.

15. Logan J, Graham ID. The Ottawa Model of Research Use. In: Rycroft-Malone J, Bucknall T, editors. Models and frameworks for implementing evidence-based practice: Linking evidence to action. edn. West Sussex: Wiley-Blackwell & Sigma Theta Tau International Honor Society of Nursing; 2010. p. 83–107.

16. Wang Y, Li Y, Yang R. Study on the status and equality of human medical care resources during 2010–2015 (in Chinese), Today Nurse; 2016. p. 22–5.

17. Sandelowski M. Whatever happened to qualitative description? Res Nurs Health. 2000;23(4):334–40.

18. FDI Invest in China [http://www.fdi.gov.cn/]

19. Hunan Provincial People's Government [http://www.enghunan.gov.cn/]

20. Graneheim UH, Lundman B. Qualitative content analysis in nursing research: concepts, procedures and measures to achieve trustworthiness. Nurse Educ Today. 2004;24:105–12.

21. China Internet Network Information Center: Thirty-ninth China Statistical Report on Internet Development 2017.

22. Prgomet M, Georgiou A, Westbrook JI. The impact of mobile handheld technology on hospital physicians' work practices and patient care: a systematic review. J Am Med Inform Assoc. 2009;16(6):792–801.

23. van Velsen L, Beaujean DJ, van Gemert-Pijnen JE. Why mobile health app overload drives us crazy, and how to restore the sanity. BMC Med Inform Decis Mak. 2013;13:23.

24. Abkowitz A, Chin J. China launches Baidu probe after the death of a student. Wall Street J. 2016. https://www.wsj.com/articles/china-launches-baidu-probe-after-the-death-of-a-student-1462209685.

25. Xu GQ. Basic quality structure in evidence-based nursing practice and current status survey (in Chinese). Lab Med Clin. 2014;11:3100–2.

26. Zhang LY. Factors influencing and measures of the development of evidence-based nursing (in Chinese). Chin J Nurs. 2003;38:57–8.

27. Kocaman G, Seren S, Lash AA, Kurt S, Bengu N, Yurumezoglu HA. Barriers to research utilisation by staff nurses in a university hospital. J Clin Nurs. 2010;19(13–14):1908–18.

28. Chen Y, Diao J, Yan TT. A bibliometric analysis of nursing papers published by Chinese authors based on SCIE from 2004 to 2013 (in Chinese). J Nurs (China). 2015;22:18–23.

29. Li Z, Chen Y, Zhu N, Li W, Wu Y. A study on status quo and strategy of nursing scientific research of clinical nurses (in Chinese), Today Nurse; 2016. p. 145–7.

30. Zhang ZY, Wu YY. Review of nurses' scientific research abilities in China (in Chinese). Chin Nurs Manag. 2012;12:37–9.

31. Wang H, Gui Y, Zhang J, Liu L, Zhao J. Current situation and influencing factors of nurses' knowledge on evidence-based nursing (in Chinese). J Nurs Adm. 2015;15:98–100.

32. Zhang J, Qin Y. Status quo and influencing factors of nursing scientific research of nurses from Peking union medical college hospital (in Chinese). Chin Nurs Res. 2010;24:59–61.

33. Squires JE, Estabrooks CA, Gustavsson P, Wallin L. Individual determinants of research utilization by nurses: a systematic review update. Implement Sci. 2011;6:1.

34. Farokhzadian J, Nayeri ND, Borhani F, Zare MR. Nurse leaders' attitudes, self-efficacy and training needs for implementing evidence-based practice: is it time for a change toward safe care? Br J Med Med Res. 2015;7(8):662–71.

35. Lai NM, Teng CL, Lee ML. The place and barriers of evidence based practice: knowledge and perceptions of medical, nursing and allied health practitioners in Malaysia. BMC Res Notes. 2010;3:279.

36. Heydari A, Mazlom SR, Ranjbar H, Scurlock-Evans L. A study of Iranian nurses' and midwives' knowledge, attitudes, and implementation of evidence-based practice: the time for change has arrived. Worldviews Evid Based Nurs. 2014;11(5):325–31.

37. Altin S, Passon A, Kautz-Freimuth S, Berger B, Stock S. A qualitative study on barriers to evidence-based practice in patient counseling and advocacy in Germany. BMC Health Serv Res. 2015;15:317.

38. Aiken LH, Sloane DM, Bruyneel L, Van den Heede K, Griffiths P, Busse R, Diomidous M, Kinnunen J, Kozka M, Lesaffre E, et al. Nurse staffing and education and hospital mortality in nine European countries: a retrospective observational study. Lancet. 2014;383(9931):1824–30.

39. Adamsen L, Larsen K, Bjerregaard L, Madsen JK. Danish research-active clinical nurses overcome barriers in research utilization. Scand J Caring Sci. 2003;17(1):57–65.

40. Kajermo KN, Unden M, Gardulf A, Eriksson LE, Orton ML, Arnetz BB, Nordstrom G. Predictors of nurses' perceptions of barriers to research utilization. J Nurs Manag. 2008;16(3):305–14.

41. Patiraki E, Karlou C, Papadopoulou D, Spyridou A, Kouloukoura C, Bare E, Merkouris A. Barriers in implementing research findings in cancer care: the Greek registered nurses perceptions. Eur J Oncol Nurs. 2004;8(3):245–56.

42. Van Weijen D. The language of (future) scientific communication. In: Research trends. Vol. 31; 2012.

43. Yang J. Learners and users of English in China. English Today. 2006;22(2):3–10.

44. Jiao H, Hu Y, Cao YL, Xu JM, Zhang BH. A survey of cognition status quo toward evidence-based nursing and its related factors of nursing staff with bachelor degree or above in shanghai area (in Chinese). Chin Nurs Res. 2009;23(19):1693–7.

45. Chau JP, Lopez V, Thompson DR. A survey of Hong Kong nurses' perceptions of barriers to and facilitators of research utilization. Res Nurs Health. 2008;31(6):640–9.

46. Liu K, You LM, Chen SX, Hao YT, Zhu XW, Zhang LF, Aiken LH. The relationship between hospital work environment and nurse outcomes in Guangdong, China: a nurse questionnaire survey. J Clin Nurs. 2012;21(9–10):1476–85.

47. Hu S, Tang S, Liu Y, Zhao Y, Escobar ML, de Ferranti D. Reform of how health care is paid for in China: challenges and opportunities. Lancet. 2008;372(9652):1846–53.

48. Dummer TJ, Cook IG. Exploring China's rural health crisis: processes and policy implications. Health Policy. 2007;83(1):1–16.

49. Yip W, Hsiao WC. Non-evidence-based policy: how effective is China's new cooperative medical scheme in reducing medical impoverishment? Soc Sci Med. 2009;68(2):201–9.

50. World Health Organization Representative in China [WHO-RC]. China, Health, Poverty and economic development. Beijing: World Health Organization Macroeconomics and Health; 2005.

51. Aarons GA, Ehrhart MG, Torres EM, Finn NK, Roesch SC. Validation of the implementation leadership scale (ILS) in substance use disorder treatment organizations. J Subst Abus Treat. 2016;68:31–5.

52. Gerrish K, Nolan M, McDonnell A, Tod A, Kirshbaum M, Guillaume L. Factors influencing advanced practice nurses' ability to promote evidence-based practice among frontline nurses. Worldviews Evid Based Nurs. 2012;9(1):30–9.

53. Ploeg J, Davies B, Edwards N, Gifford W, Miller PE. Factors influencing best-practice guideline implementation: lessons learned from administrators, nursing staff, and project leaders. Worldviews Evid Based Nurs. 2007;4(4):210–9.

54. Su SF, Jenkins M, Liu PE. Nurses' perceptions of leadership style in hospitals: a grounded theory study. J Clin Nurs. 2012;21(1–2):272–80.

55. Zhou H, Long L. A review of paternalistic leadership research (in Chinese). Adv Psychol Sci. 2014;13:227–38.

56. Chen Z. Launch of the health-care reform plan in China. Lancet. 2009;373(9672):1322–4.

57. Aarons GA, Ehrhart MG, Farahnak LR, Sklar M. Aligning leadership across systems and organizations to develop a strategic climate for evidence-based practice implementation. Annu Rev Public Health. 2014;35:255–74.

58. Ploeg J, de Witt L, Hutchison B, Hayward L, Grayson K. Evaluation of a research mentorship program in community care. Eval Program Plann. 2008;31(1):22–33.

59. Gifford W, Lefebre N, Davies B. An organizational intervention to influence evidence-informed decision making in home health nursing. J Nurs Adm. 2014;44(7/8):395–402.
60. Mokhtar IA, Majid S, Foo S, Zhang X, Theng YL, Chang YK, Luyt B. Evidence-based practice and related information literacy skills of nurses in Singapore: an exploratory case study. Health Informatics J. 2012;18(1):12–25.
61. Davies B, Edwards N, Ploeg J, Virani T. Insights about the process and impact of implementing nursing guidelines on delivery of care in hospitals and community settings. BMC Health Serv Res. 2008;8:29.
62. Rycroft-Malone J, Seers K, Chandler J, Hawkes CA, Crichton N, Allen C, Bullock I, Strunin L. The role of evidence, context, and facilitation in an implementation trial: implications for the development of the PARIHS framework. Implement Sci. 2013;8:28.

12

Communication in mental health nursing - Bachelor Students' appraisal of a blended learning training programme - an exploratory study

Merete Furnes[1]* (iD), Kari Sofie Kvaal[1] and Sevald Høye[1,2]

Abstract

Background: It is important that mental health nursing students at Bachelor level obtain effective communication skills. Many students dread the fact that in the mental health field they will encounter patients and relatives with various backgrounds and personalities. Large classes and limited teaching resources in nursing education are challenging. To prepare students for mental health nursing practice, a communication skills course based on the blended learning method was developed and carried out at two different campuses.

The aim of the study is to explore Bachelor nursing students' appraisal of blended learning methods for enhancing communication skills in mental health nursing.

Methods: This study employed an exploratory design. Teaching and information materials were available on the learning management system (LMS). Videotaped role play training was carried out in the Simulation Department. Data were collected after the course by means of a questionnaire with closed and open-ended questions. The response rate was 59.2%. Quantitative data were analysed using the Statistical package for the Social Sciences (SPSS) and the Kruskal Wallis test, while qualitative data were analysed by content analysis based on Graneheim and Lundman's approach.

Results: No impact of background variables was observed. Students appreciated teachers' participation in role play and immediate feedback was considered especially important for learning outcomes. The students perceived that their communication skills and knowledge had improved after completing the blended learning programme.

Conclusions: According to the nursing students, blended learning is an appropriate method for improving communication skills in preparation for mental health nursing. Blended learning makes it possible to build flexible courses with limited resources.

Keywords: Blended learning, Role play, Communication skills, Mental health nursing, Video, Feed-back

Background

Effective communication is a fundamental element in all nursing and forms an integral part of quality patient care [1, 2]. The National Curriculum for Nursing Education in Norway sets out requirements related to nurses' communication skills after the three-year bachelor degree programme. Nurses must be able to encounter patients and their families with sensitivity, empathy and moral accountability. They should also have the ability to communicate with people of different ethnic, religious and cultural backgrounds who have a range of personalities, as well as being able to teach and guide patients, families, staff and students [3].

Nursing students with a native language other than that of the majority of their peers, might face an additional challenge when it comes to communication skills. Language competence is described as a prerequisite for good communication skills [4].

Internationally, good communication skills are described as an important part of nurses' core competencies, crucial

* Correspondence: merete.furnes@inn.no
[1]Faculty of Health and Social Services, Inland Norway University of Applied Sciences, Elverum, Norway
Full list of author information is available at the end of the article

for nursing practice and patient-centred care [5]. The way patients are greeted by nurses and other health professionals will affect how health care is provided [6, 7].

In addition, communication is important for patient safety. The Joint Commission on Accreditation of Healthcare Organizations (JCAHO) claims that 65% of adverse events or incorrect treatment is associated with communication failure [8]. In its description of core competencies in the health profession, the US Institute of Medicine recommends increased focus on improving professional communication, cooperation and a patient-centred approach in order to strengthen patient safety [8, 9].

Nursing students encounter patients with various issues during the Bachelor Programme. During mental health nursing training, students encounter patients with dementia, anxiety, depression and other serious mental disorders. Students often do not look forward to mental health nursing practice. The field is unfamiliar to most students and the communication demands are large [10]. Many people, including nurses, have prejudices against psychiatric patients [11]. Stevens et al. (2013) describe students' dread of psychiatric patients as a stereotypical fear of people with mental illness [12]. In the interpersonal relationship between nurses and patients or their relatives, nurses encounter diverse emotions, which is also the case in mental health care. There are no difficult patients, but challenging relationships. In order to communicate effectively, nurses must acknowledge their own emotional responses [13]. Studies demonstrate that the way nurses encounter patients influences the patients' level of aggression [14]. Treating patients in an appropriate manner requires not only self-awareness on the part of nurses, but also an understanding of the specific behaviours they may find challenging [15].

Simulation of communication in nursing practice provides an opportunity to prepare for practice before encountering real patients [16–18]. Role play is a core component of the development of processing skills. The design of role play can vary. Standardized Patients (SPs), often actors trained to simulate specific illnesses or conditions, might be used. Another possibility is peer role play, a method that is easier and cheaper to implement. Both methods seem to be valuable for communication skills training [19]. However, simulation has little tradition and a short history within mental health nursing. Studies have revealed that teaching methods vary widely between different countries, academic institutions and clinical settings [20, 21]. Some studies recommend integrated therapeutic communication training in mental health care during the nursing education to increase students' confidence in their communication skills. However, it has also been stated that more research on this topic is required [21–23].

Simulation as a learning tool should be combined with other established principles of learning, such as group work and lectures. The face-to-face lecture tradition can make students passive listeners. In Norwegian Nursing Education, half of the bachelor programme takes the form of clinical training in hospitals or community health care. At Inland Norway University of Applied Sciences (INN), more resources are used for supervision in the clinical part of the programme than in the theoretical part. As higher education lectures in Norway are not mandatory, attendance at such lectures has decreased and students have called for a variety of methods. In Report no.16 (2016–2017), the Norwegian Government provides guidelines for more active and varied learning methods in higher education [24]. The use of blended learning has increased in combination with technological advancement [25]. Blended learning is a relatively new pedagogical framework that includes several methods [26]. One such method is the so-called «flipped classroom», where the time usually devoted to lectures is used in other ways. Lectures can be recorded on video and made available to students on the Learning Management System (LMS), after which the teachers meet the students for discussion, guidance and reflection on the content of the recorded lectures [27]. The advantage of asynchronous video recorded lectures is that the student can play them at any time, take breaks and watch them on several occasions [27, 28].

There is a demand for low-cost and effective methods in nursing education that lead to the desired learning outcomes. The intention of this study is to contribute an experience of blended learning to meet this demand. Students' experience of this method is described in postgraduate programmes [29]. However, few studies have explored the experience of simulation in mental health nursing as a part of the blended learning methodological framework at bachelor level [30]. In the present study we wish to investigate which background variables influence the outcome of the method.

The aim of the study is to explore Bachelor nursing students' appraisal of blended learning methods for enhancing communication skills in mental health nursing.

The research questions were:

1) Are gender and native language associated with nursing students' appraisal of learning outcomes?
2) In what way does the presence of teachers influence students' learning outcomes regarding therapeutic communication?
3) How do students appraise web-based lessons, videotaped role play and reflectiongroups in terms of learning outcomes?

Methods

Design

An exploratory design was used and a questionnaire developed to gather both quantitative and qualitative data.

Participants and setting

This study is based on students' assessments of a communication skills course with focus on mental health nursing and psychiatry at bachelor level. The course was part of the third year of the bachelor programme, thus the participants had over 2 years of experience as nursing students. The communication skills course took place during the first 3 weeks of a 20 week mental health nursing programme, including practical training at several mental health institutions. Immediately after the course, the students went to various institutions for mental health nursing practice. The nursing department at INN is divided into two classes on two different campuses, one large and one small, located in cities 100 km apart from each other. All lectures are common to both classes and are conducted by lecturers in an auditorium at the large campus. The lectures are video-taped and transmitted synchronously to the small campus, where the students watch the lecturer on a large screen.

The communication skills course was conducted simultaneously in the two campuses. The large campus, which is the main campus, has 165 nursing students in each class. The majority of teachers and the university administration are located at this campus. The small campus has 40 students in each class with only a small number of teachers. 75% of the students are aged between 21 and 30 years, and almost 20% have a native language other than Norwegian.

Learning outcome

The main learning outcome of this course was the enhancement of students' communication skills in mental health nursing. Learning outcomes were based on the European Qualification Framework (EQF) [31] . The expected learning outcomes were knowledge of basic therapeutic communication terms, knowledge of and skills in verbal and non-verbal communication between nurse and patient, and knowledge of and skills in affective awareness and tolerance when nurses encounter difficult and challenging emotions from patients and relatives. The expected learning outcomes related to competence were ability to connect theory and practice and to reflect on one's own communication in various situations.

Intervention

As there are over 40 different courses at the largest campus, and only three auditoriums in which video transfer is possible, synchronous lectures for the students presents great challenges. To solve this dilemma, a digital presentation of asynchronous content was developed, to ensure that nursing students could prepare themselves for clinical training in mental health nursing.

The programme consisted of two main areas:

– E-learning materials on the LMS, which were provided 2 weeks in advance to enable the students to prepare for the intervention (weeks one and two).
– Simulation by role play. The role play was videotaped and formed the basis for the subsequent reflection group comprising the teacher and students (week three).

The LMS E-learning materials consisted of information about the objectives, learning outcomes and time schedules. In addition, videos with lectures on communication theory and techniques, examples of communication situations and detailed descriptions of the patient cases were also available. The lectures emphasised the learning outcomes. No lectures were given in the traditional auditorium face-to-face form.

Communication training was performed as role play carried out in the Simulation Department. Four patient case "stations" were established. Each station represented one simulation situation: anxiety and depression, psychosis, dementia and relatives. The students were divided into groups of four. In each group, four roles were described. At the small campus the roles were patient, nurse, video photographer and observer. Teachers were not present during the role play at the small campus. At the large campus the roles were nurse, video photographer and observers, while the patient role was played by teachers with experience of mental health nursing. The roles changed for each patient case station, so that all students experienced different perspectives and everyone could play the nurse role. The students selected the situation in which they would play the role of nurse in advance, giving them the opportunity to prepare for the patient case they would encounter.

Every role play situation contained communicative and emotional challenges. All situations were videotaped by one of the group with a camera on a tablet or mobile device. Immediately after the role play, the person who played the patient gave feedback on how she/he experienced the communication with the nurse. The day after the simulation, each student group met a teacher for reflection at both the small and the large campus. This teacher had not participated in the role play at the large campus the previous day. Due to limited time, each group was only allowed to choose one video recording of the nurse-patient situation for reflection. Students and teacher viewed the video together, and focused on communication skills; what was positive and what could be improved.

Measurement

The questionnaire was developed, adapted and tailored to measure the extent to which the students perceived that they had achieved the learning outcomes, which is in line with the European Qualification Framework [31]. In addition, the questionnaire was designed to measure the students' assessment of the blended learning methods employed during the communication course. The face validity was critically appraised by means of discussions in a reference group, after which the authors revised the questionnaire based on consensus among the reference group members. The reference group consisted of both clinical nurses and researchers including a Professor in Mental Health Clinical Nursing and an Associate Professor in Clinical Nursing at Inland Norway University of Applied Sciences (INN University). The questionnaire was written in Norwegian, but has been translated into English by an Assistant Professor whose first language is English.

The questionnaire has seven overall themes comprising various items. The ordinal items were divided into five levels from 1 (not at all) to 5 (to a high degree). Two of the themes were formulated as statements, with five levels from 1 (totally disagree) to 5 (totally agree).

For background information, we asked for the students' age (grouped into < 20 years, 21 to 29 years and 30>), gender (dichotomized as male/female), health care work experience before starting nursing education (dichotomized as yes/no) and native language (dichotomized as Norwegian/foreign).

In addition, we used three open-ended questions; (i) Which patient case was perceived as the most useful and why? (ii) What element of the programme led to the greatest learning outcome? and (iii) Have you any suggestions or recommendations for changes to the course?

Data collection

At the conclusion of the training programme the students individually filled in a paper version of the questionnaire, which was distributed by teachers from the Institute of Nursing Sciences, INN University. Some of the students started their clinical practice immediately after the course and for that reason received the questionnaire with a stamped addressed envelope to facilitate its return to the researchers.

Data analysis

The analyses were performed using the SPSS (Statistical Package for the Social Sciences), version 23. The answers were entered into the statistical program by one of the authors (MF).

The Kruskal Wallis test was employed for comparison.

The answers to the open- ended questions were analysed by content analysis based on Graneheim and Lundman [32]. The responses were transcribed verbatim and transferred into meaning units and condensed meaning units. In addition, short comments were taken into account and categorized.

Ethical considerations

Approval was obtained from the head of the Department of Nursing at INN University, due to the desire for continuous improvement of teaching methods.

The students received oral information about the assessment of the training programme before the questionnaires were distributed. Written information was enclosed with the questionnaire. The students were guaranteed complete anonymity and informed that participation was voluntary. Furthermore, the written information contained details about the purpose of the study. The participants gave their consent by filling out the questionnaire.

The students completed the questionnaire anonymously and it was not possible to link the responses to any individual.

Approval was granted by the Norwegian Centre for Research Data (NSD). NSD Reference Number 35719. The NSD provides protection for both data and human subjects.

Results

In total, 169 questionnaires were distributed to the students and 100 were returned (response rate 59.2%), of which 88% were from women. A total of 12% of the students had a native language other than Norwegian. 69% had health care work experience before they started the nursing education. Both the small and the large campus were represented in the respondent group, 14 and 86% respectively.

Neither gender, native language nor health care work experience had significant impact on students' assessment of the course.

Assessment of learning outcomes

The results revealed that the students' communication knowledge and skills increased. They perceived that they had become familiar with the key Assisting Communication terms to a large and very large extent (73%). A similar number (71%) became familiar with the various elements of Active listening to a large and very large extent. Even more (90%) indicated that to a large and very large extent they had become familiar with and gained an understanding of how important it is for nurses to be emotionally aware and tolerant when meeting patients and relatives. In addition, 78% expressed that to a large and very large extent they could combine theoretical and practical knowledge when caring for patients suffering from psychological problems and their relatives. Almost all participants (94%) indicated that to a large and very large extent they reflected on their own communication methods when meeting patients, relatives and fellow students/colleagues.

Assessment of the importance of blended methods

The digital materials presented on the LMS were considered important to a large and very large extent by 55%, while 41% indicated that the importance was medium and 4% that they were of some importance.

The use of role play was considered to be of large and very large importance by 62%. Only 12% evaluated it as important to some extent or not at all. Assessment of role play combined with videotaping was deemed important to a large and very large extent by 57%, while 13% indicated that it was of some or no importance. The combination of training through videotaped role play and reflection on the video the following day was considered important to a large and very large extent by 62% of the students, while 15% considered it of some or no importance.

In response to the question about which simulated cases led to the best learning outcomes, it was found that psychosis had the highest score (65%), followed by anxiety and depression (17%), care givers' role (11%) and dementia (7%) (Table 1).

The presence and absence of teachers only had a significant difference on the students' assessment of learning communication skills by means of role play and video ($p < 0.01$).

Qualitative approach

The students were asked to elaborate on their answers to the following three open-ended questions: Which of the patient cases provided the greatest learning benefit? (Table 2); Which part of the programme provided the best learning outcomes? (Table 3); and Have you any suggestions for future communication courses?

When the students explained the reasons for their choice of the patient case that benefitted them the most, they appeared to emphasise the value of being prepared to encounter patients in mental health care practice. Three categories with subcategories emerged (Table 2):

Increased knowledge about the patient

Many students highlighted the importance of realistic situations for giving them an opportunity to encounter patients and situations of which they had little previous experience.

"The case involving psychosis was the most unfamiliar to me and therefore an informative and useful situation that made me better prepared for the upcoming psychiatric practice". "Had not seen psychotic patients previously. Learned a lot by meeting such a patient" ('Little previous experience of mental health').

"But I think the next of kin provided a good learning outcome as I find conversations with relatives "scary"!" ('Challenging situations').

"It was a new experience to see these situations in real life and the actor was very good at playing his role" ('Realistic situation').

Table 1 Comparison of students' assessment of methods and learning outcome when teachers were present and absent by means (95% CI) using the Kruskal Wallis test

	Teachers present	Teachers absent	p-value
1a) Assessment of the use of role play and video for communication skills training	Teachers present	Teachers absent	p-value
I learned more about how I can communicate by using role play than I would without using role play	3.9 (3.7 to 4.2)	3.1 (2.6 to 3.7)	P < 0.01
I learned more about my own communication skills through seeing myself on video than I would have done without using video	3.7 (3.5 to 4.0)	2.9 (2.2 to 3.5)	P < 0.01
1b) Assessment of learning outcomes and goals	Teachers present	Teachers absent	p-value
I am familiar with the key Assisting Communication terms	3.8 (3.7 to 3.9)	4.0 (3.6 to 4.4)	0.24
I am familiar with the various elements of Active listening	3.9 (3.7 to 4.0)	3.8 (3.7 to 3.9)	0.66
I am familiar with and have an understanding of how important it is for nurses to be emotionally aware and emotionally tolerant when meeting patients and relatives	4.2 (4.1 to 4.4)	4.3 (3.9 to 4.6)	0.80
I can combine theoretical and practical knowledge when meeting patients suffering from psychological problems and their relatives	4.0 (3.8 to 4.1)	3.9 (3.5 to 4.2)	0.52
I reflect on my own communication methods when meeting patients, relatives and fellow students/colleagues	4.4 (4.3 to 4.6)	4.2 (3.7 to 4.6)	0.13
1c) Assessment of the importance of methods used in the teaching and practice programme.	Teachers present	Teachers absent	p-value
Importance of training through role play	3.8 (3.6 to 4.0)	3.4 (2.9 to 3.9)	0.12
Importance of training through role play combined with video	3.6 (3.4 to 3.9)	3.4 (2.8 to 4.0)	0.27
Importance of training through role play, video and feedback	3.8 (3.5 to 4.0)	3.2 (2.6 to 3.9)	0.07

Table 2 Learning outcomes of patient cases

Themes	Well prepared to meet the patients							
Categories	Increased knowledge about the patient			Teachers' participation is important			Learning communication through role play	
Sub categories	Little previous experience of mental health	Challenging situation	Relevant situations	Feedback on communication	Sharing experiences	Simulated situations must be realistic	The nurse role was challenging	Have to be prepared when playing the nurse

Teacher participation is important

Students have more confidence in teachers' knowledge about the mentally ill patient than that of their fellow students. This is important for feedback, for sharing their own experiences and for making the role play realistic.

The following statements exemplify the subcategories:

"Discovered my challenges and was inspired to read more". "Got constructive feedback on what the nurse could have done better" (Feedback on communication).

"Learned how to calm the patient and divert her/his attention". "The teacher told me about her own encounter with psychotic patients" (Sharing experiences).

"VERY good that teachers played the patient!" "Great involvement on the part of the teacher, which motivated me to read more". "Felt that the day did not live up to my expectations as we were left to ourselves and the role play performed with fellow students was guesswork and false" (Simulated situations must be realistic).

Learning communication through role play

Most of the answers indicate that role play is effective for learning and developing communication skills. Playing the nurse is demanding, but educational. The subcategories are exemplified by the following statements:

"It was an ordeal taking care of the relatives and making them feel comfortable" (The nurse role was challenging).

"It was this patient situation I played as a nurse, so I had to gain knowledge of the diagnosis and communication in advance" (Have to be prepared when playing the nurse).

The most important outcome after completion of the course seems to be that the students had increased their communication and mental health nursing competence and were ready for practical studies (Table 3).

Two categories are underpinned by subcategories and exemplified by the following statements:

Increased self-awareness

"Role play with filming made me reflect on what happened during the meeting with the patient, become more confident about the fact that what I did that worked and enabled me to see what needs to be adjusted in relation to appropriate communication" (More confidence in own communication).

"Seeing myself on film was very informative, because I was able to observe my strengths and choices, which were rather bad. I could never have gained so much awareness of this had I not been able to see myself" (Awareness of own strengths and weakness).

"The main thing I got out of this was seeing how we resolve situations in different ways and can discuss and make new observations the next time." "I learned about emotional consciousness and tolerance, transference and countertransference, body language and awareness" (Techniques adapted to situations).

Table 3 Overall learning outcomes

Themes	Ready for practical studies					
Categories	Increased self-awareness			Increased knowledge awareness		
Sub categories	More confident in own communication	Awareness of own strengths and weaknesses	Techniques adapted to situations	Syllabus increased communication knowledge	Learning customized subject material in LMS	Examples increased understanding of mental health

Abbreviations: *LMS* Learning Management System

Increased knowledge awareness

"Read a lot more on theory and got a better overview of the basic concepts of communication and linked theory to practice experience." "Read the syllabus, then I could use that experience to improve my communication skills" (Syllabus increases communication knowledge).

"Teaching videos on Fronter were very elaborate and emphasised the need to be prepared for the day in the Simulation Department" (Learning customized subject material in the LMS).

Recommendations for improvement

Twenty-five students provided short comments to the last open question: 'Any suggestions for improvements?' The students had some suggestions for how to improve the course, although several pointed out the parts that are worth continuing.

"We could have had even more role play with filming. I think I would learn more with simulation of additional cases."

"Continue to have teachers as "patients". It was more real, without any nonsense! A teacher or otherwise a professional actor due to their greater experience of what a person with mental illness is like, makes it more realistic" (Large campus).

"Continue the role play, but filming leaves one very nervous and makes it difficult to learn!"

Some students mentioned the wish for feedback: *"Standardized, immediate feedback to ensure the same feedback to all students. It is important that all teachers who play the patient provide feedback on what could be improved. Also important to point out what was good."*

Discussion

This study aimed to explore Bachelor nursing students' appraisal of an educational course based on blended learning in order to enhance communication skills in mental health nursing.

The main finding is that the students were satisfied with the overall programme. They perceived that their communication skills and knowledge had improved after completing the blended teaching methods.

The result was little affected by the students' background. One might expect that a native language other than Norwegian would influence and perhaps have a negative effect on the perception of the communication learning outcome [4], but this was not the case in the present study. Other studies demonstrate that men have a more positive attitude towards digital tools than is the case with women [33, 34], while another study indicates little difference in gender attitudes [35]. The present study reveals no significant gender differences.

Teachers have a significant impact on the students' perception of increased communication skills. Students at the small campus who played the patient role themselves rated the learning outcomes of role play and filming lower than the students at the large campus. Thanks to their experience of nursing patients with mental disorders and their families, the teachers at the large campus who played the role of the patient and relative created an impression that the simulation was realistic. The students were confident that the teachers' performance of the patient and relative roles was in line with reality.

Encountering standardized patients in a safe simulation situation is a way to imitate clinical settings and can make students more prepared to meet real patients. The study shows that the situations must be considered realistic, which may explain the high score on the importance of teachers being present in the Simulation Department. Few studies have compared these two methods [19], but a previous study shows that students perceive that both alternatives are valuable preparation for practice [36]. However, the same study concludes that the use of standardized patients is rated higher by nurse supervisors. The students at the small campus were well aware that teachers played the patient role at the large campus. This might have influenced their motivation and attitude to the course, and could be a reason for the great difference in perceived learning outcome.

Immediate feedback was considered more important than the reflection group the following day. Those who played the "patient" gave immediate feedback after completing the role play, which was highlighted as valuable. Students found that the feedback was provided differently, depending on the teacher. The content of the feedback was not planned in advance. As a result, the quality of the feedback from the "patient" to the student who played the nurse was quite unsystematic. The study shows that standardized feedback is critical for optimal learning. An instruction manual about what feedback should contain was found to be important in other studies [8, 37, 38]. which may indicate that it is not the teacher's presence that is essential, but that students encounter a standardized patient. However, the present study cannot confirm this supposition.

Some statements reveal that students made new discoveries by watching themselves on video, which is confirmed by other studies [39]. Students rated role play using video somewhat lower than role play without video. This can be understood in several ways: All the students in the group want to be seen, which is an elementary, basic need. The reflection group did not reflect on all film scenarios, only one of four chosen by the group. Another explanation is that reflection on one's own communication on video is difficult, because the reflection process is removed from introspective explanations [40, 41]. Seeing each individual student in a class of 100–200 is a challenge for educators. Therefore, learning situations like those in the present study should be organized in a way that ensures feedback to each student and an opportunity to reflect on everyone's communication. Other studies pinpoint the same problem and suggest increased use of peer learning to resolve this challenge [42].

Students perceived the blended learning programme as an important preparation for practice. Several responses indicate that students had some negative expectations of mental health nursing practice. It is considered especially challenging for nursing students to cope with difficult emotions. Changing attitudes to mental health nursing practice is not explicitly measured in this study, but previous studies show that experience of working with psychiatric patients has a positive impact on health workers' attitudes [43]. A large proportion responded that their knowledge of the importance of emotional awareness and tolerance when meeting patients and their relatives increased by a large or very large extent as a result of the teaching programme. This corresponded with the percentage stating that the most unfamiliar patient situations were those that provided the greatest opportunity for learning. They learned the most from especially challenging situations, such as meeting a patient with psychosis. The situations in which the students encountered a patient with dementia were ranked as the least interesting (6%). This can provide a broad picture of the students' expectations of mental health practice. Having met patients with dementia earlier in their education programme, especially in nursing homes, they recognized these simulation situations and found no particular learning outcomes in them. It may also indicate that dementia is of little interest to nursing students, despite the fact that according to ICD-10 [44], dementia disorders constitute a mental illness. Alternatively, it can be understood as a desire for new experiences. New situations that they have not encountered before are in all likelihood more challenging than a situation with which they are more familiar.

It seems important for each student to try to play the nurse role. The statements show that the students prepared well for the patient situation when they were playing the role of the nurse, while they were less prepared for the other situations. To ensure that students prepare to face all situations, the distribution of roles can be done when students attend the Simulation Department. In this course, the students had the opportunity to distribute the roles within the group in advance. In summary, the results of the present study seem to indicate that encountering difficult situations in a safe simulation environment increases students' competence to become aware of their own affective pattern and responses.

Blended learning often consists of a combination of classroom lectures and other digital and non-digital methods [26]. This programme replaced classroom lectures by video based asynchronous lectures. Research shows that both students and healthcare workers appreciate asynchrony, digital teaching and lectures [45]. A challenge for educators is to meet 21st century students' expectations of flexible, digital teaching [46]. Although students' digital competence is described in Norwegian education ministry documents [47], there is still no corresponding qualifications required for university lecturers, despite the fact that students call for more flexible teaching methods [48].

The present study revealed that the role play in the Simulation Department was important for learning outcomes. This implies that the active learning part of blended learning should be highly valued and increased. The higher the students' activity level the greater is their learning potential [49]. Students did not participate in the planning of the course. More involvement from students in the early phase might have revealed some alternatives and logistical solutions. Perhaps active student involvement should start even earlier with an iterative process to identify what students need and involving them in the development of learning material based on their requirements. A Norwegian study has identified five important learning student learning needs during the development of new technological learning material: clarification of learning expectations, help to recognize the bigger picture, stimulation of interaction, creation of structure and context specific content [50].

This study contributes information about learning methods to enhance communication skills among nursing students preparing for mental health nursing. The results show that students in large classes with limited resources assess the blended learning method as leading to the achievement of the desired learning outcome to a high degree. Blended learning makes it possible to design courses that are more flexible than those based on ordinary lectures in auditoriums. This method is also transferable to other topics and courses.

Methodological considerations

A strength of this study is that all students who participated had the opportunity to state their opinions of the
course, not only a selected group. One hundred students
answered the questionnaire, which ensures anonymity.

The main methodological limitation is the instrument for data collection. Teachers and researchers at
the University developed the questionnaire based on
the learning outcomes for the specific course. The
questionnaire was not pre-tested or validated with
other instruments.

Some of the participants filled out the questionnaire a
few weeks after the course. This might represent another
limitation as the passage of time can affect the memory
and therefore influence the accuracy of the answers. The
time required to complete the questionnaire may also
have reduced the number of responses (59.2%).

The qualitative part of the study may have some
limitations. Only a small number of students chose to
answer the open-ended questions. Many used
keywords, making it difficult to categorize the responses
due to the risk of losing their full meaning. Furthermore,
conducting research on one's own students always involves an ethical challenge for the researcher [51]. This
challenge is primarily related to qualitative studies where
the researcher (teacher) meets the respondent (student).
In the present study, the respondents are totally anonymous despite the open-ended questions. In addition, the
researcher was not present when the students completed
the questionnaire, thus had no possibility to influence the
answers.

Evaluating one's own courses could involve a risk of
wanting the results to be better than they actually are. To
ensure analytical distance, two of the authors (M.F and S.
H) analysed the open-ended responses together [52].

Conclusion

Blended learning is a relevant method in communication
courses, especially the active learning part comprising role
play in a Simulation Department. The present findings
demonstrate that students learn more by practicing the
nurse role than being an observer. The reason for this is
that they were prepared for their own performance.
Videotaping the role play provides a unique opportunity
to reflect on one's own performance. However, the students rated this method somewhat lower than role play
alone. Our findings indicate that the method requires a
cautious and carefully planned approach with sufficient
time for each student to be seen and given feedback.

It is difficult to ignore the finding that feedback
from an experienced teacher or standardized patient
is important for the perceived learning outcome. The
students themselves recommended the use of teachers
in all role play. There might be two alternative

strategies for achieving a higher perceived learning
outcome: 1. Transferring resources from the reflection
group to allow time for standardized, immediate feedback. 2. More time for the reflection group so that all
video scenarios can be seen and discussed, thus
fulfilling the students' need to be seen individually.

Early student involvement and participation in developing the learning material is recommended, as it might
increase the quality of the digital resources by tailoring
them to the needs of the students.

Abbreviations

EQF: European qualification framework; ICD-10: International statistical
classification of diseases and related health problems; INN University: Inland
Norway University for applied sciences; JCAHO: The joint commission on
accreditation of healthcare organizations; LMS: Learning management
system; NSD: Norwegian centre for research data; SPSS: Statistical package
for the social sciences

Acknowledgements

The authors wish to acknowledge the Bachelor students at Inland Norway
University of Applied Sciences (INN) for taking the time to answer the
questionnaire, thus making this study possible. Thanks to Monique Federsel
for reviewing the English language.

Authors' contributions

MF designed the study and collected the data. MF, KK and SH analysed and
interpreted the data. MF, KK and SH prepared the manuscript. All authors
have read and approved the final manuscript.

Competing interests

The authors declare that they have no competing interests.

Author details

¹Faculty of Health and Social Services, Inland Norway University of Applied
Sciences, Elverum, Norway. ²Faculty of Nursing and Health Sciences, Nord
University, Bodø, Norway.

References

1. McGilton K, Irwin-Robinson H, Boscart V, Spanjevic L. Communication
    enhancement: nurse and patient satisfaction outcomes in a complex
    continuing care facility. J Adv Nurs. 2006;54(1):35–44.
2. O'Hagan S, Manias E, Elder C, Pill J, Woodward-Kron R, McNamara T, Webb
    G, McColl G. What counts as effective communication in nursing? Evidence

from nurse educators' and clinicians' feedback on nurse interactions with simulated patients. J Adv Nurs. 2014;70(6):1344–55.

3. Research MoEa. National Curriculum for nursing education in Norway. Oslo: Rammeplan for sykepleierutdanning; 2008.

4. Chan A, Purcell A, Power E. A systematic review of assessment and intervention strategies for effective clinical communication in culturally and linguistically diverse students. Med Educ. 2016;50(9):898–911.

5. Boykins AD. Core communication competencies in patient-centered care. ABNF J. 2014;25(2):40–5.

6. Percival J. Promoting health: making every contact count. Nurs Stand. 2014; 28(29):37–41.

7. McCance T, McCormack B, Dewing J. An exploration of person-Centredness in practice. Online J Issues Nurs. 2011;16(2):1–1.

8. Fay-Hillier TM, Regan RV, Gallagher Gordon M. Communication and patient safety in simulation for mental health nursing education. Issues Ment Health Nurs. 2012;33(11):718–26.

9. Liaw SY, Zhou WT, Lau TC, Siau C, Chan SW-C. An interprofessional communication training using simulation to enhance safe care for a deteriorating patient. Nurse Educ Today. 2014;34(2):259–64.

10. Kameg K, Mitchell AM, Clochesy J, Howard VM, Suresky J. Communication and human patient simulation in psychiatric nursing. Issues Ment Health Nurs. 2009;30(8):503–8.

11. Happell B, Gaskin CJ. The attitudes of undergraduate nursing students towards mental health nursing: a systematic review. J Clin Nurs. 2013;22(1/2):148–58.

12. Stevens J, Browne G, Graham I. Career in mental health still an unlikely career choice for nursing graduates: a replicated longitudinal study. Int J Ment Health Nurs. 2013;22(3):213–20.

13. Brownie S, Scott R, Rossiter R. Therapeutic communication and relationships in chronic and complex care. Nurs Stand. 2016;31(6):54–61.

14. Swain N, Gale C. A communication skills intervention for community healthcare workers reduces perceived patient aggression: a pretest–postest study. Int J Nurs Stud. 2014;51(9):1241–5.

15. Michaelsen JJ. Emotional distance to so-called difficult patients. Scand J Caring Sci. 2012;26(1):90–7.

16. Grant MS, Jenkins LS. Communication education for pre-licensure nursing students: literature review 2002–2013. Nurse Educ Today. 2014;34(11):1375–81.

17. Lewis D, O'Boyle-Duggan M, Chapman J, Dee P, Sellner K, Gorman S. 'Putting words into action' project: using role play in skills training. Br J Nurs. 2013;22(11):638–44.

18. Ünal S. Evaluating the effect of self-awareness and communication techniques on nurses' assertiveness and self-esteem. Contemp Nurse. 2012;43(1):90–8.

19. Bosse HM, Schultz JH, Nickel M, Lutz T, Möltner A, Jünger J, Huwendiek S, Nikendei C. The effect of using standardized patients or peer role play on ratings of undergraduate communication training: a randomized controlled trial. Patient Educ Couns. 2012;87(3):300–6.

20. Huiting X, Lei L, Jia W, Kum Eng J, Parasuram R, Gunasekaran J, Chee Lien P. The effectiveness of using non-traditional teaching methods to prepare student health care professionals for the delivery of mental state examination: a systematic review. JBI Database System Rev Implement Rep. 2015;13(7):177–212.

21. Hubbard GB. Customized role play: strategy for development of psychiatric mental health nurse practitioner competencies. Perspect Psychiatr Care. 2014;50(2):132–8.

22. Martin CT, Chanda N. Mental health clinical simulation: therapeutic communication. Clin Simul Nurs. 2016;12(6):209–14.

23. Hall K. Simulation-based learning in Australian undergraduate mental health nursing curricula: a literature review. Clin Simul Nurs. 2017;13(8):380–9.

24. Ministry of Education and Research. Report no 16 (2016-2017). Culture for Quality in Higher Education. (Meld.St.16 (2016-2017). Kultur for kvalitet i høyere utdanning). Norwegian Government.

25. McGarry BJ, Theobald K, Lewis PA, Coyer F. Flexible learning design in curriculum delivery promotes student engagement and develops metacognitive learners: an integrated review. Nurse Educ Today. 2015;35(9):966–73.

26. McCutcheon K, Lohan M, Traynor M, Martin D. A systematic review evaluating the impact of online or blended learning vs. face-to-face learning of clinical skills in undergraduate nurse education. J Adv Nurs. 2015;71(2):255–70.

27. Sams A, Bergmann J. Flip your students' learning. Educ Leadersh. 2013; 70(6):16–20.

28. Johansen F, Stadheim A, Nina T. Produksjon og bruk av digitale læringsobjekter i fleksibel ingeniørutdanning (Production and use of digital learning objects in flexible engineering education). UNIPED. 2011;34(01):21–33.

29. Smyth S, Houghton C, Cooney A, Casey D. Students' experiences of blended learning across a range of postgraduate programmes. Nurse Educ Today. 2012;32(4):464–8.

30. Rigby L, Wilson I, Baker J, Walton T, Price O, Dunne K, Keeley P. The development and evaluation of a 'blended' enquiry based learning model for mental health nursing students: "making your experience count". Nurse Educ Today. 2012;32(3):303–8.

31. European Qualitfication Framework. https://ec.europa.eu/ploteus/content/ descriptors-page.

32. Graneheim UH, Lundman B. Qualitative content analysis in nursing research: concepts, procedures and measures to achieve trustworthiness. Nurse Educ Today. 2004;24(2):105–12.

33. Anderton RS, Chiu LS, Aulfrey S. Student perceptions to teaching undergraduate anatomy in health sciences. Int J High Educ. 2016;5(3):201–16.

34. Kay RH. Examining gender differences in attitudes toward interactive classroom communications systems (ICCS). Comput Educ. 2009;52(4):730–40.

35. Cam SS, Yarar G, Toraman C, Erdamar GK. The effects of gender on the attitudes towards the computer assisted instruction: a meta-analysis. J Educ Train Stud. 2016;4(5):250–61.

36. Schlegel CMMERN, Woermann UMDMME, Shaha MPRN, Rethans J-JMDP, van der Vleuten CP. Effects of communication training on real practice performance: a role-play module versus a standardized patient module. J Nurs Educ. 2012;51(1):16–22.

37. Bokken L, Linssen T, Scherpbier A, van der Vleuten C, Rethans J. Feedback by simulated patients in undergraduate medical education: a systematic review of the literature. Med Educ. 2009;43(3):202–10.

38. Bouter S, van Weel-Baumgarten E, Bolhuis S. Construction and validation of the Nijmegen evaluation of the simulated patient (NESP): assessing simulated patients' ability to role-play and provide feedback to students. Acad Med. 2013;88(2):253–9.

39. Moon Sook Y, Sun-Mi C. Effects of peer review on communication skills and learning motivation among nursing students. J Nurs Educ. 2011;50(4):230–3.

40. Eva KW, Regehr G. Self-assessment in the health professions: a reformulation and research agenda. Acad Med. 2005;80(10 Suppl):S46–54.

41. Hulsman RL, Harmsen AB, Fabriek M. Reflective teaching of medical communication skills with DiViDU: assessing the level of student reflection on recorded consultations with simulated patients. Patient Educ Couns. 2009;74(2):142–9.

42. Stenberg M, Carlson E. Swedish student nurses' perception of peer learning as an educational model during clinical practice in a hospital setting—an evaluation study. BMC Nurs. 2015;14(1):48.

43. Happell B. The importance of clinical experience for mental health nursing – part 2: relationships between undergraduate nursing students' attitudes, preparedness, and satisfaction. Int J Ment Health Nurs. 2008;17(5):333–40.

44. World Health Organization. The ICD-10 Classification of Mental and Behavioural Disorders. Diagnostic Criteria for Research. Geneva; 1993.

45. Sinclair P, Kable A, Levett-Jones T. The effectiveness of internet-based e-learning on clinician behavior and patient outcomes: a systematic review protocol. JBI Database System Rev Implement Rep. 2015;13(1):52–64.

46. Johannesen M, Øgrim L, Giæver TH. Notion in motion: teachers' digital competence. Nordic J Digit Literacy. 2014;04:300–12.

47. The Norwegian Ministry of Education and Research (Utdannings-ogforskningsdepartementet). The Framework for basic skills. (Rammeverket for grunnleggende ferdigheter). 2012. https://www.udir.no/laring-og-trivsel/lareplanverket/grunnleggendeferdigheter/rammeverk-for-grunnleggende-ferdigheter/.

48. Norwegian Agency for Quality Assurance in Education. Student barometer. Report 2- 2017. 2017. https://khrono.no/files/2017/11/15/studiebarometeret_2016_hovedtendenser.pdf.

49. Dutra DK. Implementation of case studies in undergraduate didactic nursing courses: a qualitative study. BMC Nurs. 2013;12(1):15–23.

50. Haraldseid C, Friberg F, Aase K. How can students contribute? A qualitative study of active student involvement in development of technological learning material for clinical skills training. BMC Nurs. 2016;15(1):2.

51. Clark E, McCann TV. Researching students: an ethical dilemma. Nurs Res. 2005;12(3):42–51.

52. The Norwegian National Research Ethics Committees. General guidelines for research ethics. 2017. https://www.etikkom.no/globalassets/documents/publikasjoner-som-pdf/generalguidelines.pdf.

13

Developing and evaluating an instrument to measure Recovery After INtensive care: the RAIN instrument

Ingegerd Bergbom[1,2*], Veronika Karlsson[3] and Mona Ringdal[1,4]

Abstract

Background: Measuring and evaluating patients' recovery, following intensive care, is essential for assessing their recovery process. By using a questionnaire, which includes spiritual and existential aspects, possibilities for identifying appropriate nursing care activities may be facilitated. The study describes the development and evaluation of a recovery questionnaire and its validity and reliability.

Methods: A questionnaire consisting of 30 items on a 5-point Likert scale was completed by 169 patients (103 men, 66 women), 18 years or older (m=69, SD 12.5) at 2, 6, 12 or 24 months following discharge from an ICU. An exploratory factor analysis, including a principal component analysis with orthogonal varimax rotation, was conducted. Ten initial items, with loadings below 0.40, were removed. The internal item/scale structure obtained in the principal component analysis was tested in relation to convergent and discrimination validity with a multi-trait analysis. Items consistency and reliability were assessed by Cronbach's alpha and internal item consistency. Test of scale quality, the proportion of missing values and respondents' scoring at maximum and minimum levels were also conducted.

Results: A total of 20 items in six factors - forward looking, supporting relations, existential ruminations, revaluation of life, physical and mental strength and need of social support were extracted with eigen values above one. Together, they explained 75% of the variance. The half-scale criterion showed that the proportion of incomplete scale scores ranged from 0% to 4.3%. When testing the scale's ability to differentiate between levels of the assessed concept, we found that the observed range of scale scores covered the theoretical range. Substantial proportions of respondents, who scored at the ceiling for forward looking and supporting relations and at floor for the need of social support, were found. These findings should be further investigated.

Conclusion: The factor analysis, including discriminant validity and the mean value for the item correlations, was found to be excellent. The RAIN instrument could be used to assess recovery following intensive care. It could provide post-ICU clinics and community/primary healthcare nurses with valuable information on which areas patients may need more support.

Keywords: Recovery, Intensive care recovery, Factor analysis, Recovery questionnaire

* Correspondence: ingegerd.bergbom@gu.se
[1]Institute of Health and Care Sciences at the Sahlgrenska Academy, University of Gothenburg, Gothenburg, Sweden
[2]Faculty of Caring Science, Work Life and Social Welfare, Borås University, Borås, Sweden
Full list of author information is available at the end of the article

Background

Many aspects of health and recovery have been measured and evaluated in relation to different healthcare areas as well as in relation to certain treatments or diagnoses. Different questionnaires and instruments have been developed to measure or predict recovery time following hospital care and illnesses [1–8] focusing on different dimensions, such as cognition, physical symptoms, anxiety, depression, quality of life and health. However, spiritual and existential thoughts have not been a focus in these measurements on the recovery process. After being discharged from intensive care unit (ICU) and usually a life threatening medical condition, patients' lives may include not only lingering physical discomfort and difficulties in daily life but also thoughts about life and death and their future. Therefore, these aspects, when estimating patients' recovery following ICU care and experiences of having been seriously ill/injured, are of importance for planning and implementing care actions.

Warrén Stomberg et al. [9] have, in a literature review, described ten recovery questionnaires/instruments that assess or measure recovery following day surgical procedures. The assessed dimensions were divided into two groups: 1) physiological-physical and 2) emotional, nutritional, eliminating, nauseous and vomiting. In a systematic review by Ebrahim et al. [10], they found that 44 studies indicated that patients' positive recovery expectations predicted a quicker return to work while negative expectations predicted longer sick leave. However, few studies used a psychometrically valid instrument for measuring these recovery expectations.

Recovery following serious illness/injury and ICU care has been described and investigated in several studies, but there is no valid instrument for measuring recovery that include existential and spiritual health. Recovery has been evaluated from one to several years following IC [11–14] or during a period immediately following discharge from the hospital [15]. Measuring health related quality of life (HRQL) has been one method to estimate patients' recoveries [12, 13]. Discomforting delusional memories [12, 14] have been found in patients after hospital and ICU discharge. Kelly and McKinley [16] reported that patients, six months following discharge, still suffered from mobility difficulties and sleep disturbances. Muscle weakness and loss of body weight have also been reported following critical illness and ICU care [17–20]. In an Australian qualitative interview study, six months following ICU [21] most patients reported having returned to a healthy state even if they continued to report pain, sleeping disturbances, tiredness, depression, feeling of loneliness, and financial problems. Post-Traumatic Stress Disorder (PTSD), as a complication following critical illnesses and IC, has also been reported

in several studies since the 1980s [19, 22–25]. Based on such research, Åkerman et al [26] developed the 3-SET 4P questionnaire for evaluating recovery after ICU, which focused on physical and psychosocial problems but not existential or spiritual issues. The questionnaire consists of 53 items on a 5-point Likert scale with 16 physical, 26 psychosocial, and 11 follow-up care items. In the pilot study, 39 patients answered the questionnaire, and 17 of those did the retest. Physical problems revealed four factors (11 questions), psychosocial five factors (22 items), and follow-up four factors (10 items). They concluded that patients following IC described several discomforts, disabilities, and symptoms during the recovery process.

The recovery concept and theoretical framework

The word recovery consists of "re" and "cover", which could have three meanings: 1) recovery (from something) – the process of becoming well again after illness/injury; 2) recovery (in something) – the process of improving or becoming stronger again; 3) recovery (of something) – the action or process of getting something back that has been stolen or lost. As each of these meanings contain a process, an aspect of time is inherently involved [27]. Based on these meanings recovery and experiences of health, well-being, as well as quality of life can be seen as both connected and interrelated. According to Gadamer [28], health is connected to the rhythm of life: breathing, sleeping, and metabolic processes. When equilibrium is lost in these, it is not only a medical-biological state but also a social and life-historical transformation the patients go through as they will no longer return to the same people they were before falling ill. Loss of health and illness itself may also be a loss of one's physical and/or mental freedom, which affects life as a whole, evoking existential issues. Therefore, recovery could be seen as the challenge to restore one's own sense of self-identity. Based on the thought that recovery and health are interrelated, recovery could be viewed as a movement from illness towards health, involving both objective and subjective dimensions [29]. Objective dimensions contain symptoms and signs that can be assessed by other people, such as physicians and nurses. Subjective dimensions contain self-reported experiences or feelings. From the patient's perspective, the experiences and feelings of being recovered or feeling well or not is of interest, as this may affect their need for care and support/help. People's experience of health and recovery always includes their perception based on their previous experience and personal values on what quality of life means.

Recovery and regaining health can be seen as a movement from disintegration towards integration and of wholeness [29, 30]. Integration means coordinating

separate parts into something more functional wholeness, where the parts remain qualitatively separated. The
wholeness is seen as multidimensional and consists of
the individual and his/her whole environment, where the
meaning of life, life motivation, will and a perspective
for a future is vital. The word "integrate" means to make
whole. Being recovered or being healthy is understood
as an integrated condition of freshness, soundness and
well-being. Disintegration is the opposite, which means
dissolution [29, 30]. Issues concerning the patients' experiences of their illness, the care event and maybe lingering symptoms and discomfort have been integrated
into their lives and, in some sense, been given meaning.
For example patients claim that they feel well, despite
reporting discomforting symptoms. They can claim that
they could live with these discomforts, and that they feel
lucky to have survived [20]. Thus, a movement towards
integration means becoming "whole" again, re-covered,
where the suffering becomes bearable. This means being
able to look forward, to yearn, to be open and ready to
interact with others, give or find meaning in the past
and present. These issues refer to spiritual or existential
dimensions of recovery. In terms of this study, we define
recovery as a process towards integration or wholeness
even if setbacks are experienced.

It can be concluded that health and recovery are complex phenomena and, therefore, difficult to measure
[28]. There are several areas, such as spiritual, existential, and social, that are not covered in many health and
recovery questionnaires. A questionnaire that takes these
issues in consideration could be useful in clinical follow-
up care of patients who have been cared for in the ICU,
but it could also be a useful tool for the patients themselves to evaluate changes throughout their recovery
process.

Objectives
The aim was to describe the development and evaluation
of the Recovery after Intensive Care questionnaire's
(RAIN) validity and reliability.

Development of the questionnaire
Based on previous research on patients' recovery following ICU care [11–13, 31, 32], patient interviews [20] and
the thoughts and ideas about integration, health and recovery [28, 30], basic elements in the recovery process
and condition were identified by the authors. These elements were: 1) bodily – when the body has returned to
an acceptable condition, and it works as it should again,
thus regaining a form of freedom; 2) mentally-socially –
when a person transitions from being excluded from the
world of healthy people to becoming included by reaching out and interacting; 3) existentially – when a normal
daily world, including routines, has developed and a

revaluation of life takes place, reviewing the past but also
looking forward to the future by evaluating what is
meaningful; and 4) Spiritual – when they have the will
to live again, are looking forward or longing for something, and are also able to share their own experiences
in order to cope with their pain or suffering. Based on
these elements, 30 items were constructed by the
authors.

In the next phase, these items were evaluated and analyzed by an independent expert group of four faculty
members. The criteria for inviting these experts were
that they should be registered nurses, have a specialist
nurse education in intensive care and be experienced in
caring for patients in ICU before, during or after ser-
ious/critical/acute illness/injuries. At least one of them
should have conducted research in ICU. These experts
evaluated the items to determine if they were clear and
easy to understand and items logical order. This resulted
in four open ended and two yes/no questions being
added. In the end, the questionnaire consisted of 36
questions, and of these, 30 were on a Likert type scale.

Patient pilot-test and evaluation of reliability and validity
In phase three, a pilot test of the questionnaire (36
items) was conducted. Four patients were recruited by
one of the authors and another four patients were recruited by an IC nurse to participate. All patients were
recruited six months after discharge from two hospital
ICUs in Sweden. Thus, a total of eight patients of different ages and gender answered the questionnaire. They
were asked to judge and assess the questions' relevancy,
clarity, and ease of answering. One patient reported that
the two questions about the relationship to relatives and
sharing thoughts with relatives were repetitive. All patients had the opinion that the questions were easy to
answer.

Content validity test
In the fourth phase, seven faculty members, who were
experts within healthcare and/or IC were invited to
evaluate and assess the relevancy and clarity of the 36
items using a dichotomous scale. At this meeting, one of
the authors had asked one of the attendants to be in
charge of the meeting. A content validity index (CVI)
[33] was conducted and found to be acceptable.

The final questionnaire
The final questionnaire consisted of a total of 36 items.
The 30 Likert type questions, ranging from 1-No/Never
to 5-Yes, very much/often, meaning that the higher the
number, the higher recovery, constituted the foundation
for testing the instrument's properties. The four open-
ended questions about present discomforts or symptoms, which symptom or discomfort was the most

troubling, what the patient was longing for, and how the patient felt about their situation at the moment in relation to the reason for needing IC were excluded when analyzing the answers. The two financial questions were Yes/No, and they were considered part of the demographic data and thus not included in the analysis. Thus, the instrument RAIN consists of 30 items.

Participants and procedure

Patients were recruited consecutively by a critical care nurse (CCN) from an eight-bed general ICU in a county hospital in Sweden. In this ICU, patients were treated for surgical and medical conditions and trauma. The study inclusion criteria were that all patients were at least 18 years old, had received care at the ICU for at least 24 hours, and could read and write in Swedish. The CCN from the post-ICU patient reception and another CCN phoned eligible patients consecutively around one month after being discharged from the ICU and asked if the researchers could call them regarding the study. At the same time, the patients were informed about the study. The patients were then phoned by the researchers and invited to participate in the study, which would require them to answer a questionnaire. The authors obtained the patients' addresses, and then sent the questionnaire package, which included RAIN, a prepaid envelope, a written consent letter, and information about the study. The patients were to answer the questionnaire and send the questionnaire and informed consent letter back. The questionnaires were sent out approximately 2, 6, 12, or 24 months after the patient had left the ICU. The reason for evaluating and measuring recovery at different points of time was that recovery has a time aspect, meaning that patients may adapt to any lingering discomfort over a period of time. Prior to each mailing, the authors contacted the national registration authority to ensure that the patient was alive and the address was valid. The data were collected between 2013 and 2016. This length of time period was due to the fact that we wanted to investigate recovery even one and two years after ICU discharge. This meant that the questionnaire was sent 1-2 years after patients had agreed to participate in the study.

Ethical approval

The Regional Ethical Review board at the University of Gothenburg approved the study (Dnr 695-10, 2010) before data collection commenced.

Methods

Analyses of factor structure

Initially, a potential factor structure of the 30-item scale was tested by means of exploratory factor analysis. The method used was a principal component analysis with orthogonal varimax rotation [34]. All statistical analyses were run on PASW/SPSS Statistics version 22. More items were removed based on this principal component analysis. Thus, items with low loadings (below 0.40) across all the suggested factors as well as items that loaded equally on several factors were removed. Overall, this resulted in the removal of 10 items. The remaining 20 items were thereafter analyzed a second time with the same type of principal component analysis. In this second analysis, three criteria for factor extraction were applied: Eigen values above one, the scree plot and homogeneity, and meaningfulness of items building up each factor (Fig. 1).

A multi-trait analysis performed after the final principal component analysis demonstrate construct validity of the scale in relation to convergence and discrimination. These tests could be regarded as a simple form of confirmatory factor analyses to measure latent factors [34, 35].

Convergent validity demonstrate the related stability in the scale. It was tested by a correlation between items and the expected scale corrected for overlap, where the correlation should be more than 0.40[36] to show convergent validity. The scale was also tested for discriminant validity by taking the items that correlated higher with the hypothesized scale compared to all other scales.

Item consistency and reliability were further assessed by internal item consistency and Cronbach's alpha. According to conventional rules, the Cronbach alpha coefficient should exceed 0.70 [34]. Internal item consistency (Table 2) should not be lower than 0.40 [36]. Both of these values were reached for all items that remained in the questionnaire.

The quality of a scale also depend on maximum (ceiling) or minimum (floor) levels of respondents scoring. Furthermore the proportion of missing values should be taken into consideration. The half-scale criterion was used to handle missing items within a scale [35]. Thus, if a respondent answered all items connected to a scale, a sum score was calculated to form the scale score. If a respondent answered 50% or more (but not all) of the items, a mean value of the answered questions was calculated. This mean value was then imputed to form a sum score of all missing items. Finally, if a respondent answered fewer than 50% of the items connected to a scale, the missing values were treated as missing.

Results

During a period of three years in one ICU, 169 patients answered the questionnaire. Of the 169 respondents, 61% (103) were male, 39% (66) were female, and the mean age was 69±12.5 years. Regarding their financial situation, 78% of the patients reported that their situation was acceptable, but 31% found that it had worsened since their critical illness and stay in the ICU.

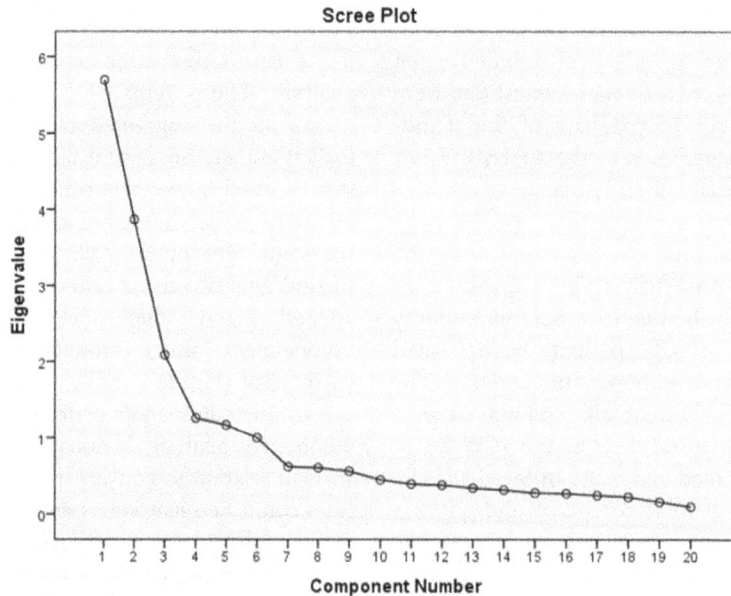

Fig. 1 A scree plot showing factors (component number) above one in eigenvalue

Exploratory factor analysis

The principal component analysis performed on the 20 remaining items showed a very clear factor structure (see Table 1). All items loaded satisfactorily high and clear on a corresponding factor. Table 1 shows the rotated pattern matrix from the analysis. Six factors were extracted with eigen values above one, and together they explained 75% of the variance of the 20 items. The factors were labelled: forward looking, supporting relations, existential ruminations, revaluation of life, physical and mental strength, and need of social support.

Tests of internal structure, reliability, and scale properties

The results of these tests are displayed in Table 2. All 20 items surpassed the criterion for satisfactory convergent validity, i.e., item-scale correlations > 0.40 when corrected for overlap. The mean values for these correlations ranged from 0.57 to 0.78, and no separate correlation was lower than 0.53. The Cronbach alpha coefficient, a related measure of item consistency, was accordingly very good for all scales, ranging from 0.75 to 0.90. Likewise, the tests of item discriminant validity also revealed satisfactory results.

Another examined scale property was the proportion of incomplete scale scores. When using the half-scale criterion, the proportion of scales scores treated as missing ranged from 0 percent to 4.3 percent, and the proportion of calculated scale scores ranged from 0.6 percent to 5.3 percent (see Table 2). Furthermore, there were no single items that clearly stood out as considerably more "missed" than others. Out of the 169 respondents, the frequency of non-answered items ranged from

zero (one item) to eight (two items). Together, these data imply that the respondents in general understood and were able to respond to all items.

Further tests concerned the observed range of scale scores compared with the theoretical range. An important property of a scale is its ability to differentiate between levels of the assessed concept. The extent to which observed scale scores cover the theoretical score range is an indication of that ability. As can be seen in Table 2, the theoretical range was very well covered by the observed scale scores.

The percent of responses at the floor and ceiling levels showed the proportion of responses at the extreme endpoints of the scales. Substantial proportions of respondents who scored at the ceiling were found for the scales labelled forward looking (19.6%) and supporting relations (32.3%). The opposite was found for the need of social support scale. Here, 48.1% scored at the floor. Such high ceiling/floor effects could depend on two aspects. First, the study sample could be among those who have recovered best, are forward looking, and have little need for further support. Second, the scales in question could be less efficient at discriminating on the more positive ends of the ability to look forward and the need for further social support.

Discussion

This study aimed to describe the development and evaluate the validity and reliability of a new instrument to measure recovery among patients after ICU treatment. As mentioned earlier, several instruments measuring postoperative recovery have been developed and

Table 1 Results of the Principle Component Analysis and factor loading of the 20-item Version of the RAIN instrument

	Forward looking	Supporting relations	Existential ruminations	Revaluation of life	Physical and mental strength	Need of social support
Can you look forward?	.866					
Feel hope for the future	.862					
Plan for the future	.806					
Prepare to go forward	.680					
Share thoughts with relatives		.887				
Energy to be together with relatives		.885			.328	
Share thoughts about critical illness		.803				
Someone to speak to about difficulties		.617				
Thoughts about the closeness to death			.830			
Thoughts about your critical illness			.828			
Thoughts about your disease			.770			
Thoughts about hospital stay			.729			
Revalue life				.897		
Appreciate different things in life				.869		
Discover new characteristics of yourself				.716		
Recovered physically	.411				.746	
Recovered mentally					.719	
Sleeping well					.700	
Talk to someone outside of your family						.878
Need to talk to a professional						.836

used in many countries, but no instrument for post ICU care recovery which includes existential questions has been available to the best of our knowledge. Evaluating and measuring recovery following IC is complicated as many factors may influence the patients' own opinions about their recovery. In post-surgical and ICU follow ups, HRQL has been used in order to measure patients' opinions on their quality of life [12, 13]. For the recovery instruments that are used, most have focused simply on physical symptoms and mental issues, omitting many other facets of recovery.

The questions in the RAIN questionnaire were based upon previous empirical research, thoughts and theory models of health as a feeling of wholeness, where body, soul and spirit are in unity [30]. Moreover, the questionnaire was developed upon the understanding that recovery is seen as a process of regaining health, a movement towards integration even if setbacks sometimes occur. Therefore, dimensions that also reflect existential, social and spiritual

life issues were seen as important as previous studies have stated these aspects impact patients' recoveries [11–13, 20, 32]. For example, patients expressed that they felt well but, at the same time, were in need of help from family members [20] or suffered from thoughts of death and could not look forward to anything in life [31]. This might reflect thoughts about life and what life means, which Cöster [37] describes as 'livsförståelse,' meaning understanding of life/to view life. If life has no meaning, there is no health or well-being [38]. Such thoughts are also expressed in Morse's theory Responding to Threats to Integrity of Self [39].

The analysis resulted in six clear factors. This supports the idea that recovery depends on several factors, not only physical symptoms and discomforts. Such factors are close relationships, thoughts and beliefs, and what is seen as important and meaningful in life. A wide range of issues are represented in the instrument, and the discriminant validity and the mean value of the item

Table 2 Summary of Multi-trait Scaling Analyses of the RAIN-instrument (N = 169)

	Forward looking	Supporting relations	Existential ruminations	Revaluation of life	Physical and mental strength	Need of social support
Number of items	4	4	4	3	3	2
Number of scale levels	16	16	16	12	12	8
Theoretical range	4-20	4-20	4-20	3-15	3-15	2-10
Observed range	4-20	4-20	4-20	3-15	3-15	2-10
Mean (SD)[a]	16.12 (3.8)	16.96 (3.6)	12.41 (3.7)	9.12 (3.8)	11.73 (2.9)	4.10 (2.5)
% incomplete scale score[b]	4.3	1.1	2.4	4.3	0.0	3.7
% at ceiling	19.6	32.3	2.5	5.7	15.2	5.1
% at floor	1.3	1.3	1.9	12.7	0.6	48.1
Mean (R) internal consistency[c]	0.78 (.68-.89)	0.72 (.59-.80)	0.66 (.58-.71)	0.68 (.61-.72)	0.57 (.52-.64)	0.73 (.73-.73)
Item-scale discriminant validity[d]	0/0/0/100	0/0/10/90	0/0/0/100	0/0/0/100	0/0/13/87	0/0/0/ 100
Cronbach's α	0.90	0.86	0.84	0.83	0.75	0.82
% calculated scale scores[e]	1.2	5.3	0.6	0.6	1.2	0.6

[a]Mean(SD) of summed scores.
[b]Missing according to half scale criterion.
[c]Pearson correlations between items and hypothesized scale, corrected overlap. Mean of correlations for each scale and range.
[d]Percent correlations that are significantly lower/lower/higher/significantly higher with hypothesized scale compared to other scales.
[e]Calculated according to the half-scale criterion

correlations found satisfactory results, suggesting this new scale could prove useful to measure recovery in patients who received IC treatment.

The dimension "supporting relations" contained four items concerning issues that showed the importance of sharing thoughts and experiences with relatives and/or others. This is in line with findings in a study by Ringdal et al [40]. It was found that all concern and care given by family members as well as healthcare professionals made the patients feel accepted even if they were in need of help and felt weak. If recovery is facilitated by patients sharing their thoughts and experiences with others, nurses and physicians might either ask about patients' thoughts and experiences or encourage relatives and family members to listen to their loved ones concerns. Experiences from critical illness/injury, ICU treatment and care can be seen as belonging to each individual's life history. Ringdal and Rose [41] discuss that patients' discomforting memories belonging to the ICU period as well as difficulties to remember parts of their lives may affect their present and future life and thus recovery.

It was found that most patients answered that they did not need to talk to any professionals about their thoughts and feelings. It could be discussed if this question "Do you need to talk to a professional?" evokes thoughts about the need of psychological or psychiatric expertise rather than another medical professional. Also, the question, "Do you need to talk to someone outside the family?" may further indicate that illness, suffering, and recovery from illness/injury are seen as a private matter. The need of talking and sharing thoughts about

the illness/injury and the ICU stay could be considered exclusively a family/relative concern as the mean value for factor two about the family is relatively high. These factors could be influencing the results.

Other explanations may also be connected to the fact that those patients that agreed to participate in the study may have had a successful recovery and were probably feeling relatively well. Patients who did not accept the invitation may have felt worse or did not have the strength to participate, potentially skewing our results. Unfortunately, we do not have any statistics on how many denied participation or how many were not reachable; therefore, we cannot determine the response rate. This could be seen as a limitation when assessing the recovery of the population. However, in this study, our focus was to describe the questionnaire and its properties and not the recovery of the 169 patients at this early stage of questionnaire development.

Despite these limitations, the participants were heterogeneous and represented both genders, a wide range of ages, and lapsed time, after ICU discharge. The sample size (N = 169), in relation to the number of the 30 items, met the recommended criteria of five respondents for each item [42].

There were few missing items, which indicate that either the questions were not difficult to answer or were all found relevant enough to be answered. The conceptual framework with a six-factor solution explained 75% of the variance, which is satisfactory. However, the ceiling and floor levels must be investigated in future studies to determine their impact on the overall scale. The floor and/or ceiling effects can result because of two circumstances: 1) the study group was not representative in some way by either containing patients that were too sick or too healthy. If this is the case, the questionnaire can only be tested with a new study with new patients. 2) The scale cannot cover all aspects, and this can only be tested by adding items that cover the shortcomings of the scale. This will be tested in a future study where we will continue this project and then add items to avoid potential floor and ceilings effects.

While the RAIN instrument provides an opportunity to quantify recovery, it also provides nurses with useful and valuable information for follow-up communications with former patients at so called post-ICU clinics. The RAIN instrument can also facilitate for primary and community healthcare nurses to communicate and follow-up with patients who have been seriously ill/injured and cared for at ICUs.

Conclusion

The factor analysis including discriminant validity and the mean value of the item correlations were found satisfactory. The Cronbach alpha coefficient, a related measure of item consistency, was accordingly very good for all scales, ranging from 0.75 to 0.90. Based on these findings we recommend nurses and/or caregivers use the RAIN instrument for follow-up or post-ICU services on patients who received intensive care to get a more holistic view of their recovery.

Acknowledgements

We are very grateful to all the patients who agreed to participate in this study and all the colleagues at the intensive care units who provided us with information about eligible patients. We would also like to thank the healthcare experts, researchers and nurses who contributed to the development of the questionnaire over several years. A special thanks to Associate Professor Lars-Olof Persson, who provided feedback and guidance as well as reviewing the statistical analyses, Assistant Professor Annikki Jonsson, who contacted patients and collected data and Cecilia Glimelius Pettersson RN, MScN, who recruited patients for the pilot study. We would lastly like to thank Christie Tetreault at That Editing Touch for the excellent editing of the manuscript.

Funding

This study was supported by the Agneta Prytz-Folkes and Gösta Folkes foundation. There had not been any conditions connected to the research regarding design of the study data collection, analysis, interpretation of data or in writing the manuscript.

Availability of data and materials

Patients' data are not publicly available due to the potential of an invasion of privacy since the data contain unique social security numbers along with some demographic information that would jeopardize the patients' anonymity. The raw data (SPSS files and the answered questionnaires with no personal data about patients) used and which support our findings are free and available on request, please contact author Ingegerd Bergbom (ingegerd.bergbom@gu.se). All data generated and analyzed during this study are included and presented in this article. The RAIN questionnaire is available to other researchers free of charge. Please contact ingegerd.bergbom@gu.se for more information.

Authors' contributions

All authors have read and made significant contributions to the design, data collection, data analyses and critical revisions of the manuscript at every step of each version. All authors have agreed to the final version that is being submitted. IB was responsible for developing and constructing the questionnaire and drafted the manuscript and revised it through the whole process. However, all authors participated in the final construction of the questionnaire and at the meetings with experts for evaluating the questions. MR conducted the focus group meeting. IB and VK have recruited patients and sent out the questionnaire. The patient pilot study was conducted by VK and another researcher (not author), mentioned in acknowledgement. MR has performed the statistical analysis and these have been discussed with all authors during the whole process. IB edited the first draft of the manuscript, and the text about the results from the factor analysis has been drafted by MR. However all authors have read and comment the manuscript throughout the whole process. All authors have agreed to the final version and have contributed to design, acquisition of data and analysis as well as revising the manuscript critically for important intellectual content. All authors read and approved the final manuscript.

Ethics approval and consent to participate

The Regional Ethical Review Board at the University of Gothenburg approved the study (Dnr 695-10, 2010) before data collection commenced. The development and evaluation of the RAIN instrument was one of several studies in the research program that focused on the recovery among patients cared for in intensive care units. All patients were verbally and written informed about the study, which included a questionnaire and thereafter they, who accepted to participate in the study signed a consent form. All authors confirm that they have read and agreed to the content in this article. Participants' data are not presented in this article, as the aim was to describe the development and evaluation of the RAIN questionnaire.

Competing interests

The authors declare that they have no competing interests.

Author details

[1]Institute of Health and Care Sciences at the Sahlgrenska Academy, University of Gothenburg, Gothenburg, Sweden. [2]Faculty of Caring Science, Work Life and Social Welfare, Borås University, Borås, Sweden. [3]Department of Health Sciences, University West, Trollhättan, Sweden. [4]Department of Anesthetic and Intensive Care, Kungälvs hospital, Kungälv, Sweden.

References

1. Royse CF, Newman S, Williams Z, Wilkinson DJ. A human volunteer study to identify variability in performance in the cognitive domain of the postoperative quality of recovery scale. Anesthesiology. 2013;119:576–81.
2. Lizana FG, Bota DP, De Cubber M, Vincent J-L. Long-term outcome in ICU patients: What about quality of life? Intensive Care Med. 2003;29:1286–93.
3. Lippa SM, Lange RT, Bailie JM, Kennedy JE, Brickell TA, Psych D, French LM. Utility of the Validity-10 scale across the recovery trajectory following traumatic brain injury. JRRD. 2016;53:379–90.
4. Allvin R, Svensson E, Rawal N, Ehnfors M, Kling A-M, Idwall E. The Postoperative Recovery Profile (PRP) – a multidimensional questionnaire for evaluation of recovery profiles. J Eval Clin Pract. 2011;17:236–43.
5. Meuser KT, Gingerich S, Salyers MP, McGuire AB, Reyes RU, Cunningham H. The illness management and recovery (IMR) scales. (Client and Clinician version). New Hampshire-Dartmouth Psychiatric Research Center: Concord NH; 2004.
6. Myles PS, Weitkamp B, Jones K, Melick J, Hensen S. Validity and reliability of a postoperative quality of recovery score: the QoR-40. Brit J Anaesthesia. 2000;84:11–5.

7.   McIntosh S, Adams J. Anxiety and quality of recovery in day surgery: A questionnaire study using Hospital Anxiety and Depression Scale and Quality of Recovery Score. Internat J Nurs Pract. 2011;17:85–92.

8.   Hancock N, Newton SJ, Honey A, Bundy AC, O'shea K. Recovery Assessment Scale – Domain and Stages (RAS-DS). Its feasibility and outcome measurement capacity. Aust NZ J Psychiatry. 2015;49:624-633.

9.   Warrén Stomberg M, Saxborn E, Gambreus S, Brattwall M, Jakobsson JG. Tools for the assessment of the recovery process following discharge from day surgery: a literature review. Clinical Feature. 2015;25:219–24.

10. Ebrahim S, Malachowski C, Kamal el Din M, Mulla SM, Montoya L, Bance S, Busse JW. Expectations of one's own recovery. Measures of patients' expectations about recovery. A systematic review. Journal Occup Rehab. 2015;25:240–55.

11. Olsson U, Bosaeus I, Bergbom I. Patients' experiences of the recovery period 12 months after upper gastrointestinal surgery. Gastroenterology Nurs. 2010; 33:422–31.

12. Ringdal M, Plos K, Örtenwall P, Bergbom I. Memories and health related quality of life after intensive care – a follow-up study. Crit Care Med. 2010; 38:38–44.

13. Pettersson M, Bergbom I, Mattsson E. Health related quality of life after treatment of Adominal Aortic Aneurysm with open repair and endovascular techniques – a two-year follow-up. Surg Sci. 2012;3:436–44.

14. Zetterlund P, Plos K, Bergbom I, Ringdal M. Memories from Intensive Care unit persists for several years – A longitudinal prospective multi-centre study. Intensive & Crit Care Nurs. 2012;28:159–67.

15. Glimelius Pettersson C, Ringdal M, Bergbom I. Diaries and memories following an ICU stay; a 2-months follow-up study. Nurs Crit Care. 2015; https://doi.org/10.1111/nic.12162.

16. Kelly AM, McKinley S. Patients' recovery after critical illness at early follow up. J Clin Nurs. 2010;19:691–700.

17. Herridge MS, Cheung AM, Tansey CM. One year outcomes in survivors of the acute respiratory distress syndrome. NEngl J Med. 2003;348:683–93.

18. Bercker S, Weber-Carstens S, Deja M, Grimm C, Wolf S, Behse F. Critical illness polyneuropathy and myopathy in patients with acute respiratory distress syndrome. Crit Care Med. 2005;33:711–5.

19. Deacon K. Re-building life after ICU: A qualitative study of the patients' perspective. Intensive & Crit Care Nurs. 2012;28:114–22.

20. Karlsson V, Bergbom I, Ringdal M, Jonsson A. After discharge home: a qualitative analysis of older ICU patients' experiences and care needs. Scand J Caring Sci. 2016;30:749–56.

21. Daffurn K, Bishop GF, Hillman KM, Bauman A. Problems following discharge after intensive care. Intensive & Crit Care Nurs. 1994;10:244–51.

22. Kuch K, Swinson RP. Post-traumatic stress disorder. In: Vincent J-L, editor. Updates in intensive care and emergency medicine. Berlin: Springer-Verlag, Berlin 1988. p. 548-555.

23. Jones C, Griffiths RD, Macmillan RR, Palmer TEA. Psychological problems occurring after intensive care. Brit J Intensive Care. 1994;4:46–53.

24. Schandl A, Brattström O, Svensson-Raskha A, Hellgren E, Falkenhav M, Sackeya P. Screening and treatment of problems after intensive care: A descriptive study of multidisciplinary follow-up. Intensive & Crit Care Nurs. 2011;27:94–101.

25. Jones C. Recovery Post ICU. Intensive & Crit Care Nurs. 2014;30:239–45.

26. Åkerman E, Fridlund B, Ersson A, Granberg-Axéll A. Development of the 3-SET 4P questionnaire for evaluating former ICU patients' physical and psychosocial problems over time: A pilot study. Intensive & Crit Care Nurs. 2009;25:80–9.

27. Oxford Learner's Dictionaries. 2017-12-16. https://oxfordlearnersdictionaries. com/definition/english/recovery?

28. Gadamer H-G. The enigma of health. Standford California:Stanford University Press. 1996;

29. Eriksson K. Hälsans idé. [The idea of health]. 2nd ed. Stockholm: Almqvist & Wiksell;1986.

30. Eriksson K, Bondas-Salonen T, Herberts S, Lindholm L, Matilainen D. Den mångdimensionella hälsan – verklighet och visioner. [The multidimensional health –reality and visions]. Slutrapport, pp 1–62. Vasa Sjukvårdsdistrikt SKN, Institutionen för vårdvetenskap. Åbo Akademi: Vasa; 1995.

31. Bergbom I. The process of recovery from severe illness, injury or surgical treatment. Rec Adv Research Updates. 2008;9:419–31.

32. Ringdal M, Johansson L, Lundberg D, Plos K, Bergbom I. Outcomes After Injury – Memories, Health-Related Quality of Life, Anxiety and Symptoms of Depression After Intensive Care. Journal of Trauma. 2009;66:1226–33.

33. Yaghmale F. Content validity and its estimation. J Med Educ. 2003;3:25–7.

34. Nunnally JC. Bernstein, IH. Psychometric theory. 3rd ed. New. York: McGraw-Hill; 1994.

35. Fayers PM, Machin D. Quality of Life – The assessment, analysis and reporting of patient reported outcomes. 3rd ed. Oxford: Wiley-Blackwell. 2016;

36. Hays RD, Hayashi T, Carson S, Ware JE. User's guide for the Multi-trait Analysis Program (MAP). Santa Barbara CA: The Rand Publication series; 1988.

37. Cöster H. Att kunna tala allvar med sig själv. [To be able to seriously talk to yourself]. Karlstad: Karlstad University Studies; 2003:10.

38. Eriksson K. The suffering human being. Chicago USA: Nordic Studies Press; 2006.

39. Morse JM. Responding to threats to integrity of self. Adv Nurs Sci. 1997;19: 21–36.

40. Ringdal M, Plos K, Bergbom I. Memories of being injured and patients' care trajectory after physical trauma. BMC Nursing. 2008;7:8.

41. Ringdal M, Rose L. Recovery after critical illness: The role of follow-up services to improve psychological well-being. Crit J Nurs Res. 2012;44:7–17.

42. Pett MA, Lackey NR, Sullivan JJ. Making sense of factor analysis: The use of factor analysis for instrument development in health care research. Thousand Oaks: Sage Publications; 2003.

14

Perceived organizational support and moral distress among nurses

Navideh Robaee[1], Foroozan Atashzadeh-Shoorideh[2*] ⓘ, Tahereh Ashktorab[3], Ahmadreza Baghestani[4] and Maasoumeh Barkhordari-Sharifabad[5]

Abstract

Background: Moral distress is prevalent in the health care environment at different levels. Nurses in all roles and positions are exposed to ethically challenging conditions. Development of supportive climates in organizations may drive nurses towards coping moral distress and other related factors. This study aimed at determining the level of perceived organizational support and moral distress among nurses and investigating the relationship between the two variables.

Methods: This was a correlational-descriptive study. A total of 120 nurses were selected using random quota sampling method. A demographic questionnaire, Survey of Perceived Organizational Support, and Moral Distress Scale were used to collect the data which were analyzed using descriptive and analytical tests in SPSS20.

Results: The mean perceived organizational support was low (2.63 ± 0.79). The mean moral distress was 2.19 ± 0.58, which shows a high level of moral distress. Moreover, Statistical analysis showed no significant relationship between perceived organizational support and moral distress ($r = 0.01$, $p = 0.86$).

Conclusion: Given the low level of perceived organizational support and high moral distress among nurses in this study, it is necessary to provide a supportive environment in hospitals and to consider strategies for diminishing moral distress.

Keywords: Ethics, Morals, Perceived organizational support, Moral distress, Nurses

Background

Moral distress is a common problem among the professionals employed in health care settings [1]. It occurs when the individuals feel that they cannot act according to the pivotal values and duties or when the measures taken to achieve the intended results fail to succeed so that the totality of individual's ethical principles is seriously endangered [2]. In other words, moral distress can be considered as the stress tolerated by professionals at a time when, despite an awareness of the right performance, they cannot achieve the correct performance due to some barriers [1, 3–5]. Moral distress has been described as a major problem in the nursing profession [5, 6].

The particular characteristics of nursing and the different work cultures generated in different health care institutions expose nurses to a higher risk of moral distress than other professionals [7]. Moral distress has undesirable outcomes for both nurses and patients, and can have direct and indirect effects on nurses. Physical disorders such as nightmares, headache and anxiety and a dysfunctional personal life have been reported among nurses at risk for moral distress [8].

Moreover, feeling of anger, failure, sin, and disability are among the consequences of moral distress. Some studies have demonstrated that moral distress is correlated with personnel burnout, deteriorated team work, reduced quality of care, and challenges related to patient safety [2, 9, 10]. It will further lead to occupational stress and turnover [11].

Various factors contribute to moral distress in nurses among them are invasive procedures on patients with incurable diseases, orders for unnecessary tests or examinations,

* Correspondence: f_atashzadeh@sbmu.ac.ir
[2]Department of Nursing Management, School of Nursing and Midwifery, Shahid Beheshti University of Medical Sciences, Vali-Asr Avenue, Cross of Vali-Asr and Hashemi Rafsanjani Highway, Opposite to Rajaee Heart Hospital, Tehran 1996835119, Iran
Full list of author information is available at the end of the article

insufficient and inefficient treatment by colleagues, lack of balance in power among the health specialists, and lack of organizational support [12].

When exposed to stressful environments and high job demands, the employees need the financial and spiritual support of their organization. Perceived organizational support is a condition based on how much the organization considers employees' values and needs [13]. Organizational support is one of the important indices of nursing work environment [14], and can be considered an influential moral factor [15].

Additionally, one aspect of ethical competency of nurse leaders is their supportive behavior [14]. The leaders' supportive behavior will be compensated for by the followers' proper compliance. The organization is less likely to face a situation in which the staff's behavior disturbs the leader's or group's work [14, 16–20]. This perception of level of organizational support especially about ethical practice is a vital element of the constraints upon nurses' actions [21].

Perceived organizational support reduces stressors in the workplace and is potentially involved in dealing with work-related fatigue, excitement, and depression [22]. Supportive occupational environments are the most important factor in creating job satisfaction for nurses that influences positively the patients' treatment, absorption and maintenance of manpower in the organization. A climate with high levels of support diminishes occupational tension and maintains the nurses in the organization [23].

Moreover, some studies have revealed that perceived organizational support is negatively correlated with work absenteeism [24], and intent to turnover [25], while it is positively correlated with award expectation, role of performance and social behavior, preventive and civil behaviors [26], and also organizational commitment and subsequently self-competency [27]. Nurse leaders' supportive behavior plays a key role in productivity and promoting nurses' professional performance [20, 28].

Iran is a developing country located in the south-west of Asia with a population of about 80,000,000 people. The nursing manpower at different levels is estimated to be about 150,000. As it is the case in many other developing countries, nurses in Iran encounter many challenges such as long working hours, changing work shifts, limited vacation, abundant occupational wants and wishes, unsatisfactory payment or salary, and inappropriate behavior towards some patients or their families [29, 30]. These challenges often result from deficient techniques of manpower management in hospitals [30], shortage of manpower, job dissatisfaction, nurses' low social status, absence of a satisfactory student acceptance system at the universities, and shortage of ethics course in the nursing curriculum [31–36], leading to increased workload, fostered medical and nursing errors, and subsequently, moral distress in nurses [36].

There are some controversies about the level of moral distress among Iranian nurses [37–40]. A review of literature related to the two variables "perceived organizational support" and "moral distress" indicated that the investigation of these two variables has been very limited on Iranian nurses. Furthermore, no comprehensive study has been found on determining the correlation between "perceived organizational support" and "moral distress" among Iranian nurses. Development of supportive organizations may lead nurses to better cope with moral distress and other problems such as job dissatisfaction [5, 21, 41–43].

Aim

The purpose of this research was to determine the level of perceived organizational support and moral distress among nurses and to investigate the relationship between these two variables.

Methods

Research design

This correlational descriptive study used random quota sampling to select the participants. First, considering the distribution of hospitals affiliated to Shahid Beheshti University of Medical Sciences in different regions of Tehran (north, south, east, west and center), one hospital was randomly selected from each region and the required number of nurses was selected from each hospital in proportion to the total number of nurses working in it. Considering the number of hospitals surveyed, 120 questionnaires were distributed among all the qualified nurses selected from the morning, evening, and night shifts using random sampling.

The sample size was calculated by the following formula to explore correlation between moral distress and perceived organizational support.

$$N = \left[\frac{Z_\alpha + Z_\beta}{c}\right]^2 + 3$$

Where N is the desired sample size, Z_α is the standard normal score of 95% of confidence interval = 1.96, Z_β = statistical power at 90%, which is 1.28 and $c = 0/5 \times Ln[(1 + r)(1 - r)]$ with being the correlation coefficient, which is 0.3 according to a study by Jay Maningo-Salinas [15].

Considering a participant attrition of 10%, 120 nurses were selected for the study. However, 110 completed questionnaires were analyzed. The study inclusion criteria consisted of having a bachelor's degree or higher in nursing and at least 1 year of work experience.

Data collection tools

In this study, a demographic questionnaire, Eiesenberger's Survey of Perceived Organizational Support (SPOS), and nurses' Moral Distress Scale (MDS) were used to collect the data.

Demographic information questionnaire

The demographic questionnaire examined participants' demographic data including age, gender, marital status, level of education, work experience, work shifts, and history of attendance in ethics workshops.

Survey of Perceived Organizational Support

The 8-item SPOS was developed by Eisenberger et al. [13]. Each item in this survey is scored based on a 7-point Likert scale from strongly disagree (zero) to strongly agree (six). The range of scores in each item varies from zero to six while on a total scale is zero to 48. A higher score indicates more perceived organizational support. This scale is a unidimensional measure and has been widely used in research studies. Evidence of its validity and reliability has been reported in numerous studies [44–46]. The Cronbach's alpha coefficient of perceived organizational support was calculated as 0.74 in this study.

Moral distress scale

The nurses' MDS is a native scale developed by Atashzadeh-Shoorideh et al. [40]. It contains 30 items in three dimensions, namely "inappropriate competencies and responsibilities", "errors", and "not respecting the ethical principles". All the items in this scale are scored based on a 5-point Likert scale from 0 (not at all) to 4 (very much). The score of moral distress is then calculated as the mean of the total score of the items. The score of moral distress obtained is then classified into four categories: 0–1 is low, 1.01–2 is moderate, 2.01–3 is high, and 3.01–4 is very high moral distress. The Cronbach's alpha coefficient for the "Moral Distress Scale" and all of its dimensions designed by Atashzadeh-Shoorideh et al. was calculated in this study as 0.77.

Data collection

The participants were oriented on how to answer the questionnaires and were informed about the voluntary nature of participation in the study. The questionnaires were distributed among nurses working in different shifts and were collected within 2 days.

Data analysis

The collected data was analyzed via SPSS 20 using the descriptive statistics of data as absolute and relative frequency report, and inferential statistics as a determination of correlation between the variables under study via Pearson product moment correlation coefficient.

Results

The study participants consisted of 110 nurses with a mean age of 34.1 ± 7.4 years and a mean work experience of 9.6 ± 6.5 years, 90% of them were female, 55.5% were married and 95.5% held a bachelor's degree in nursing. The majority of the nurses (48.2%) were working in rotating shifts. The majority (51.8%) had not attended ethics workshops in the past (Table 1).

As shown in Table 2, the mean perceived organizational support was low (2.63 ± 0.79) and the mean moral distress was high (2.19 ± 0.58). The highest mean of moral distress pertained to the dimension of errors (2.43 ± 0.65). No relationships were observed between perceived organizational support and moral distress ($p = 0.86$) or its dimensions ($p > 0.05$); (Table 3).

There was a statistically significant relationship between moral distress and work shifts. Also, relationship between the dimension of errors and work shifts was statistically significant. The significance level set for the work shift test was $p = 0.04$ for moral distress and $p = 0.00$ for the dimension of errors. A significant relationship was also observed between the inappropriate competencies and responsibilities dimension of moral distress and work experience ($p = 0.04$) as shown in Table 4.

Discussion

This study was conducted to determine the level of perceived organizational support and moral distress among nurses and to investigate the relationship between these two variables.

The results revealed low perceived organizational support in the nurses, this finding supports the results of previous studies. In a study by Kwak conducted on nurses in South Korea, organizational support was investigated using corrected nursing work index with a rate assessed as falling in the low limits [47]. Another

Table 1 Sociodemographic characteristics of study participant

Variables		M (SD)	n (%)
Age		34.1 (7.4)	
Gender	Female		99 (90)
	Male		11 (10)
Marital Status	Single		49 (44.5)
	Married		61 (55.5)
Level of Education	Bachelor's Degree		105 (95.5)
	Master's Degree		5 (4.5)
Work Experience		9.6 (6.5)	
Work Shifts	Fixed		35 (31.8)
	Rotating		75 (68.2)
History of attendance in ethics workshops.	Yes		53 (48.2)
	No		57 (51.8)

Table 2 Mean and standard deviation of perceived organizational support, moral distress, and the associated dimensions

Variable	Mean(SD)	Range of Score
Perceived organizational support	2.63 (0.79)	0.75–4.25
Total moral distress	2.19 (0.58)	1–3.40
Inappropriate competencies and responsibilities	2.12 (0.54)	1–3.70
Errors	2.43 (0.65)	1–3.73
Not respecting the ethical principles	1.96 (0.76)	1–3.56

No relationships were observed between perceived organizational support and moral distress ($p = 0.86$) or its dimensions ($p > 0.05$); (Table 3)

study carried out on nurses in Italy reported the mean score of perceived organizational support as 2.26 ± 0.78 which is lower than the central point value reported by Eisenberger et al.'s scale [48]. This is inconsistent with other studies that reported moderate perceived organizational support [15, 29]. Jay Maningo-Salinas investigated the perceived organizational support level among oncology nurses using Eisenberg et al.'s scale and reported it at the moderate level of 3.70 ± 0.86.16. Moreover, the study by Gorji et al. reported the perceived organizational support among the emergency room nurses as moderate [29].

The dissimilarity of results between these studies and the present one may be due to the differences in the instruments used, the research populations, the climate of the organization and how their respective managers managed the research populations. The lack of a supportive environment in hospitals may cause further moral and work conflicts, job dissatisfaction, and reduced employees' trust in the organization [48].

The current study reported the intensity of moral distress as high among the nurses, which is consistent with the results obtained by Woods et al. conducted on nurses in New Zealand [49]. Also, Cummings found that the prevalence of moral distress was high among nurses and proposed this phenomenon as responsible for nurses' turnover rates [50].

Moral distress has been reported as moderate in some studies [37–39, 53], while it is reported to be lower than moderate in a number of other studies [51, 52]. A study on Swedish nurses elucidated the point that moral distress was at the low range [54]. Additionally, the studies carried out in America reported the nurses' moral distress scores at rather low levels [5, 55]. Another study

undertaken in Turkey showed that nurses had low-level moral distress [1], a finding which is inconsistent with our results.

This inconsistency may be attributed to differences in organizational, cultural, educational, geographical, and individual factors and beliefs. For instance, mention can be made of the existence of the required standards of care in hospitals, level of knowledge and awareness, high participation of the health staff, and ethical traits of the participants. Also, it may be speculated that the extreme differences in moral distress between this study and other endeavors may be attributed to variations in the study population and measurement instruments used in the present study. The scale used in this study to measure moral distress includes three dimensions while the moral distress instrument used in other studies has been one-dimensional with some items not appropriately working in the Iranian context. For example, the item of "discharge a patient when he has reached the maximum length of stay based on diagnostic related grouping although he has many teaching needs" in Corley Moral Distress Scale isn't appropriate in Iranian nurses. Comparing the findings of this research with other studies has shown that moral distress for most nurses is moderate to high.

In this study, the highest level of moral distress pertained to the dimension of "errors", while the lowest level belonged to the aspect of "not respecting ethical principles". In numerous studies, the most common causes of moral distress among nurses have been reported to be working with incompetent staff [1, 40, 49, 56], useless care [1, 40], and inappropriate intra-team relations [1, 49]. On the basis of the results of these studies, high level of distress in the dimension of "errors" seems to be logical compared to other dimensions.

The results of this study showed no statistically significant relationships between perceived organizational support and moral distress and any of its' dimensions, A study by Maningo-Salinas, conducted on oncology nurses, expunged upon the correlation between moral distress and inclination for turnover and also determined the mediating effect of perceived organizational support on these two variables. Their findings suggested that perceived organizational support does not mediate the correlation between moral distress and inclination for turnover and that the interaction between moral distress and perceived organizational support was not statistically significant [15]. They point out no statistically

Table 3 Correlation between perceived organizational support and moral distress and its dimensions

	Inappropriate competencies and responsibilities		Errors		No respect for ethics		Total moral distress	
	r	p	r	p	r	p	r	p
Perceived organizational support	0.048	0.61	0.062	0.52	−0.062	0.52	0.017	0.86

Table 4 Correlation between organizational support and moral distress and its dimensions with Sociodemographic characteristics

Variable		Perceived organizational support		Total moral distress		Inappropriate competencies and responsibilities		Errors		Not respecting the ethical principles	
		r	p	r	p	r	p	r	p	r	p
Age		−0.10	0.25	−0.04	0.67	0.12	0.20	−0.17	0.07	0.00	1.00
Gender	Female	0.01	0.89	0.06	0.51	0.07	0.43	0.06	0.54	−0.03	0.70
	Male										
Marital Status	Single	0.07	0.42	−0.07	0.42	0.08	0.40	−0.17	0.06	−0.01	0.86
	Married										
Level of Education	Bachelor's Degree	0.10	0.27	0.10	0.28	0.18	0.06	0.08	0.40	0.76	0.43
	Master's Degree										
Work Experience		−0.14	0.12	0.00	0.98	0.19	0.04^*	−0.14	0.13	0.00	0.95
Work Shifts	Fixed	0.07	0.44	0.18	0.04^*	0.07	0.41	0.25	0.00^*	0.13	0.15
	Rotating										

$^*p < 0.05$

significant relationship, this possibility suggests that Eisenberg's perceived organizational support scale may not be the best instrument for measuring perceived organizational support among the nurses. Hence, it is necessary to carry out a more comprehensive study regarding the use of a perceived organizational support tool in nursing [15].

Of course, several studies have reported the effect of ethical work climate on moral distress. The ethical climate does not often lead to personnel's' perceived organizational support. The reason for this can be the creation of a work environment which is reliable in the organization [57]. Fogel showed that ethical climate agents have a moderating effect on the moral distress, turnover, poor patient care, and justice subjects [58]. In the study by Fogel, the relations between managers and Fnurses induced significant effects on ethical work climate [58]. This, in turn, affects moral distress. Silen's study showed that ethical climate is an important factor in nurses' work setting [54]. But in some articles, it has been indicated that a negative relationship exists between ethical climate and moral distress [50–53, 59].

In the current study, perceived organizational support was not significantly correlated with any of the demographic variables examined, while a significant relationship was observed between the inappropriate competencies and responsibilities dimension of moral distress and the variable of work experience. The present study found a statistically significant relationship between total moral distress and the dimension of errors and work shifts. This is inconsistent with the results obtained by Atashzadeh-Shoorideh et al. [40]. The inconsistency between the findings of the present study and the study of Atashzadeh-Shoorideh et al. may be due to the differences in the research setting and work environment, which may have led to lower rates of error and

moral distress in the nurses examined by Atashzadeh-Shoorideh et al. [40].

The limitations of this research are the descriptive design and data collection with a questionnaire and reliance on self-report data. As a result, some people may refuse to provide real responses and give unrealistic responses. A further limitation is the potential impact of confounding factors such as high occupancy, fatigue, and lack of readiness of nurses to complete the questionnaire. This study used a cross-sectional design. For this reason, it makes the conclusion about cause-effect relations difficult. Therefore, a closer examination can be done by conducting in-depth and longitudinal studies. A further limitation of this research was the selection of nurses from just one city. With the implementation of national and international studies, the possibility of generalizing these findings will increase.

Conclusion

The results of this study showed that the level of perceived organizational support was low in nurses and moral distress was high. Therefore, it is necessary to provide a supportive environment in hospitals and to consider strategies for diminishing moral distress.

Also, the findings indicated that there was no significant correlation between perceived organizational support and moral distress. These results are not consistent with the findings of other studies on moral distress. It is recommended that a similar study be carried out with other measurement scales of organizational support and the results be compared and contrasted with our findings.

Abbreviations
ICU: Intensive Care Unit; MDS: Moral Distress Scale; RN: Registered Nurse; SPOS: Survey of Perceived Organizational Support

Acknowledgments
The authors would like to express their gratitude to all the hospitals affiliated to the Ministry of Health and its medical sciences universities, to all the participating nurses and finally to Dr. Eisenberger for allowing us to use the Survey of Perceived organizational support.

Funding
This research project was funded by Shahid Beheshti University of Medical Sciences in Tehran, Iran (Project code: 7582). Shahid Beheshti University of Medical Sciences had no part in the design of the study and collection, analysis, and interpretation of data and in writing the manuscript.

Authors' contributions
All authors (NR, FA, TA, AB and MB) have participated in the conception and design of the study. NR contributed the data collection and prepared the first draft of the manuscript. FA and TA critically revised and checked closely the proposal, the analysis and interpretation of the data and design the article. AB carried out the analysis, interpretation of the data and drafting the manuscript. MB has been involved in revising the manuscript critically. All authors read and approved the final manuscript.

Competing interests
The authors declare that they have no competing interests.

Author details
[1]Student Research Committee of Nursing and Midwifery, International Branch of Shahid Beheshti University of Medical Sciences, Tehran, Iran. [2]Department of Nursing Management, School of Nursing and Midwifery, Shahid Beheshti University of Medical Sciences, Vali-Asr Avenue, Cross of Vali-Asr and Hashemi Rafsanjani Highway, Opposite to Rajaee Heart Hospital, Tehran 1996835119, Iran. [3]School of Nursing and Midwifery, Shahid Beheshti University of Medical Sciences, Tehran, Iran. [4]Department of Biostatistics, School of Allied Medical Sciences, Shahid Beheshti University of Medical Sciences, Tehran, Iran. [5]Department of Nursing, School of Medical Science, Yazd Branch, Islamic Azad University, Yazd, Iran.

References
1. Karagozoglu S, Yildirim G, Ozden D, Çınar Z. Moral distress in Turkish intensive care nurses. Nurs Ethics. 2017;24(2):209–24.
2. Wallis L. Moral distress in nursing. AJN Am J Nurs. 2015;115(3):19–20.
3. Johnstone M-J, Hutchinson A. "Moral distress"–time to abandon a flawed nursing construct? Nurs Ethics. 2015;22(1):5–14.
4. McCarthy J, Gastmans C. Moral distress: a review of the argument-based nursing ethics literature. Nurs Ethics. 2015;22(1):131–52.
5. Corley MC, Minick P, Elswick RK, Jacobs M. Nurse moral distress and ethical work environment. Nurs Ethics. 2005;12(4):381–90.
6. Gallagher A. Moral distress and moral courage in everyday nursing practice. Online J Issues Nurs. 2011;16(2):1–8.
7. Hamric AB, Borchers CT, Epstein EG. Development and testing of an instrument to measure moral distress in healthcare professionals. AJOB Prim Res. 2012;3(2):1–9.
8. Lazzarin M, Biondi A, Di Mauro S. Moral distress in nurses in oncology and haematology units. Nurs Ethics. 2012;19(2):183–95.
9. Rodney PA. What we know about moral distress. AJN Am J Nurs. 2017; 117(2):S7–10.
10. Burston AS, Tuckett AG. Moral distress in nursing: contributing factors, outcomes and interventions. Nurs Ethics. 2013;20(3):312–24.
11. Corley MC, Elswick RK, Gorman M, Clor T. Development and evaluation of a moral distress scale. J Adv Nurs. 2001;33(2):250–6.
12. McCarthy J, Deady R. Moral distress reconsidered. Nurs Ethics. 2008;15(2): 254–62.
13. Eisenberger R, Jones JR, Aselage J, Sucharski IL. Perceived organizational support. J Appl Psychol. 1986;71(3):500–7.
14. Barkhordari-Sharifabad M, Ashktorab T, Atashzadeh-Shoorideh F. Ethical competency of nurse leaders A qualitative study. Nurs Ethics. 2016; Epub ahead of print 14 Jun 2016. DOI: https://doi.org/10.1177/0969733016652125.
15. Maningo-Salinas MJ. Relationship between moral distress, perceived organizational support and intent to turnover among oncology nurses. Minneapolis, MN: Capella University; 2010.
16. Den Hartog DN, De Hoogh AHB. Empowering behaviour and leader fairness and integrity: studying perceptions of ethical leader behaviour from a levels-of-analysis perspective. Eur J Work Organ Psychol. 2009; 18(2):199–230.
17. Mayer DM, Kuenzi M, Greenbaum R, Bardes M, Salvador RB. How low does ethical leadership flow? Test of a trickle-down model. Organ Behav Hum Decis Process. 2009;108:1–13.
18. Neubert MJ, Carlson DS, Kacmar KM, Roberts JA, Chonko LB. The virtuous influence of ethical leadership behavior: evidence from the field. J Bus Ethics. 2009;90(2):157–70.
19. Resick CJ, Hanges PJ, Dickson MW, Mitchelson JK. A cross-cultural examination of the endorsement of ethical leadership. J Bus Ethics. 2006;63(4):345–59.
20. Barkhordari-Sharifabad M, Ashktorab T, Atashzadeh-Shoorideh F. Ethical leadership outcomes in nursing: A qualitative study. Nurs Ethics. 2017; Epub ahead of print 18 Jan 2017. doi: https://doi.org/10.1177/0969733016687157.
21. Erlen JA. Moral distress: a pervasive problem. Orthop Nurs. 2001;20(2):76–80.
22. Liu L, Hu S, Wang L, Sui G, Ma L. Positive resources for combating depressive symptoms among Chinese male correctional officers: perceived organizational support and psychological capital. BMC Psychiatry. 2013;13:89.
23. AbuAlRub RF. Job stress, job performance, and social support among hospital nurses. J Nurs Scholarsh. 2004;36(1):73–8.
24. Adebayo SO, Nwabuoku UC. Conscientiousness and perceived organizational support as predictors of employee absenteeism. Park J Soc Sci. 2008;5(4):363–7.
25. Tumwesigye G. The relationship between perceived organisational support and turnover intentions in a developing country: the mediating role of organisational commitment. African J Bus Manag. 2010;4(6):942–52.
26. Uymaz AO. Prosocial organizational behavior: is it a personal trait or an organizational one. Eur J Bus Manag. 2014;6(2):124–9.
27. Battistelli A, Galletta M, Vandenberghe C, Odoardi C. Perceived organisational support, organisational commitment and self-competence among nurses: a study in two Italian hospitals. J Nurs Manag. 2016;24(1):E44–53.
28. Dehghan Nayeri N, Nazari AA, Salsali M, Ahmadi F, Adib HM. Iranian staff nurses' views of their productivity and management factors improving and impeding it: a qualitative study. Nurs Health Sci. 2006;8(1):51–6.
29. Gorji HA, Etemadi M, Hoseini F. Perceived organizational support and job involvement in the Iranian health care system: a case study of emergency room nurses in general hospitals. J Educ Health Promot. 2014;3:58.
30. Sabokroo M, Kalhorian R, Kamjoo Z, Taleghani G. Work-family conflict: the role of organizational support on intention to leave the job (case study of Tehran hospital nurses). J Public Manag. 2011;3(6):111–26.
31. Shahriari M, Mohammadi E, Abbaszadeh A, Bahrami M, Fooladi MM. Perceived ethical values by Iranian nurses. Nurs Ethics. 2011;19(1):30–44.
32. Esmaelzadeh F, Abbaszadeh A, Borhani F, Peyrovi H. Ethical sensitivity in nursing ethical leadership: a content analysis of Iranian nurses experiences. Open Nurs J. 2017;11:1–13.
33. Atashzadeh-Shorideh F, Ashktorab T, Yaghmaei F. Iranian intensive care unit nurses' moral distress a content analysis. Nurs Ethics. 2012;19(4):464–78.

34. Farsi Z, Dehghan Nayeri N, Negarandeh R, Broomand S. Nursing profession in Iran: an overview of opportunities and challenges. Japan J Nurs Sci 2010; 7(1):9–18.

35. Sadeghi A, Goharloo Arkawaz A, Cheraghi F, Moghimbeigi A. Relationship between head nurses' servant leadership style and nurses' job satisfaction. Q J Nurs Manag. 2015;4(1):28–38.

36. Cheraghi MA, Salsali M, Safari M. Ambiguity in knowledge transfer: the role of theory-practice gap. Iran J Nurs Midwifery Res. 2010;15(4):155–66.

37. Poladi F, Atashzadeh-Shoorideh F, Abaaszade A, Moslemi A. The correlation between moral distress and burnout in nurses working in educational hospitals of Shahid Beheshti University of Medical Sciences during 2013. Iran J Med Ethics Hist Med. 2015;8(4):37–45.

38. Joolaee S, Jalili H, Rafiee F, Haggani H. The relationship between nurses' perception of moral distress and ethical environment in Tehran University of Medical Sciences. Iran J Med Ethics Hist Med. 2011;4(4):56–66.

39. Ameri M, SafaviBayat Z, Ashktorab T, Kavoosi A. Atefeh Vaezi. Moral distress: evaluating nurses' experiences. Iran J Med Ethics Hist Med. 2013;6(1):64–73.

40. Atashzadeh-Shoorideh F, Ashktorab T, Yaghmaei F, Alavi MH. Relationship between ICU nurses' moral distress with burnout and anticipated turnover. Nurs Ethics. 2015;22(1):64–76.

41. Cassells JM, Silva MC, Chop RM. Administrative strategies to support staff nurses as moral agents in clinical practice. Nursingconnections. 1990;3(4):31–7.

42. Corley MC. Nurse moral distress: a proposed theory and research agenda. Nurs Ethics. 2002;9(6):636–50.

43. Olson LL. Ethical climate as the context for nursing retention. J Illinois Nurs. 2002;99(6):3–7.

44. Lee J, Peccei R. Discriminant validity and interaction between perceived organizational support and perceptions of organizational politics: a temporal analysis. J Occup Organ Psychol. 2011;84(4):686–702.

45. Francis CA. The mediating force of "face" supervisor character and status related to perceived organizational support and work outcomes. J Leadersh Organ Stud. 2012;19(1):58–67.

46. Gillet N, Colombat P, Michinov E, Pronost A, Fouquereau E. Procedural justice, supervisor autonomy support, work satisfaction, organizational identification and job performance: the mediating role of need satisfaction and perceived organizational support. J Adv Nurs. 2013;69(11):2560–71.

47. Kwak C, Chung BY, Xu Y, Eun-Jung C. Relationship of job satisfaction with perceived organizational support and quality of care among south Korean nurses: a questionnaire survey. Int J Nurs Stud. 2010;47(10):1292–8.

48. Bobbio A, Bellan M, Manganelli AM. Empowering leadership, perceived organizational support, trust, and job burnout for nurses: a study in an Italian general hospital. Health Care Manag Rev. 2012;37(1):77–87.

49. Woods M, Rodgers V, Towers A, La Grow S. Researching moral distress among New Zealand nurses: a national survey. Nurs Ethics. 2015;22(1):117–30.

50. Cummings CL. The effect of moral distress on nursing retention in the acute care setting. Jacksonville, FL:University of North Florida; 2009.

51. Maiden JM. A quantitative and qualitative inquiry into moral distress, compassion fatigue, and medication error in critical care nurses. San Diego, CA: University of San Diego; 2008.

52. Fernandez-Parsons R, Rodriguez L, Goyal D. Moral distress in emergency nurses. J Emerg Nurs. 2013;39(6):547–52.

53. Pauly B, Varcoe C, Storch J, Newton L. Registered nurses' perceptions of moral distress and ethical climate. Nurs Ethics. 2009;16(5):561–73.

54. Silén M, Svantesson M, Kjellström S, Sidenvall B, Christensson L. Moral distress and ethical climate in a Swedish nursing context: perceptions and instrument usability. J Clin Nurs. 2011;20(23–24):3483–93.

55. O'Connell CB. Gender and the experience of moral distress in critical care nurses. Nurs Ethics. 2015;22(1):32–42.

56. Vaziri MH, Merghati-Khoei E, Tabatabaei S. Moral distress among Iranian nurses. Iran J Psychiatry. 2015;10(1):32–6.

57. Valentine S, Greller MM, Richtermeyer SB. Employee job response as a function of ethical context and perceived organization support. J Bus Res. 2006;59(5):582–8.

58. Fogel KM. The relationships of moral distress, ethical climate, and intent to turnover among critical care nurses. Chicago, IL: The University of Chicago; 2007.

59. Mathumbu D, Dodd N. Perceived organisational support, work engagement and organisational citizenship behaviour of nurses at Victoria Hospital. Aust J Psychol. 2013;4(2):87–93.

15

Challenges faced by nurses in using pain assessment scale in patients unable to communicate

Kolsoum Deldar[1], Razieh Froutan[2]* (iD) and Abbas Ebadi[3]

Abstract

Background: One helpful strategy adopted for pain management in non-verbal, intubated patients is the use of a proper pain assessment scale. The purpose of the present study is to achieve a better and deeper understanding of the existing nurses' challenges in using pain assessment scales among patients unable to communicate.

Methods: This qualitative study was conducted using content analysis. Purposive sampling was used to select the participants and continued until data saturation. The participants included 20 nurses working in intensive care units. Data was collected using semi-structured interviews and analysis was done using an inductive approach.

Results: Four categories and ten sub-categories were extracted from the experiences of the nurses working in the intensive care units in terms of nursing challenges in using non-verbal pain assessment scales. The four categories included "forgotten priority", "organizational barriers", "attitudinal barriers", and "barriers to knowledge".

Conclusions: The findings of the present study have shown that various factors might influence on the use of non-verbal pain assessment scales in patients unable to communicate. Identifying these challenges for nurses can help take effective steps such as empowering nurses in the use of non-verbal pain assessment scales, relieving pain, and improving the quality of care services.

Background

Pain is an unpleasant sensory and emotional experience associated with actual or potential tissue damage or described in terms of such damage [1]. It is a common phenomenon and a major stressor in intubated patients [2–4]. Various reasons other than the original disease, e.g. endotracheal tube suctioning, chest tube insertion, respiratory exercises, coughs, and certain positions on the bed, can cause pain [5–7]. Despite advances in theories related to pain control [8–11], pain is still a major problem in critically ill patients admitted to intensive care units (ICU) and 40–77.4% of ICU patients complain about the experience of pain [12, 13]. Since these patients may suffer from numerous neurological, physiological, and communicative disabilities arising from a variety of reasons including dependence on a mechanical ventilator (MV) and concurrent use of sedatives, they may not be able to accurately estimate the level of their pain [14, 15]. Inappropriate diagnosis of pain experienced by ICU patients is also associated with complications such as increased risk of infection, prolonged MV, hemodynamic disorders, paranoia, immune-suppression, and even death [16–18].

Some researchers believe that the most reliable method of pain evaluation is the patient's self-report [16]. But if patient doesn't have enough ability to provide verbal self-report of pain (e.g. ICU patients), it is recommended to use other available methods for pain management [14].

The first step in the management of pain is its diagnosis and evaluation [19], i.e. a reliable pain assessment tool is essential to efficient pain management [14, 20–22]. Such a tool can contribute to correct decision-making during pain management [23, 24] and promote pain diagnosis and evaluation [25]. Therefore, an effective pain assessment scale should be a part of the recording process system. Since evaluation is a basic principle in nursing care and it can form the foundation for nursing interventions, each

* Correspondence: Froutanr@mums.ac.ir
[2]Department of Medical-Surgical Nursing, School of Nursing and Midwifery, Mashhad University of Medical Sciences, Mashhad, Iran
Full list of author information is available at the end of the article

hospital should have a practical approach to pain measurement [26]. A variety of pain measurement tools, including the Visual Analogue Scale (VAS), Numeric Rating Scale (NRS), Verbal Descriptor Scale (VDS), Smiling Face Scale (SFS), and Numeric Descriptor Scale (NDS), can be used to determine the severity of pain and its related behaviors [27–30]. In addition, the Behavioral Pain Scale (BPS), Critical-Care Pain Observation Tool (CPOT), and Nonverbal Pain Scale (NVPS) can be administered to screen pain in critically ill ICU patients who are unable to communicate [31, 32]. This group of patients may include unconscious, sedated, or intubated patients, as well as those with reduced consciousness levels, communication barriers, or head trauma [10, 33]. However, there are few documents on the use of such scales. According to G'elinas et al. (2004), pain assessment scales were only employed in 1.6% of the 183 events recorded for intubated patients. Although evaluation of pain behaviors was common (reported in 73% of cases), such evaluations and observations were conducted without any valid and reliable tools [34]. In a study on 3601 critically ill intubated patients, Payen et al. (2007) found that pain was not assessed in 53% of the patients who had received pain-killers. Moreover, only 28% of pain evaluations were performed through appropriate and specific pain assessment tools [35].

Since all patients under MV receive analgesics or sedatives, mostly narcotic drugs, pain assessment scales for these patients have not received adequate attention [36]. It seems that efficient pain evaluation and management for critically ill patients has become a major challenge for ICU nurses [21]. Therefore, considering the role of nurses as the main individuals involved in pain evaluation and management, this study sought to address the nurses' challenges in the use of pain assessment tools in patients unable to communicate.

Methods

Study design

This qualitative study was conducted using content analysis. The researchers performed an in-depth direct analysis of experiences of ICU nurses. The findings are presented as codes, subcategories, and categories using an inductive approach [37].

Participants and study setting

The selection of participants was performed using a purposeful sampling method. 20 interviews were conducted with nurses working in ICUs. Subject selection was conducted with maximum variation in personal factors (age, education level, duration of work experience, and organizational role). Data was collected using semi-structured interviews, and analysis was done using an inductive approach. All study participants were interested in sharing their experiences.

Ethical considerations

This study was approved by the Ethics Committee of Mashhad University of Medical Sciences in May 2016 (code: IR.MUMS.REC.1395.159). Moreover, the participants were ensured of data confidentiality and autonomy. They were informed of the purpose of the study and the voluntary nature of their participation. A written consent was obtained from all participants before recording the interviews.

Data collection and analysis

Content analysis was performed on Persian transcripts, before translation. The interviews were started with a number of general questions (e.g. "Please describe one of your experiences of one day working in the ICU.") and continued with more specific questions (e.g. "Please speak about your own experiences of pain management in patients unable to communicate.", "Please describe your experiences of using non-verbal pain scales.", and "What problems and issues do you face?"). Individual semi-structured interviews were conducted in a private room at the participants' workplace.

Based on the Graneheim and Lundman's method [37], the analysis process consisted of the following steps:

1. The recorded interviews were transcribed and read to get an overall understanding.
2. The texts were divided into meaningful units.
3. The meaningful units were extracted and encoded.
4. Based on their similarities and differences, the initial codes were classified into subcategories.

During the open coding stage, all the transcripts were reread closely and thoroughly for several times and the keywords, expressions, incidents, and actualities were noted. The basic codes were taken, and the codes and all extracted data were compared to identify the existing similarities and differences. Afterward, the categories and subcategories were created. A preparatory arrangement of codes, categories, and subcategories was framed from the first interview, and the developing codes were considered as the outcomes.

Trustworthiness

Maximum variation sampling, member checking, and peer questioning and cross-examination were used to ensure the trustworthiness, dependability, and credibility of the data, respectively. In order for member checking, each participant was provided with the transcript of his/her coded interview along with a summary of the extracted themes and asked to determine whether the codes are representative of and matched with their experiences. Peer checking of the transcripts was conducted by two faculty members with a PhD in nursing. They received the transcripts and followed the above-mentioned process to reach the core themes. The obtained inter-rater agreement was equal to or above 90%.

The long presence of the authors in the field (from May 2016 to Apr 2017) enabled them to win the participants' trust and develop strong communication links with the interviewees. This facilitated precise data collection.

Results

The study sample consisted of 20 ICU nurses (nine men and 11 women). The mean age and mean work experience were 35.7 ± 6.1 and 12.3 ± 6.1 years, respectively. Other details are available in Table 1.

The factors inhibiting the use of pain assessment scales in patients unable to communicate were grouped into four categories including "forgotten priority", "organizational barriers", "attitudinal barriers", and "barriers to knowledge" (Table 2).

The findings along with their related quotes are shown below:

Forgotten priority

One of the concepts extracted from data analysis based on the experiences of our participants was "forgotten priority". This category consisted of four subcategories including: "non-routine pain assessment/evaluation", "inadequate physician-nurse interaction regarding patient pain", "absence of non-verbal pain assessment scales in the nursing flowchart", and "lack of relevant policies and clinical guidelines".

Due to non-routine pain assessment/evaluation in patients unable to communicate, nurses did not use pain measurement scales for these patients. As participant #8 stated:

"... I have been working in the ICU for about 7 years... almost all the duties in our shifts are routine... care for the airway and attention to the alarms of the mechanical ventilators... during this time I have not performed evaluation of pain for patients with decreased level of consciousness (LOC)... Well, until now, pain evaluation and recording have not been conducted routinely for these patients... therefore, there has been no necessity to use non-verbal pain assessment scales..."

Table 1 Summary of participant characteristics

Variables	Status	Percent
Gender	Females	55%
	Males	45%
Educational Degree	Bachelor's	90%
	Master's or higher	10%

Table 2 The main categories and related sub-categories

Category	Sub-category
Forgotten priority	Non-routine pain assessment/evaluation
	Inadequate physician-nurse interaction in terms of patient pain
	Absence of non-verbal pain assessment scales in the nursing flowchart
	Lack of policies and clinical guidelines
Organizational barriers	Inadequate nurse-patient ratio
	Presence of less experienced personnel
Attitudinal barriers	Adequacy of sedatives
	Failure to understand pain in unconscious patients
	No belief in non-verbal pain assessment scales
Barriers to knowledge	Unfamiliarity with the use of non-verbal pain assessment scales
	Insufficient training for clinical use of pain assessment scales

The second category of "forgotten priority" was inadequate physician-nurse interaction regarding patient pain. Despite the fact that pain management is an important patient right and a health-care priority, patient pain is seldom mentioned during the visit time. Participant #13 mentioned that:

"...during the visits of intubated patients experiencing decreased LOC; test results, respiratory mode, and so on are discussed and there are not talks about patient pain and its evaluation results... well, this situation can impact the use of non-verbal pain assessment scales for such patients..."

Given the absence of non-verbal pain assessment tools in the nursing flowchart, the nurses believed that no place (in patient record or nursing flowchart) was specified for the use of these standardized tools despite the importance of pain relief in patients under MV. Participant #20 indicated that:

"... We can record the results of arterial blood gases, blood tests, vital signs, and nursing reports in the nursing flowchart... however, no place has been specified for non-verbal pain assessment tools..."

Lack of relevant policies and clinical guidelines was the fourth subcategory obtained from the analysis of "forgotten priority". The participating ICU nurses highlighted the absence of clinical guidelines on the selection and use of various non-verbal pain assessment tools. Participant #17 stated that:

"... It is definitely important to me to relieve pain in patients who cannot self-report it... however, the hospital has never introduced a standardized scale to us even though there are various scales in this context to help the personnel to act in the same manner, but not based on their tastes."

Organizational barriers

The participants underscored "organizational barriers" as other challenges faced by ICU nurses. This category contains two subcategories including "inadequate nurse-to-patient ratio" and "presence of less experienced personnel".

The participants argued that heavy workload and time limitations, consequent to inadequate nurse-to-patient ratio, prevented them from providing constant high-quality care. Participant #12 indicated that:

"Due to the high workload in the ICU, being responsible for two or more patients admitted into the ICU in each shift, health information system recordings, and paperwork; there is no possibility to use non-verbal pain assessment scales."

Analyzing the viewpoints of less experienced nurses (newly employed) showed that their attention and energy was mainly focused on acquiring skills such as working with ICU equipment, doing procedures, and calculating drug dosage. They, hence, had no opportunity to work with non-verbal pain assessment scales. Therefore, the "presence of less experienced personnel" served as another organizational barrier. Participant #9 said that:

"... My incentives in the ICU are to learn about the mechanical ventilators... I significantly focus on the calculation and regulation of infusion of medicines, the alarms of mechanical ventilators,..."

Attitudinal barriers

"Attitudinal barriers" in nurses was another concept derived from data analysis. This category consisted of three subcategories including "adequacy of sedatives", "failure to understand pain in unconscious patients", and "no belief in non-verbal pain assessment scales". Nurses are responsible for pain assessment and should adopt pain-reducing procedures if pain is not relieved. However, the participating nurses believed that there was no need to use pain assessment scales when a patient received sedative infusions. Participant #7 argued that:

"...there is no need to use pain assessment scales for patients with decreased LOC when drugs such as fentanyl are used in the form of infusion... because they are taking sedatives..."

Moreover, the subcategory "failure to understand pain in unconscious patients" was extracted from the participants' statements indicating that patients with decreased LOC could not feel pain. Participant #2 reiterated that:

"...patients with impaired consciousness have no pain... in fact; they do not feel pain... so it is not necessary to use pain assessment scales for such patients..."

The participants believed that non-verbal scales could not measure and evaluate pain correctly. They, thus, had "no belief in non-verbal pain assessment scales". They considered their personal judgments of patient pain as the best pain assessment method. Participant #5 discussed that:

"... Lots of these pain scales are out of use... they are not 100% correct... I feel that I can evaluate and assess pain... an example is the scale developed for embolism... we had cases in which negative embolism was reported using these scales, but the patient was affected with embolism clinically..."

Barriers to knowledge

Another category extracted from data analysis was "barriers to knowledge". This category contained two subcategories including "unfamiliarity with the use of non-verbal pain assessment scales" and "insufficient training on the clinical use of pain assessment scales".

Based on the participants' statements, undergraduate education did not provide nursing students with adequate knowledge on pain assessment. Therefore, unfamiliarity with pain assessment accounted as a major barrier to pain assessment and measurement. Most participating nurses stated that they had not received adequate training on pain assessment and measurement scales in either school or workplace (hospital). Participant #13 said that:

".. well, it is natural that we are kind of familiar with these standardized pain assessment scales... because my colleagues and I, who are working in the ICU, hold undergraduate degrees... well, pain assessment scales are not very often included in the undergraduate programs."

Participant #7 highlighted "insufficient training for the clinical use of pain assessment and measurement scales" and argued that:

"...we have never taken certified training classes in the hospital to become familiar with pain assessment scales as well as the necessity to employ them for patients in the ICU and for those connected to the mechanical ventilator up until now... there have been just sporadic classes in this unit..."

Discussion

Four main categories, including "forgotten priority", "organizational barriers", "attitudinal barriers", and "barriers to knowledge" were extracted from the analysis of the experiences of ICU nurses. Specific subcategories of each category were also determined based on unique and integrated properties. This study was among the first Iranian studies to adopt a qualitative approach to explore the experiences of ICU nurses about the use of pain assessment scales. It sought to answer the question: "What challenges are experienced by ICU nurses when using pain assessment tools in patients unable to communicate?"

The findings of this study indicated that although ICU nurses perform routine practices for patients unable to communicate during each shift; they do not follow a routine pain management protocol in this group of patients. Nevertheless, pain management is a major determinant of nursing care quality, i.e. pain should be evaluated when vital signs are measured and its relief should be considered as the core and essence of nursing care [38]. Nurses are also responsible for the prevention or reduction of pain [39]. They are, in fact, one of the important healthcare team members with proper opportunities to assess, identify, and evaluate pain management. They are, hence, required to play an active role in pain management. However, few studies have shown that nurses are actually playing such roles [40].

While nurses' efforts for pain management mainly aim to improve patient outcomes, there is no appropriate non-verbal pain assessment scale to evaluate pain in ICU patients. It seems that failure in this respect can lead to decreased quality of pain management in patients unable to communicate. According to Bucknall et al. (2007), nurses can only make effective decisions for pain management through the repeated and regular evaluation of pain intensity and related behaviors [41]. Erdek et al. (2004) concluded that there was not an appropriate form of pain assessment in ICU patients and such patients were unable to self-report their pain [42]. A study in Jordan reported that the existing pain assessment methods applied in the ICUs of the country only focused on pain management among patients suffering from cancer. In fact, no particular pain assessment tools were used for ICU patients who are unable to communicate

[43]. Similar barriers were reported by ICU nurses in the United States [42].

The experiences of the ICU nurses in this study indicated that physicians' inattention to pain monitoring, decreased nurse's attention to pain and its relief. Our participants reported physicians focused on several complications, such as fever, but failed to evaluate pain. Nevertheless, pain relief is an essential human right and a major nursing priority [44].

The absence of non-verbal pain assessment scales in nursing flowcharts is another challenge which ICU nurse's face while adopting pain management strategies. Currently, the nursing flowchart in these units only uses VAS and SFS to record patient pain. However, there is a need for a standardized form of non-verbal pain assessment and measurement for patients unable to communicate. In the absence of such scales, as well as a specific system for the analysis of their results, the effectiveness of treatments cannot be accurately determined [10]. However, the inclusion of the pain management section in the ICU checklist, as a part of daily activities, can be considered as a valuable scale for reducing patient discomfort [45].

The ICU nurses participating in this study used infusions of sedatives and narcotic drugs for patients unable to communicate without following any pain assessment scales and specific guidelines. Lack of relevant policies and guidelines on pain control was also reported by Keykha et al. (2013) [46]. Nevertheless, lack of access to clinical pain management guidelines can negatively affect pain management [29, 47], i.e. the use of guidelines and non-verbal pain assessment scales would have positive effects on the experience of pain reduction in ICU patients.

Based on the findings of the present study, the undesirable nurse-to-patient ratio in the ICUs and nurses' heavy workload forced nurses to disregard some clinical practices and prevented them from the frequent use of pain assessment tools. The time limits could also interfere with the quality of care and were thus considered as a barrier to optimal care [48]. On the other hand, limited time forced nurses to prioritize duties of equal importance [49]. Unfortunately, the alarming shortage of nurses is considered as an important challenge in healthcare systems [50, 51]. In Iran, there is a need for over100 thousand more nurses [52].

Apart from the issue of time, experiences and skills of the nurses are similarly critical in pain diagnosis [53]. The less experienced ICU nurses recruited in this study had no opportunities for performing pain measurement and working with non-verbal pain assessment tools because they were mostly interested in the acquisition of other skills (e.g. working with the MV and other equipment).

The findings of this study highlighted the viewpoints of ICU personnel's as other factors influencing the use of pain assessment scales. In fact, pain management often depends on the viewpoints, culture, and beliefs of the health-care team [54]. The ICU nurses in this study believed that there was no need to use pain assessment scales for patients receiving sedatives. Examining their viewpoints and experiences also revealed that the personnel did not feel any need to assess pain in patients when they were receiving pain-killers and sedatives prior to performing invasive and painful procedures. The findings of a study in this respect also showed that most patients under an MV received sedatives and pain-killers without any particular pain assessment [35]. However, prescribing the correct dosage of sedatives in patients with decreased LOC requires the routine administration of pain assessment tools [55]. Enskar et al. (2007) showed that Swedish nurses had more knowledge about pain assessment and more positive attitudes towards pain. These factors could lead to better pain relief [56].

"Failure to understand pain in unconscious patients" was another concept derived from the experiences of the ICU personnel in this study. The nurses argued that patients with decreased LOC had no pains, i.e. pain assessment and scales were not necessary for these patients. Likewise, nurses in other investigations mainly neglected pain in unconscious patients. They did not actually consider pain as a serious issue since they assumed that patients with decreased LOC did not have a sense of pain [57]. However, the point of importance is that the state of sleep and sedation is not equal to the absence of pain or its relief [14]. It is difficult to evaluate pain in such patients due to the inability to communicate following decreased LOC, receiving sedatives, and using the MV. Consequently, inadequate pain management and control in unconscious patients has been raised as a challenge in nursing care [58].

The final concept obtained from this category of experiences by ICU nurses was "no belief in pain management scales". The nurses did not believe in pain scales and argued that personal judgment of the patient's pain was the best method of pain assessment because they had experiences of ineffective use of other tools such as the scale for embolism. Given their high workload and time limits, these nurses also believed that they could assess patients' pain only through the patient's face and observation of their hemodynamics. Other studies have also mentioned personal beliefs and viewpoints as major barriers in this respect. The personnel's lack of belief can thus lead to treating patients based on their personal opinions [59]. Given that nurses need tools to correctly assess pain [39, 60], they should avoid personal assessment and judgment in this respect.

The concept of "barriers to knowledge" indicates that "unfamiliarity with non-verbal pain assessment scales" and "inadequate ability to use non-verbal pain assessment scales" are among the main challenges in this domain. In the present study, the ICU nurses did not use pain measurement scales because they received little information in their undergraduate programs or in-service re-training courses about pain assessment scales. Most nurses believed that they were not well prepared for this function during their training courses presented in nursing education centers [61].

Moreover, Rose et al. (2012) examined the performance of ICU nurses regarding pain management and control. They reported that nurses were not willing to use pain assessment scales in non-verbal patients and that they had little information about such scales, which could negatively affect their performance in terms of patient pain management [62].

In this regard, Farahani et al. (2008) stated that inadequacy of training courses for pain measurement was one of the significant barriers to its use [63]. Therefore, training pain assessment scales, their use and the related guidelines are of utmost importance for improving systematic pain assessment in ICU patients and ultimately for increasing nurses' knowledge of pain care.

Conclusion

The findings of the present study indicate that various factors such as "forgotten priority", "organizational barriers", "attitudinal barriers", and "barriers to knowledge" could affect the use of scales for pain assessment and management in patients unable to communicate. Given the inability to self-report in these patients, pain cannot be properly assessed and treated in such patients. The existing barriers to using non-verbal pain assessment scales in these patients can also lead to false evaluations of pain by nurses and consequently unrealistic perception of pain and inadequate medication. Identifying these challenges for nurses can help take effective steps such as empowering nurses in the use of non-verbal pain assessment scales, relieving pain, and improving the quality of care services.

Abbreviations
ICU: Intensive care unit; LOC: Decreased level of consciousness; MV: Mechanical ventilator

Acknowledgements
We are grateful to Research deputy of Mashhad University of Medical Sciences for great cooperation on this research. Also we would like to thank all the ICU nurses who participated in our study and gave up their valuable time to be interviewed.

Funding
No funding.

Authors' contributions
RF led the study; RF, KD and AE contributed to the design of the study; RF and AE analyzed the data; all authors interpreted the findings; RF and KD compiled the first draft of the paper; all authors commented on drafts of the paper and approved the final draft of the paper.

Competing interests
The authors declare that they have no competing interests.

Author details
[1]Department of Medical Informatics, Faculty of Medicine, Mashhad University of Medical Sciences, Mashhad, Iran. [2]Department of Medical-Surgical Nursing, School of Nursing and Midwifery, Mashhad University of Medical Sciences, Mashhad, Iran. [3]Behavioral Sciences Research Center, Faculty of Nursing, Baqiyatallah University of Medical Sciences, Tehran, Iran.

References
1. IASP Taxonomy [https://www.iasp-pain.org/Taxonomy?navItemNumber=576#Pain]. Accessed June 2017.
2. Campbell GB, Happ MB. Symptom identification in the chronically critically ill. AACN advanced critical care. 2010;21(1):64.
3. Pandharipande PP, Patel MB, Barr J. Management of pain, agitation, and delirium in critically ill patients. Pol Arch Med Wewn. 2014;124(3):114–22.
4. Stanik-Hutt JA, Soeken KL, Belcher AE, Fontaine DK. Pain experiences of traumatically injured patients in a critical care setting. Am J Crit Care. 2001;10(4):252.
5. Arroyo-Novoa CM, Figueroa-Ramos MI, Puntillo KA, Stanik-Hutt J, Thompson CL, White C, Wild LR. Pain related to tracheal suctioning in awake acutely and critically ill adults: a descriptive study. Intensive and Critical Care Nursing. 2008;24(1):20–7.
6. Bergeron DA, Leduc G, Marchand S, Bourgault P. Descriptive study of the evaluation process and documentation of postoperative pain in a university hospital [in French]. Pain Res Manag. 2011;16:81–6.
7. Li D, Miaskowski C, Burkhardt D, Puntillo K. Evaluations of physiologic reactivity and reflexive behaviors during noxious procedures in sedated critically ill patients. J Crit Care. 2009;24(3):472. e479-472. e413.
8. Gélinas C, Johnston C. Pain assessment in the critically ill ventilated adult: validation of the critical-care pain observation tool and physiologic indicators. Clin J Pain. 2007;23(6):497–505.
9. Pudas-Tähkä SM, Axelin A, Aantaa R, Lund V, Salanterä S. Pain assessment tools for unconscious or sedated intensive care patients: a systematic review. J Adv Nurs. 2009;65(5):946–56.
10. Shannon K, Bucknall T. Pain assessment in critical care: what have we learnt from research. Intensive and critical care nursing. 2003;19(3):154–62.
11. Watt-Watson J, Stevens B, Garfinkel P, Streiner D, Gallop R. Relationship between nurses' pain knowledge and pain management outcomes for their postoperative cardiac patients. J Adv Nurs. 2001;36(4):535–45.
12. Gélinas C. Management of pain in cardiac surgery ICU patients: have we improved over time? Intensive and Critical Care Nursing. 2007;23(5):298–303.
13. Li DT, Puntillo K. A pilot study on coexisting symptoms in intensive care patients. Appl Nurs Res. 2006;19(4):216–9.
14. Herr K, Coyne PJ, Key T, Manwarren R, McCaffery M, Merkel S, Pelosi-Kelly J, Wild L. Pain assessment in the nonverbal patient: position statement with clinical practice recommendations. Pain Management Nursing. 2006;7(2):44–52.
15. Rose L, Haslam L, Dale C, Knechtel L, Fraser M, Pinto R, McGillion M, Watt-Watson J. Survey of assessment and management of pain for critically ill adults. Intensive and Critical Care Nursing. 2011;27(3):121–8.
16. Puntillo K, Pasero C, Li D, Mularski RA, Grap MJ, Erstad BL, Varkey B, Gilbert HC, Medina J, Sessler CN. Evaluation of pain in ICU patients. CHEST Journal. 2009;135(4):1069–74.
17. Sacerdote P, Bianchi M, Gaspani L, Manfredi B, Maucione A, Terno G, Ammatuna M, Panerai AE. The effects of tramadol and morphine on immune responses and pain after surgery in cancer patients. Anesth Analg. 2000;90(6):1411–4.
18. Skrobik Y, Ahern S, Leblanc M, Marquis F, Awissi DK, Kavanagh BP. Protocolized intensive care unit management of analgesia, sedation, and delirium improves analgesia and subsyndromal delirium rates. Anesth Analg. 2010;111(2):451–63.
19. IASP curriculum outline on pain for nursing [https://www.iasp-pain.org/Education/CurriculumDetail.aspx?ItemNumber=2052]. Accessed June 2017.
20. Assessment and management of pain (3[ed].) [http://rnao.ca/sites/rnao-ca/files/AssessAndManagementOfPain_10_FINAL_WEB_Dec_24.pdf]. Accessed June 2017.
21. Barr J, Fraser GL, Puntillo K, Ely EW, Gélinas C, Dasta JF, Davidson JE, Devlin JW, Kress JP, Joffe AM. Clinical practice guidelines for the management of pain, agitation, and delirium in adult patients in the intensive care unit. Crit Care Med. 2013;41(1):263–306.
22. Herr K, Coyne PJ, McCaffery M, Manworren R, Merkel S. Pain assessment in the patient unable to self-report: position statement with clinical practice recommendations. Pain Management Nursing. 2011;12(4):230–50.
23. Gélinas C. Pain assessment in the critically ill adult: recent evidence and new trends. Intensive and Critical Care Nursing. 2016;34:1–11.
24. Wøien H, Bjørk IT. Intensive care pain treatment and sedation: nurses' experiences of the conflict between clinical judgement and standardised care: an explorative study. Intensive and Critical Care Nursing. 2013;29(3):128–36.
25. Arbour C, Gélinas C, Michaud C. Impact of the implementation of the critical-care pain observation tool (CPOT) on pain management and clinical outcomes in mechanically ventilated trauma intensive care unit patients: a pilot study. Journal of Trauma Nursing. 2011;18(1):52–60.
26. Buffum MD, Hutt E, Chang VT, Craine MH, Snow AL. Cognitive impairment and pain management: review of issues and challenges. J Rehabil Res Dev. 2007;44(2):315.
27. Chanques G, Viel E, Constantin JM, Jung B, de Lattre S, Carr J, Cisse M, Lefrant JY, Jaber S. The measurement of pain in intensive care unit: comparison of 5 self-report intensity scales. Pain. 2010;151(3):711–21.
28. Egan M, Cornally N. Identifying barriers to pain management in long-term care: Mary Egan and Nicola Cornally discuss to what extent patient, organisational and caregiver factors hamper the delivery of best practice. Nursing Older People. 2013;25(7):25–31.
29. Hjermstad MJ, Fayers PM, Haugen DF, Caraceni A, Hanks GW, Loge JH, Fainsinger R, Aass N, Kaasa S. Studies comparing numerical rating scales, verbal rating scales, and visual analogue scales for assessment of pain intensity in adults: a systematic literature review. J Pain Symptom Manag. 2011;41(6):1073–93.
30. Souza RC, Garcia DM, Sanches MB, Gallo AM, Martins CP. IL S: [nursing team knowledge on behavioral assessment of pain in critical care patients]. Revista gaucha de enfermagem. 2013;34(3):55–63.
31. Chen J, Lu Q, Wu X-Y, An Y-Z, Zhan Y-C, Zhang H-Y. Reliability and validity of the Chinese version of the behavioral pain scale in intubated and non-intubated critically ill patients: two cross-sectional studies. Int J Nurs Stud. 2016;61:63–71.
32. Sole ML, Klein DG, Moseley MJ. Introduction to critical care nursing. 6th ed. St. Louis: Elsevier Health Sciences; 2013.
33. Aissaoui Y, Zeggwagh AA, Zekraoui A, Abidi K, Abouqal R. Validation of a behavioral pain scale in critically ill, sedated, and mechanically ventilated patients. Anesth Analg. 2005;101(5):1470–6.
34. Gélinas C, Fortier M, Viens C, Fillion L, Puntillo K. Pain assessment and management in critically ill intubated patients: a retrospective study. Am J Crit Care. 2004;13(2):126–36.
35. Payen J-F, Chanques G, Mantz J, Hercule C, Auriant I, Leguillou J-L, Binhas M, Genty C, Rolland C, Bosson J-L. Current practices in sedation and analgesia for mechanically ventilated critically ill PatientsA prospective multicenter patient-based study. The Journal of the American Society of Anesthesiologists. 2007;106(4):687–95.

36. Burry LD, Williamson DR, Perreault MM, Rose L, Cook DJ, Ferguson ND, Lapinsky SC, Mehta S. Analgesic, sedative, antipsychotic, and neuromuscular blocker use in Canadian intensive care units: a prospective, multicentre, observational study. Canadian Journal of Anesthesia/Journal canadien d'anesthésie. 2014;61(7):619–30.

37. Graneheim UH, Lundman B. Qualitative content analysis in nursing research: concepts, procedures and measures to achieve trustworthiness. Nurse Educ Today. 2004;24(2):105–12.

38. Idvall E, Ehrenberg A. Nursing documentation of postoperative pain management. J Clin Nurs. 2002;11(6):734–42.

39. Layman Young J, Horton FM, Davidhizar R. Nursing attitudes and beliefs in pain assessment and management. J Adv Nurs. 2006;53(0034):412–21.

40. Dihle A, Bjølseth G, Helseth S. The gap between saying and doing in postoperative pain management. J Clin Nurs. 2006;15(4):469–79.

41. Bucknall T, Manias E, Botti M. Nurses' reassessment of postoperative pain after analgesic administration. Clin J Pain. 2007;23(1):1–7.

42. Erdek MA, Pronovost PJ. Improving assessment and treatment of pain in the critically ill. Int J Qual Health Care. 2004;16(1):59–64.

43. Batiha A-M, Bashaireh I, AlBashtawy M, Shennaq S. Exploring the competency of the Jordanian intensive care nurses towards endotracheal tube and oral care practices for mechanically ventilated patients: an observational study. Global Journal of Health Science. 2013;5(1):203.

44. Sein E, Groh K. Help your patients beat their pain with preoperative education. Pain management: special interest group newsletter. 2004;14(2). Available at: http://onsopcontent.ons.org/Publications/SIGNewsletters/pm/pm14.2.html#home. Accessed Nov 2017.

45. Mularski RA, Osborne ML. Palliative care and intensive care unit care: daily intensive care unit care plan checklist# 123. J Palliat Med. 2006;9(5):1205–6.

46. Keykha A, Abbaszadeh A, Enayati H, Borhani F, Rafiei H, Hoseini BMK. Applying the instruction of pain control and sedation of the patients hospitalized in intensive care unit. Iran J Crit Care Nurs. 2013;6(4):249–58.

47. Borgsteede SD, Rhodius CA, De Smet PAGM, Pasman HRW, Onwuteaka-Philipsen BD, Rurup ML. The use of opioids at the end of life: knowledge level of pharmacists and cooperation with physicians. Eur J Clin Pharmacol. 2011;67(1):79–89.

48. Batiha A-M. Pain management barriers in critical care units: a qualitative study. International Journal of Advanced Nursing Studies. 2014;3(1):1.

49. Gunther M, Thomas SP. Nurses' narratives of unforgettable patient care events. J Nurs Scholarsh. 2006;38(4):370–6.

50. Duvall JJ, Andrews DR. Using a structured review of the literature to identify key factors associated with the current nursing shortage. J Prof Nurs. 2010;26(5):309–17.

51. McMurtrie LJ, Cameron M, Oluanaigh P, Osborne YT. Keeping our nursing and midwifery workforce: factors that support non-practising clinicians to return to practice. Nurse Educ Today. 2014;34(5):761–5.

52. Zarea K, Negarandeh R, Dehghan-Nayeri N, Rezaei-Adaryani M. Nursing staff shortages and job satisfaction in Iran: issues and challenges. Nursing & health sciences. 2009;11(3):326–31.

53. Sohrabi MB, Aghayan SM, Zolfaghari P, Delmoradi F, Amerian F, Ghasemian Aghmashhadi M. Study on Signs of Pain in Neonatals Knowledge & Health. 2011;6(3):50–3.

54. Albertyn R, Rode H, Millar AJW, Thomas J. Challenges associated with paediatric pain management in sub Saharan Africa. Int J Surg. 2009;7(2):91–3.

55. Gordon DB, Dahl JL, Miaskowski C, McCarberg B, Todd KH, Paice JA, Lipman AG, Bookbinder M, Sanders SH, Turk DC. American pain society recommendations for improving the quality of acute and cancer pain management: American pain society quality of care task force. Arch Intern Med. 2005;165(14):1574–80.

56. Enskär K, Ljusegren G, Berglund G, Eaton N, Harding R, Mokoena J, Chauke M, Moleki M. Attitudes to and knowledge about pain and pain management, of nurses working with children with cancer: a comparative study between UK, South Africa and Sweden. J Res Nurs. 2007;12(5):501–15.

57. Urden LD, Stacy KM, Thelan LA, Lough ME: Thelan's critical care nursing: diagnosis and management: Mosby Inc. 2006.

58. Urden LDSK, Lough ME. Critical care nursing diagnosis and management. 6th ed. London: Mosby; 2010.

59. Topolovec-Vranic J, Canzian S, Innis J, Pollmann-Mudryj MA, McFarlan AW, Baker AJ. Patient satisfaction and documentation of pain assessments and management after implementing the adult nonverbal pain scale. Am J Crit Care. 2010;19(4):345–54.

60. Kohr R, Sawhney M. Advanced practice nurses' role in the treatment of pain. Canadian Nurse. 2005;101(3):30–4.

61. Manias E, Botti M, Bucknall T. Observation of pain assessment and management – the complexities of clinical practice. J Clin Nurs. 2002;11(6):724–33.

62. Rose L, Smith O, Gélinas C, Haslam L, Dale C, Luk E, Burry L, McGillion M, Mehta S, Watt-Watson J. Critical care nurses' pain assessment and management practices: a survey in Canada. Am J Crit Care. 2012;21(4):251–9.

63. Farahani P, Alhani F. Barriers to the use of pain assessment tools for children by nurses. Journal of Nursing and Midwifery. 2008;18:40–4.

16

Nursing education challenges and solutions in Sub Saharan Africa

Thokozani Bvumbwe[1]* ⓘ and Ntombifikile Mtshali[2]

Abstract

Background: The Lancet Commission and the Global Health Workforce Alliance reported that professional education has generally not kept up the pace of health care challenges. Sub Saharan Africa needs an effective and efficient nursing education system to build an adequate, competent and relevant nursing workforce necessary for the achievement of Sustainable Development Goals. The Plan of Action for Scaling up Quality Nursing and Midwifery Education and Practice for the African Region 2012 - 2022 provided a framework for scale up of nurses and midwives. This integrative review examined literature on nursing education challenges and solutions in Sub Saharan Africa to inform development of a model for improving the quality, quantity and relevance of nursing education at local level.

Methods: A search of PubMed, Medline on EBCSOhost and Google Scholar was conducted using key words: nursing education, challenges, solutions and/ or Africa. Published works from 2012 to 2016 were reviewed to explore reports about challenges and solution in nursing education in Sub Saharan Africa. Full texts of relevant studies were retrieved after reading the tittles and abstracts. Critical appraisal was undertaken and the findings of the relevant studies were analysed using thematic analysis.

Results: Twenty articles and five grey sources were included. Findings of the review generally supports World Health Organisation framework for transformative and scale up of health professions education. Six themes emerged; curriculum reforms, profession regulation, transformative teaching strategies, collaboration and partnership, capacity building and infrastructure and resources. Challenges and solutions in nursing education are common within countries. The review shows that massive investment by development partners is resulting in positive development of nursing education in Sub Saharan Africa. However, strategic leadership, networking and partnership to share expertise and best practices are critical.

Conclusion: Sub Saharan Africa needs more reforms to increase capacity of educators and mentors, responsiveness of curricula, strongly regulatory frameworks, and availability of infrastructure and resources. The review adds to the body of knowledge to enhance efforts of stakeholders in the improvement of the quality, quantity and relevance of nursing education in Sub Saharan Africa.

Background

Sub Saharan Africa continues to report poor health indicators with challenged health systems due to growing burden of diseases including HIV/ AIDS and non-communicable diseases and a severe shortage of health care workers [1–4]. Shortage of healthcare workers threatens the sustainability of health care systems and negatively affects the achievement of newly launched Sustainable Development Goals (SDGs) in many countries [5, 6]. Sub Saharan Africa is

worst hit region with a shortfall of more than 600,000 nurses needed to scale up priority interventions [7]. The Lancet Commission and the Global Health Workforce Alliance reported that professional education has generally not kept up the pace of health care challenges [8–10]. The commission noted challenges with health professional education namely; mismatch of competencies to patient and population needs, poor teamwork, persistent gender stratification of professional status, narrow technical focus without broader contextual understanding, predominantly hospital orientation at the expense of primary care and weak leadership to improve health system performance [11].

* Correspondence: bvumbwe.tm@mzuni.ac.mw
[1]Faculty of Health Sciences, Mzuzu University, P/ Bag 201, Luwinga, Mzuzu, Malawi
Full list of author information is available at the end of the article

There is a global consensus that nurses and midwives constitute the majority of the global health workforce and the largest health care expenditure [8]. Nurses form the universal access point for almost 90% of healthcare users [12, 13]. Considering the significance of nursing workforce within the health care systems, efficient production, successful deployment, and ongoing retention are key to ensuring improvements in the functioning and impact of health care system including ensuring universal health coverage [9, 14]. Efficient production of nurses with relevant competencies remains a critical role of nursing education. Improvements in nursing and midwifery education are recognized as essential in increasing workforce numbers and enhancing the quality of health care and health systems.

Traditionally, nursing and midwifery education has been offered at stand-alone training institutions with more emphasis of production of lower level cadre. Many countries including Malawi, Zambia, Kenya, Zimbabwe still have majority of their nurses at technician level than registered nurse level. However, nursing and midwifery education in Africa has shown signs of development over the past two decades. World Health Organization [15] reported that many countries have now including Masters or Doctoral levels studies in their programs. Nursing colleges in many countries are affiliating their programmes to universities. The Geneva Declaration of the SIDIEF adopted in 2012 urges Francophone countries to introduce university education system for nurses and make undergraduate programme an entry requirement for the nursing profession [16]. Similarly, the Plan of action for Scaling Up Quality Nursing and Midwifery Education and Practice for the African Region 2012 – 2022 provides a framework for WHO member states to improve nursing and midwifery education and training and produce well trained nurses and midwives [17].

However, literature still report lack of necessary competencies among graduates due to lack of strategic leadership to drive transformation [9], unresponsive curricula [18, 19], shortage of nursing faculty and shortage of teaching and learning resources resulting into inadequate productive capacity of training institutions. Globally, nursing education continues to experience underinvestment, static and rigid curriculum, lack of inter-professional preparation of nurses and lack of co-ordinated collaboration and support from stakeholders.

The Plan of Action for Scaling up Quality Nursing and Midwifery Education and Practice for the African Region 2012 – 2022 provided a framework for scale up of nurses and midwives in the region. The purpose of this study was to review literature on status of nursing education in Sub Saharan Africa to inform development of a model for improvement of quality, quantity and relevance of nursing education at local level.

Methods

The researchers were informed by the works of Whittemore and Knafl [20] which has five stages; problem identification, literature search, data evaluation, data analysis and presentation.

Problem identification

The research problem emanated from a Norwegian Church Aid (NCA) funded National Nursing Education Research Conference and anecdotal notes from nursing education stakeholders who identified shortage of nursing workforce and growing concerns of poor quality of nursing care because of inefficiencies in the nursing education system. The review was guided by the following research questions: what is the status of nursing education in Sub Saharan Africa, and what are the solutions or innovations being taken to improve nursing education?

Literature search

A search of PubMed, MEDLINE, Academic search complete, health sources on EBCSOhost and Google scholar was conducted using the key words; nursing education, challenges, solutions, innovations AND Africa. The inclusion criteria for electronic records included primary source and peer reviewed reports on nursing education in Sub Saharan Africa. The review included literature from 2012 to 2016 to capture what has been reported during the period after the Plan of action for Scaling up Quality Nursing and Midwifery Education and Practice for the African Region 2012 – 2022. Peer reviewed records were targeted to ensure integrity of findings because they already have a level of scrutiny. The review also included a search of grey literature as well as extensive consultation with nursing education experts to identify relevant documents. Key stakeholders including nurse educators, nursing education policy makers were individually approached to voluntarily provide material they knew would be relevant including program documents, project reports and progress reports on nursing education. The process of the integrative review is presented in Fig. 1.

Data evaluation

Records were evaluated for their authenticity, methodological quality and informational value. A structured data extraction and quality appraisal checklist was utilized on each record for information extraction based on the Critical Appraisal Skills programme Checklist. Initially records were selected based on their titles. Abstracts of selected titles were analysed to assess their relevance to the study question. Only abstracts that

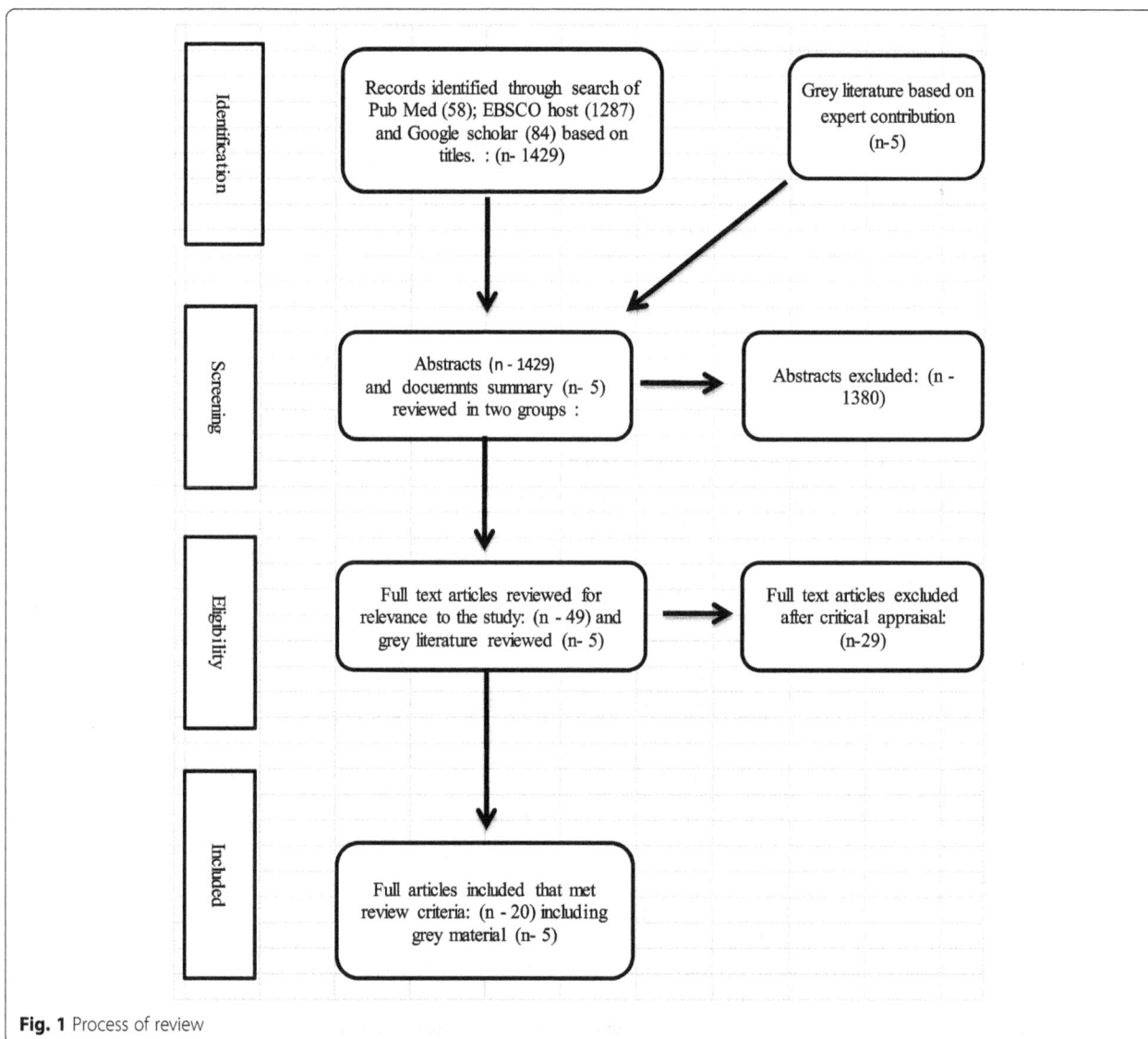

Fig. 1 Process of review

addressed nursing education challenges and solutions in Africa after 2012 were subjected to a full text review. Full text records that did not meet the appraisal process were excluded from the review. Relevant bibliographies from the identified records were also reviewed.

Data analysis

Thematic analysis was used to analyse data. Data was extracted and coded into manageable framework. This was then displayed to convert extracted data from individual sources into a display that assembles around particular variables or subgroups. Extracted data was compared item by item so that similar data was categorised and grouped together. An iterative process of examining data displays to facilitate distinction of patterns, themes, variations and relationships was done using a comparison method. Conclusions were then

drawn from the data. To ensure reliability of the review, the articles and the appraisal forms were independently reviewed by two colleagues. Findings from the researchers and the independent evaluators were compared and discussions were held to reach an agreement.

Results

The search conducted yielded a total of 1434 records. One thousand two hundred and eighty seven (1287) records were obtained from EBSCOhost database, 58 records from PubMed and 84 from Google scholar and 5 grey records obtained from experts. One thousand three hundred and eighty (1380) abstracts were excluded either because they addressed nursing education outside Sub Saharan Africa or addressed education of health professions in general. Twenty nine (29) full text reports were excluded from the study because they neither addressed the challenges nor the solutions of nursing education. Majority of the records addressed perceptions and experiences of nursing students with the nursing training. Finally, twenty (20) records and five (5) grey material were finally included in the review (Table 1).

Six themes emerged from the review namely; curriculum reforms, professional regulation, transformative teaching strategies, collaboration and partnership, capacity building and infrastructure and resources.

Theme 1: Curriculum reforms

Health care reforms alter the environment in which nurses and other health care workers practice. The review found that in Sub Saharan Africa, emphasis on primary care, emerging of new health challenges, increasing burden of disease significantly demand need for curriculum reforms [21–23]. Mthembu et al. [22] reported that reforms in curricula are necessary to ensure that nursing education produces graduates who influence the quality of the health care system and are relevant to the needs of the population.

Mtshali and Gwele [21] developed a middle range model that would guide the practice of community based education in basic nursing education in South Africa. This curriculum reform in nursing education reported community based education as relevant, responsive education and education for social justice that consciously and deliberately socialize health delivery towards primary health care. We also found that countries within Sub Saharan Africa are prioritizing curriculum reforms from content driven curriculum to competence based curriculum that are responsive to the primary health care [23]. We also found that prevalence of chronic illnesses and co-morbidities that are emerging demands an inter-professional approach and collaboration to manage health [24].

Theme 2: Profession regulation

Within the changing face of nursing education, key issues in Sub Saharan Africa related to professional regulation include notions of specialist and advanced practice, accountability and autonomy, competence, supervision, continuing education and delegation [25]. McCarthy et al. [25] highlighted that nursing education should complement, advocate and lend technical support to regulatory bodies as regulatory frameworks change due to health care adaptation. The review highlighted that strengthening nursing councils and professional associations helps to improve regulatory activities. Licensure, accreditation, continuing professional development, and scope of practice influence the quality of care provided by the nursing workforce as well as pre-service education program [26].

Theme 3: Transformative teaching strategies

Appiagyei et al. [27] observed that congestions of students in clinical sites will demand innovative ways to train the growing numbers. As student populations and methods of learning continue to increase in diversity, nurse educators and administrators must be flexible and responsive with effective and innovative solutions to complex market demands. The review found that innovative approaches to teaching and learning are significant for teaching future professions [28]. The complexity of health care demands requires critical thinking as well as competencies that are relevant to these demands. Thus demands for the use of innovative methods of teaching that engage students as active learners, continue to grow. Technology facilitates students' exposure to clinical scenarios that they would normally not encounter in their normal clinical setting [29–31].

Theme 4: Collaboration and partnerships

We found that the complexity of healthcare demands and practice environment require a coordinated and collaborative approach to training of health professionals including nurses. However, the review show that nurses' engagement in policy making is still complex and contested [32]. Evidence based practice requires decisions about healthcare based on best available, current, valid and relevant evidence. Goosby and von Zinkernagel [33] highlighted that partnerships form a strong foundation for planning and delivery of evidence based health services.

We found that the changing learning environment, competition for learning opportunities and limitations in terms of clinical support pose challenges for professional nurses to perform their multifaceted role [34]. Professional nurses play dual roles of service delivery and clinical teaching and mentoring. Careful planning of students learning experiences is imperative to ensure that students get maximum benefits from their training. Middleton et al. [35] reported that current reforms in nursing education demands sharing of knowledge and information. National and regional networks increase opportunities for sharing best practice in nursing.

Themes 5: Capacity building

Challenges facing nursing education in Sub Saharan Africa demands strong committed leadership to see mutual goals and strategic contribution and effective use of resources [36]. Building management capacity of nursing training institutions is one strategy that various countries have put in place to ensure adequate and quality education of nurses to strengthen their weak healthcare system. Nursing education operates within a complex environment which has to constantly be put under vigorous evaluation in order to encourage innovations that will

Table 1 Summary of records reviewed

Author and year	Country	Tittle	Contribution to nursing education
Middleton, L., Howard, A, Dohrn, J, Von Zinkernagel, D. et al., 2014	Sub Saharan	The Nursing Education Partnership Initiative (NEPI): Innovations in nursing and midwifery education.	Building on existing country leadership and government planning to increase the number and competencies of new nurses entering the profession. Country-level leadership, support for faculty workforce development and key educational processes and practices, and scaling up of proven educational methods and interventions at nursing educational institutions are key to ensuring sustainability and will help to achieve priority health goals for the countries of this region.
Mthembu, S., Mtshali, N., Frantz, J. 2014	South Africa	Contextual determinants for community-based learning programmes in nursing education in South Africa	Community Based Learning has emerged as a political instrument that has influenced not only a change in the country's health system but has responded to the needs of the South African population at large
Goosby, E.P, von Zinkernagel, D. 2014	Sub Saharan	The Medical and Nursing Education Partnership Initiatives.	The MEPI and NEPI focus on strengthening learning institutions is central to the vision for expanding the pool of health professionals to meet the full range of a country's health needs. A robust network of exchange between education institutions and training facilities, both within and across countries, is transforming the quality of medical and nursing education and augmenting a platform for research opportunities for faculty and clinicians, which also serves as an incentive to retain professionals in the country.
Jooste, K. & Jasper, M. 2012	South Africa	A South African perspective: current position and challenges in health care service management and education in nursing.	Different role players are involved in critical issues regarding the management and education of nursing in South Africa. Nurse managers are central to the success of service redesign, delivery and education. Nurse managers need to influence policy decisions regarding nursing service design and delivery, and the education required to prepare the next generation of practitioners for these new services.
Armstrong, S. & Rispel, L. 2015	South Africa	Social accountability and nursing education in South Africa	Social accountability, which is an essential component of transformative education, necessitates that attention be paid to the issues of governance, responsive curricula, educator preparedness, and appropriate student recruitment and selection
Adejumo, O., Fakude, L. & Linda, N., 2014	South Africa	Revisiting innovative approaches to teaching and learning in nursing programmes: Educators' experiences with the use of a case-based teaching approach at a nursing school.	Concerns raised included issues about the facilitation role of the teacher; the role of the student; curriculum alignment; assessment methods; and the role of the environment in case-based teaching and learning settings.
Marchi-Alves, L.M., Ventura, A., Trevizan, M.A., Mazzo, A. et al. 2013	Angola	Challenges for nursing education in Angola: the perception of nurse leaders affiliated with professional education institutions.	Lack of infrastructure, absence of trained human resources experts, bureaucratic problems to regularize the schools and lack of material resources hinder improvements. Public health education policies need to be established in Angola, including action guidelines that permit effective nursing activities. Professional education institutions need further regularizations and nurses need to be acknowledged as key elements for the qualitative enhancement of health services in the country.
Mutea, N. & Cullen, D., 2012	Kenya	Kenya and distance education: A model to advance graduate nursing.	A collaborative model is presented as a potential solution to advance graduate nursing. Four major constituents are identified including hospitals and agencies, communities of interest, Kenyan universities and international education partners. Each has a part to play

Table 1 Summary of records reviewed *(Continued)*

Author and year	Country	Tittle	Contribution to nursing education
			including contributions to information, communication of opinion and expertise, money and support, infrastructure and in-kind resources. Distance education is cost-effective and will help in building capacity at various levels of nursing including leadership in clinical practice, teaching, administration and research.
McCarthy, C.F., Voss, J., Salmon, M.E., Gross, J.M., Kelley, M.A. & Riley, P.L, 2013	East, Central, and Southern Africa	Nursing and midwifery regulatory reform in East, Central, and Southern Africa: a survey of key stakeholders.	Information regarding effectively engaging leaders in regulatory reform by clarifying their roles, responsibilities, and activities regarding regulation overall as well as their specific perspectives on task shifting and pre-service reform.
Daniels, F.M., Linda, N.S., Bimray, P. & Sharps, P., 2014	South Africa	Effect of increased student enrolment for a Bachelor of Nursing programme on health care service delivery.	The changing learning environment, competition for learning opportunities and limitations in terms of clinical support posed challenges for professional nurses to perform their multifaceted role which includes clinical teaching and mentoring, and affected service delivery. Therefore, careful planning of students' learning experiences in both theory and practice is imperative to ensure that teaching and learning and service delivery are not negatively affected
Wilson, L.L., Somerall, D., Theus, L., Rankin, S., Ngoma, C. & Chimwaza, A., 2014	Malawi, Zambia,	Enhancing global health and education in Malawi, Zambia, and the United States through an inter-professional global health exchange program	Program promoted inter-professional and cross-cultural understanding; fostered development of long-term sustainable partnerships between health professionals and educators in Zambia and the US; and created increased awareness and use of resources for global health education
Livingston P., Bailey J, Ntakiyiruta G, Mukwesi C, Whynot, S. & Brindley, P., 2014	Rwanda	Development of a simulation and skills centre in East Africa: a Rwandan-Canadian partnership.	Developed an adaptable model for simulation and skills centre development in low-resources settings.
Jacob, S., Holman, J., Msolomba, R., Wasili, R., Langdon, F., Levine, R., Mondiwa, M., Bateganya, M. & MacLachlan, E, 2015	Malawi	Using a task analysis to strengthen nursing and midwifery pre-service education in Malawi	Using task analysis, the identified gaps in clinical training and faculty supervision of students. The task analysis provided a robust approach to curriculum revision through identifying key content gaps. Other countries might consider adopting this approach to improving the content and relevancy of nursing and midwifery syllabi and curricula.
Kurth, A., Jacobs, S., Squires, A., Sliney, A., Davis, Stalls. & Portillo, C. 2016	Rwanda	Investing in nurses is a prerequisite for ensuring universal health coverage	The World Health Organization endorses task sharing to ensure universal health coverage in HIV and maternal health, which requires an investment in nursing education, retention, and professional growth opportunities.
Mtshali, N.G. & Gwele, N.S., 2016	South Africa	Community-based nursing education in South Africa: A grounded-middle range theory	The input from the community enhances the relevance of the curriculum to the priority needs of the surrounding community. It also ensures that the CBE curriculum is dynamic and is based on the present, because of the changes taking place in the community.
Botma, Y., 2014	Botswana	How a monster became a princess: Curriculum development.	Changing content driven curriculum to competence based curriculum improved training on nurses with a primary care focus
Bell, S.A., Rominski, S., Bam,V., Donkor, E. & Lori, J., 2013	Ghana	An analysis of nursing education in Ghana: Priorities for scaling-up the nursing workforce	Faculty and infrastructure shortages are common issues in nursing education and workforce expansion, these issues are compounded by high rates of preventable disease and injury.
Kiarie, J., Farquhar, C., Redfield, R., Bosire, K., Nduti, Mwanda, W., M'lmunya, J. & Kibwage, I., 2015	Kenya	Strengthening health systems by integrating health care, medical education, and research: University of Nairobi experience.	The study suggested innovation building capacity of healthcare workers and students through the eBNM program. Students felt they had more opportunities to practice clinical skills, closer mentoring, and closer interactions with

Table 1 Summary of records reviewed *(Continued)*

Author and year	Country	Tittle	Contribution to nursing education
			patients at the at the non-tertiary facilities than at the tertiary hospital. Health workers at the non-tertiary hospitals also reported improved quality of patient care, increased job satisfaction, and greater interest in research. County hospitals have retained employees and the nurses are upgrading their skills without losing income.
Blaauw, D., Ditlopo, P. & Rispel, L. 2014	South Africa	Nursing education reform in South Africa – lessons from a policy analysis study	The study found significant weaknesses in the policy capacity of the main institutions responsible for the leadership and governance of nursing in South Africa, which will need to be addressed if important nursing education reforms are to be realised
Appiagyei, A.A. Kiriinya, R.N., Gross, J.M., Wambua, D.N., Oywer, E.O., Kamenju, A.K., Higgins, M.K., Riley, P.L. & Rogers, M.F. 2014	Kenya	Informing the scale-up of Kenya's nursing workforce: a mixed methods study of factors affecting pre-service training capacity and production	To scale-up the nursing workforce in Kenya, concurrent investments in expanding the number of student nurse clinical placement sites, utilizing alternate forms of skills training, hiring more faculty and clinical instructors, and expanding the dormitory and classroom space to accommodate new students are needed to ensure that increases in student enrolment are not at the cost of quality nursing education.

allow flexibility and effective advancement. ICAP through the Global Nurse capacity Building Program (GNCBP) in six Sub Saharan African countries embarked on building capacity of faculty in nursing education [35, 37].

The complex environment in nursing education demands that academic managers, leaders and players continually monitor the ever- evolving, complex system of the professional tripartite: nursing education, research and practice. Nursing leaders have been challenged to spearhead a successful translation of scientific knowledge that links nursing education to professional practice in the delivery of high quality health care. Jooste and Jasper [38] reported that nurse managers need to influence policy decisions regarding nursing services design and delivery.

Capacity building also surrounds around the issue of faculty ability to prepare a generation of relevant graduates [35, 37]. The review noted that to improve the quality and quantity of nursing, it is necessary to increase the number of nursing faculty and clinical educators who have both expertise in nursing care and commensurate education.

Theme 6: Infrastructure and resources
We found that lack of infrastructure, absence of trained human resources experts and lack of material resources posed big challenges to nursing education among Sub Saharan African countries [39, 40]. With the continuing growth in the world's population and the growing disease burden, there is a critical need for increased numbers of qualified health-care personnel and increasingly more efficient healthcare systems. The review shows that the shortage of nurses and midwives has led to increased

student enrolment in most countries [34, 39]. Increase in student enrolment has resulted in a strained clinical learning environment, competition for learning opportunities among students [35]. We found that infrastructure investment will facilitate better quality education [39]. The strategy involved providing infrastructure development for the nursing training institutions to accommodate more students and to provide student training fees.

Discussion
This integrative review has attempted to synthesize relevant published work on nursing education in Africa and made recommendations towards improving the quality, quantity and relevance of nursing education in Su Saharan Africa. Despite the reported severe shortage and maldistribution of nurses between and within countries, nurses remain the single largest available group of available health workers. This positions nurses to be global leaders in driving the quality of health care delivery especially in low –resource settings [41]. Numerous literature report a very significant relationship between nursing and patient safety, patient satisfaction and quality care [42–44]. However, nursing education programs have failed to produce the required graduates who are responsive to the local health policies and programs [45] and the needs of the health care users [46–48].

Curriculum reforms
A curriculum is at the heart of every educational enterprise [49]. The change in the global health care landscape is putting much pressure for reforms on how

the health care workforce practices. Forbes and Hickey [50] highlighted four themes within the need for curriculum reform namely incorporating safety and quality in nursing education, re-designing conceptual frameworks, strategies to address content laden curricula and teaching using alternative pedagogies. Jacobs et al. [51] used a task analysis to reform curriculum identified gaps in clinical teaching and faculty supervision. Task analysis provided a robust approach to curriculum revising through identifying content gaps. The healthcare system in Sub Saharan Africa is getting more complex. Demand for adequate and quality teamwork among stakeholders in increasing. Approaches that transform systems and encourage the move away from the traditional focus on tertiary care hospitals to initiatives that foster community engagement are needed.

Nursing plays a key role in the coordination and integration of care and services from other providers [52]. Reforms that embrace inter-professional education will help to remove challenges that come about between professions and this facilitates coordinated care [53]. Liaw et al. [54] supports that inter-professional learning is essential to enhance team collaboration and communication necessary for patient safety and effective healthcare. Therefore, curriculum reform that enhances relevance of nursing programs within multidisciplinary teams and inter-professional collaboration is very significant in Sub Saharan Africa.

Profession regulation

Nursing as a profession has a unique system of rules an principles to regulate its members and demonstrate its responsibility to society [55]. The changing healthcare landscape such as an ageing society, double burden of disease with an emerging burden of non-communicable diseases, coupled with shortage of nursing specialist cadres in remote areas, the gap between healthcare supply and demand, task shifting and the perception that nurses and midwives do not work to their full potential, is necessitating changes in the scope of practice frameworks [56, 57].

International Council of Nurses [58] identified fundamental responsibilities of nurses to promote health, prevent illness, restore health and alleviate suffering. These responsibilities deal with challenges of determining the scope of professional nursing practice. Schluter et al. [59] argue that the changing pattern of healthcare delivery ultimately leads to a reconsideration on how nurses manage their work in line with associated legislation. Many countries in Sub Saharan Africa have regulatory nursing bodies which are responsible for developing and implementing a regulatory framework. However, several study across the region reported that regulatory bodies do not always have sufficient capacity and resources to face reform demands [9, 60].

Transformative teaching strategies

Many health professional training programs have mostly maintained classroom teaching. These short term lectures and seminars have proved not to be effective in diversifying skills md competencies of health workers including nurses [9]. The review indicates that Sub Saharan Countries have increased healthcare training intakes to solve the shortage of human resource crisis. This has led to congestion of students in clinical sites. Increased intakes demand innovative ways to train these growing numbers. King [61] reported that further expansion of distance education is an innovative and cost effective way of advancing nursing and midwifery in Sub Saharan Africa.

Nurse educators need to examine what they do in and out of classroom to continue to be effective, current and relevant. With the focus on community health demands, training initiatives should prioritise the acquisition of competencies through sustained mentorship and supervision, simulation rather than through ad hoc short term lectures and seminars [62, 63].

Collaboration and partnerships

In some instances a disjuncture between nursing leadership and front line nurses has been reported [64, 65]. World Health Organization [66] advocates that educational and training institutions should foster and enhance the relational activity, interaction and planning between education, health and other sectors. Both academia and practice have the overall goal of attaining optimal health for their countries.

Careful planning of students learning experiences between academia and practice is imperative to ensure that students get maximum benefits from their training. Current reforms in nursing education demands sharing of knowledge and information. Partnerships between academia and practice can contribute significantly towards a vibrant healthcare system. Effective academic practice partnerships can reduce the theory practice-gap thereby improving patient safety, reducing medical errors, strengthening practice setting and cushioning faculty shortage [67, 68]. Academia and practice are dissimilar but share values regarding nursing education. An academic practice partnership can therefore be best understood from a view point where the academic and the practice players come together and work collaboratively for a common goal [69]. Implementation of the shared goal should involve specific responsibilities for the educators, hospital administrators, students and the nurse practitioners through a systems approach [70].

Academic practice partnerships provide a platform for partners to capitalize on each other's expertise. This also improves access to a broader array of clinical experiences for students. Students receive adequate clinical support that is blended with expertise from both academic knowledge and practice competencies. Evidence supports that mentorship provided by clinical personnel is critical to students' training outcomes [71]. Quality clinical practice outcome is dependent on preparation and willingness of practice partners. Narasimhan et al. [72] noted that lack of mutual planning results in over-expenditure on unimportant activities within the effort to improve quality of nursing education.

Capacity building
World Health Organization [60] highlighted that significant investment will be required to strengthen educational infrastructure, faculty and staff development, curriculum review and clinical instruction. To improve the quality and quantity of nursing, it is necessary to increase the number of nursing faculty and clinical educators who have both expertise in nursing care and commensurate education. Evidence from South Africa indicated that the education and training system for the health sector has not grown sufficiently to meet health needs and health system requirements. This is in part due to lack of integrated planning between the health and education sectors on the development of health professionals in relation to health care need, and inadequate financing mechanisms for health professional development.

Infrastructure and resources
Health worker shortage in Sub Saharan Africa is a result of many causes which include past investment shortfalls in pre- service training, international migration, career changes among health workers, premature retirement and morbidity and mortality [7]. Experience shows that despite the increased enrolment in most countries, the number of quality clinical environment has remained the same. The review has highlighted that clinical learning environment is been strained. There is need to deliberately invest in infrastructure both at training institutions and practice levels.

Strengths and limitations of the study
This review shares useful information for improving nursing education among stakeholders worldwide. The major limitation of the study was that it only focused on literature from Sub Saharan Africa.

Implication for practice
Nursing and midwifery remains the backbone of the healthcare system worldwide. Continued efforts to improve training of nurses and midwives will ensure improved health outcomes. Effective nursing education will ensure provision of competence based practice among nurses. More research on nursing education will help to improve practice standards in nursing and midwifery.

Conclusion
The integrated review highlights that majority of countries within Sub Saharan Africa are experiencing common challenges ranging from strained training institutions due to increased enrolments, inadequate faculty capacity, lack of infrastructure and resources, high demand for clinical training sites. To ensure improved quality and quantity of production, developmental partners have increased allocation of financial resources for infrastructure and teaching and learning material. Efforts are being done to expand number of clinical sites, build faculty capacity and increase collaboration with clinical institutions for clinical instructors and mentors. Curriculum reforms are being implemented to reposition the nursing workforce for a competence based approach, community based education and inter-professional training. Clinical simulation and technology based teaching strategies are on the increase to accommodate the demands for new ways of teaching and learning.

Abbreviations
HIV/AIDS: Acquired Immunodeficiency Syndrome/ Human Immunodeficiency Virus; NCA: Norwegian Church Aid; SDGs: Sustainable Development Goals

Acknowledgements
Thanks go to all nursing students at Mzuzu University who participated in the abstract appraisal during the review.

Funding
Not Applicable

Authors' contributions
TB and NM conceptualized the study, collected and analysed data. Both authors drafted and approved the final manuscript.

Competing interests
The authors declare that they have no competing interests

Author details
[1]Faculty of Health Sciences, Mzuzu University, P/ Bag 201, Luwinga, Mzuzu, Malawi. [2]School of Nursing, University of KwaZulu Natal, Durban 4041, Republic of South Africa.

References

1. Mooketsane KS, Phirinyane MB. Health governance in Sub-Saharan Africa. Globl Soc Policy. 2015;15(3):345–8.
2. Negeri KG, Halemariam D. Effect of health development assistance on health status in sub-Saharan Africa. Risk Manag Healthc Policy. 2016;9:33.
3. Akinyemi JO, Chisumpa VH, Odimegwu CO. Household structure, maternal characteristics and childhood mortality in rural sub-Saharan Africa. Rural Remote Health. 2016;16(2):3737.
4. Keino S, Plasqui G, Ettyang G, van den Borne B. Determinants of stunting and overweight among young children and adolescents in sub-Saharan Africa. Food Nutr Bull. 2014;35(2):167–78.
5. Scheffler RM, Tulenko K, et al. The deepening global health workforce crisis: forecasting needs, shortages, and costs for the global strategy on human resources for health (2013-2030). Ann Glob Health. 2016;82(3):510.
6. Tangcharoensathien V, Mills A, Palu T. Accelerating health equity: the key role of universal health coverage in the sustainable development goals. BMC Med. 2015;13:101.
7. Kinfu Y, Dal Poz MR, Mercer H, Evans DB. The health worker shortage in Africa: are enough physicians and nurses being trained? Bull World Health Organ. 2009;87(3):225–30.
8. Global Health Workforce Alliance W. A universal truth: no health without a workforce. Geneva: World Health Organization; 2013.
9. Frenk J, Chen L, Bhutta ZA, Cohen J, Crisp N, Evans T, et al. Health professionals for a new century: transforming education to strengthen health systems in an interdependent world. Lancet. 2010;376(9756):1923–58.
10. Crisp N. A global perspective on the education and training of primary care and public health professionals. London J Prim Care. 2012;4(2):116–9.
11. Frenk J, Chen L, Bhutta ZA, Cohen J, Crisp N, Evans T, et al. Health professionals for a new century: transforming education to strengthen health systems in an interdependent world. Lancet. 2010;376:1923–58.
12. Mosadeghrad A. Factors influencing healthcare service quality. Int J Health Policy Manag. 2014;3(2):77–89.
13. Rich ML, Miller AC, Niyigena P, Franke MF, Niyonzima JB, Socci A, et al. Excellent clinical outcomes and high retention in care among adults in a community-based HIV treatment program in rural Rwanda. J Acquir Immune Defic Syndr. 2012;59(3):e35–42.
14. Institute of Medicine Committee. The future of nursing: leading change, advancing health. Washington (DC): National Academies Press (US). Copyright 2011 by the National Academy of Sciences. All rights reserved; 2011.
15. World Health Organization. Global standards for the initial education of professionals nurses and midwives. Geneva: WHO; 2009. Available from: http://www.who.int/publications
16. SIDIIEF. Declaration in favor of university education for nurses in the French-speaking countries. Geneva; 2012. Available from: https://www.sidiief.org/wp-content/uploads/Declaration-Geneve-Anglais.pdf. Accessed 15 July 2015.
17. WHO. Plan of action for scaling up Quality Nursing & Midwifery Education & practice for the African region 2012 – 2022. Region Office for Africa: WHO; 2012.
18. Brown RA, Crookes PA. What are the 'necessary' skills for a newly graduating RN? Results of an Australian survey. BMC Nurs. 2016;15:1–8.
19. Ulrich B, Krozek C, Early S, Ashlock CH, Africa LM, Carman ML. Improving retention, confidence, and competence of new graduate nurses: results from a 10-year longitudinal database. Nursing economic. 2010;28(6):363–76.
20. Whittemore R, Knafl K. The integrative review: updated methodology. J Adv Nurs. 2005;52(5):546–53.
21. Mtshali NG, Gwele NS. Community-based nursing education in South Africa: a grounded-middle range theory. J Nurs Educ Pract. 2016;6(2):55.
22. Mthembu S, Mtshali N, Frantz J. Contextual determinants for community-based learning programmes in nursing education in South Africa. S Afr J High Educ. 2014;28(6):1795–813.
23. Botma Y. How a monster became a princess: curriculum development. S Afr J High Educ. 2014;28(6):1876–93.
24. Wilson LL, Somerall D, Theus L, Rankin S, Ngoma C, Chimwaza A. Enhancing global health and education in Malawi, Zambia, and the United States through an interprofessional global health exchange program. Appl Nurs Res. 2014;27(2):97–103.
25. McCarthy CF, Voss J, Salmon ME, Gross JM, Kelley MA, Riley PL. Nursing and midwifery regulatory reform in east, central, and southern Africa: a survey of key stakeholders. Hum Resour Health. 2013;11:29.
26. McCarthy CF, Riley PL. The African health profession regulatory collaborative for nurses and midwives. Hum Resour Health. 2012;10(1):1.
27. Appiagyei AA, Kiriinya RN, Gross JM, Wambua DN, Oywer EO, Kamenju AK, et al. Informing the scale-up of Kenya's nursing workforce: a mixed methods study of factors affecting pre-service training capacity and production. Hum Resour Health. 2014;12:47.
28. Adejumo O, Lorraine F, Linda NS. Revisiting innovative approaches to teaching and learning in nursing programmes: educators' experiences with the use of a case-based teaching approach at a nursing school. 2014.
29. Livingston P, Bailey J, Ntakiyiruta G, Mukwesi C, Whynot S, Brindley P. Development of a simulation and skills centre in East Africa: a Rwandan-Canadian partnership. Pan Afr Med J. 2014;17(1):315.
30. Kiarie JN, Farquhar C, Redfield R, Bosire K, Nduati RW, Mwanda W, et al. Strengthening health systems by integrating health care, medical education, and research: University of Nairobi experience. Acad Med. 2014; 89(8 Suppl):S109–10.
31. Mutea N, Cullen D. Kenya and distance education: a model to advance graduate nursing. Int J Nurs Pract. 2012;18(4):417–22.
32. Armstrong SJ, Rispel LC. Social accountability and nursing education in South Africa. Glob Health Action. 2015;8:27879.
33. Goosby EP, von Zinkernagel D. The medical and nursing education partnership initiatives. Acad Med. 2014;89(8 Suppl):S5–7.
34. Daniels FM, Linda NS, Bimray P, Sharps P. Effect of increased student enrolment for a bachelor of nursing programme on health care service delivery. S Afr J High Educ. 2014;28(6):1750–61.
35. Middleton L, Howard AA, Dohrn J, Von Zinkernagel D, Parham Hopson D, Aranda-Naranjo B, et al. The nursing education partnership initiative (NEPI): innovations in nursing and midwifery education. Acad Med. 2014;89(8 Suppl):S24–8.
36. Blaauw D, Ditlopo P, Rispel LC. Nursing education reform in South Africa – lessons from a policy analysis study. Glob Health Action. 2014:7. https://doi.org/10.3402/gha.v7.26401.
37. Kurth AE, Jacob S, Squires AP, Sliney A, Davis S, Stalls S, et al. Investing in nurses is a prerequisite for ensuring universal health coverage. J Assoc Nurses AIDS Care. 2016;27(3):344–54.
38. Jooste K, Jasper M. A south African perspective: current position and challenges in health care service management and education in nursing. J Nurs Manag. 2012;20(1):56–64.
39. Bell SA, Rominski S, Bam V, Donkor E, Lori J. An analysis of nursing education in Ghana: priorities for scaling-up the nursing workforce. Nurs Health Sci. 2013;15(2):244–9.
40. Marchi AL, Ventura CA, Trevizan M, Mazzo A, de Godoy S, Mendes IC. Challenges for nursing education in Angola: the perception of nurse leaders affiliated with professional education institutions. Hum Resour Health. 2013;11(1):1.
41. Dall TM, Chen YJ, Seifert RF, Maddox PJ, Hogan PF. The economic value of professional nursing. Med Care. 2009;47(1):97–104.
42. Bruyneel L, Li B, Aiken L, Lesaffre E, Van den Heede K, Sermeus W. A multi-country perspective on nurses' tasks below their skill level: reports from domestically trained nurses and foreign trained nurses from developing countries. Int J Nurs Stud. 2013;50(2):202–9.
43. Cho E, Lee N, Kim E, Kim S, Lee K, Park K, et al. Nurse staffing level and overtime associated with patient safety, quality of care, and care left undone in hospitals: a cross-sectional study. Int J Nurs Stud. 2016;60:263–71.
44. You L, Aiken LH, Sloane DM, Liu K, He G, Hu Y, et al. Hospital nursing, care quality, and patient satisfaction: cross-sectional surveys of nurses and patients in hospitals in China and Europe. Int J Nurs Stud. 2013;50(2):154–61.
45. Kaye DK, Muhwezi WW, Kasozi AN, Kijjambu S, Mbalinda SN, Okullo I, et al. Lessons learnt from comprehensive evaluation of community-based education in Uganda: a proposal for an ideal model community-based education for health professional training institutions. BMC Med Educ. 2011;11(1):1.
46. Farsi Z, Dehghan-Nayeri N, Negarandeh R, Broomand S. Nursing profession in Iran: an overview of opportunities and challenges. Jpn J Nurs Sci. 2010;7(1):9–18.
47. Tanner CA. Transforming prelicensure nursing education: preparing the new nurse to meet emerging health care needs. Nurs Educ Perspect. 2010;31(6):347–53.

48. Kabore I, Bloem J, Etheredge G, Obiero W, Wanless S, Doykos P, et al. The effect of community-based support services on clinical efficacy and health-related quality of life in HIV/AIDS patients in resource-limited settings in sub-Saharan Africa. AIDS Patient Care STDs. 2010; 24(9):581–94.

49. Karseth B. Curriculum changes and moral issues in nursing education. Nurse Educ Today. 2004;24(8):638–43.

50. Forbes MO, Hickey MT. Curriculum reform in baccalaureate nursing education: review of the literature. Int J Nurs Educ Scholarsh. 2009;6:Article27.

51. Jacob S, Holman J, Msolomba R, Wasili R, Langdon F, Levine R, et al. Using a task analysis to strengthen nursing and midwifery pre-service education in Malawi. Int J Nurs Midwifery. 2015;7(5):84–103.

52. Robson W. Eliminating avoidable harm: time for patient safety to play a bigger part in professional education and practice. Nurse Educ Today. 2014; 34(5):e1–2.

53. Bridges DR, Davidson RA, Odegard PS, Maki IV, Tomkowiak J. Interprofessional collaboration: three best practice models of interprofessional education. Med Educ Online. 2011;16 https://doi.org/10.3402/meo.v16i0.6035.

54. Liaw SY, Zhou WT, Lau TC, Siau C, Chan SW. An interprofessional communication training using simulation to enhance safe care for a deteriorating patient. Nurse Educ Today. 2014;34(2):259–64.

55. Flook DM. The professional nurse and regulation. J PeriAnesth Nurs. 2003; 18(3):160–7.

56. Fairman JA, Rowe JW, Hassmiller S, Shalala DE. Broadening the scope of nursing practice. N Engl J Med. 2011;364(3):193–6.

57. Riegel B, Sullivan-Marx E, Fairman JA. Meeting global needs in primary care with nurse practitioners. Lancet. 2012;380(9840):449–50.

58. International Council of Nurses. The ICN code of ethics for nurses 2012 Available from: http://www.icn.ch/images/stories/documents/about/icncode_english.pdf. Accessed 15 July 2015.

59. Schluter J, Seaton P, Chaboyer W. Understanding nursing scope of practice: a qualitative study. Int J Nurs Stud. 2011;48(10):1211–22.

60. World Health Organization. Transformative scale up of health professional education: an effort to increase the numbers of health professionals and to strengthen their impact on population health. 2011.

61. King L. Distance education: the solution for nursing and midwifery in Africa? Int Nurs Rev. 2000;47(2):63.

62. Celletti F, Reynolds TA, Wright A, Stoertz A, Dayrit M. Educating a new generation of doctors to improve the health of populations in low-and middle-income countries. PLoS Med. 2011;8(10):e1001108.

63. Körükcü Ö, Kukulu K. Innovation in nursing education. Procedia Soc Behav Sci. 2010;9:369–72.

64. Akunja E, Kaseje D, Obago I, Ochieng B. Involvement of hub nurses in HIV policy development: case study of Nyanza Province, Kenya. Res Humanit Soc Sci. 2012;2:124Á34.

65. Shariff N, Potgieter E. Extent of east-African nurse leaders' participation in health policy development. Nurs Res Pract. 2012;2012:504697.

66. World Health Organization. WHO guidelines approved by the guidelines review committee. Transforming and scaling up health Professionals' education and training: World Health Organization guidelines 2013. Geneva: WHO; 2013.

67. Murray TA, James DC. Evaluation of an academic service partnership using a strategic alliance framework. Nurs Outlook. 2012;60(4):e17–22.

68. Chan EA, Chan K, Liu YJ. A triadic interplay between academics, practitioners and students in the nursing theory and practice dialectic. J Adv Nurs. 2012;68(5):1038–49.

69. Bvumbwe T. Enhancing nursing education via academic–clinical partnership: an integrative review. Int J Nurs Sci. 2016;3(3):314–22.

70. Missal B, Schafer BK, Halm MA, Schaffer MA. A university and health care organization partnership to prepare nurses for evidence-based practice. J Nurs Educ. 2010;49(8):456–61.

71. Lofmark A, Thorkildsen K, Raholm MB, Natvig GK. Nursing students' satisfaction with supervision from preceptors and teachers during clinical practice. Nurse Educ Pract. 2012;12(3):164–9.

72. Narasimhan V, Brown H, Pablos-Mendez A, Adams O, Dussault G, Elzinga G, et al. Responding to the global human resources crisis. Lancet. 2004; 363(9419):1469–72.

17

Registered nurses' and older people's experiences of participation in nutritional care in nursing homes

Katarina Sjögren Forss[1]* ⓘ, Jane Nilsson[2] and Gunilla Borglin[1]

Abstract

Background: The evaluation and treatment of older people's nutritional care is generally viewed as a low priority by nurses. However, given that eating and drinking are fundamental human activities, the support and enhancement of an optimal nutritional status should be regarded as a vital part of nursing. Registered nurses must therefore be viewed as having an important role in assessing and evaluating the nutritional needs of older people as well as the ability to intervene in cases of malnutrition. This study aimed to illuminate the experience of participating in nutritional care from the perspectives of older people and registered nurses. A further aim is to illuminate the latter's experience of nutritional care per se.

Methods: A qualitative, descriptive design was adopted. Data were collected through semi-structured interviews ($n = 12$) with eight registered nurses and four older persons (mean age 85.7 years) in a city in the southern part of Sweden. The subsequent analysis was conducted by content analysis.

Result: The analysis reflected three themes: 'participation in nutritional care equals information', 'nutritional care out of remit and competence' and 'nutritional care more than just choosing a flavour'. They were interpreted to illuminate the experience of participation in nutritional care from the perspective of older people and RNs, and the latter's experience of nutritional care in particular per se.

Conclusions: Our findings indicate that a paternalistic attitude in care as well as asymmetry in the nurse-patient relationship are still common characteristics of modern clinical nursing practice for older people. Considering that participation should be central to nursing care, and despite the RN's awareness of the importance of involving the older persons in their nutritional care this was not reflected in reality. Strategies to involve older persons in their nutritional care in a nursing home context need to take into account that for this population participation might not always be experienced as an important part of nursing care.

Keywords: Care, Content analysis, Interviews, Malnutrition, Nursing interventions, Older people, Patient involvement, Registered nurse

* Correspondence: katarina.sjogren.forss@mau.se
[1]Department of Care Science, Faculty of Health and Society, Malmö University, SE-205 06 Malmö, Sweden
Full list of author information is available at the end of the article

Background

Registered Nurses (henceforth abbreviated 'RN') must be seen as an important player in assessing, evaluating and intervening in cases of malnutrition among older people. However, research shows that malnutrition in older people often goes unrecognised by RNs regardless of care context, for example, in nursing homes and/or hospitals [1, 2]. Although the prevalence of malnutrition is known to range from 15 to 40% in nursing homes [3–6], in terms of evaluation and treatment [7, 8], nutritional care in general is not a highly prioritised issue. This is noteworthy, as food and drink are essential human needs hence, a vital part of the fundamentals of care [9] and consequently a mandatory competency practice skill within the remit of the RNs role in care. Thus, the support and promotion of the optimal nutritional status of older people should be a prioritised area in nursing. A plausible explanation may be that RN's responsibility within nutritional nursing care is unclear [10, 11]. Another explanation may be that RNs need further in-depth knowledge about nutritional nursing care issues [1], as this has been shown to increase their awareness of nutritional nursing care [12], and the nutritional status of older people living in nursing homes [13, 14].

Maintaining an optimal nutritional status is important for the wellbeing of older people and for promoting independent living [15]. However, despite this knowledge, malnutrition is a common and serious problem that contributes significantly to morbidity and mortality in this population group [16]. Malnutrition is associated with a decline in, for example, overall functional status as well as impaired muscle function and reduced cognitive function; in addition, malnutrition causes decreased bone mass, immune dysfunction, and anaemia [17]. The cause of malnutrition is often multifactorial and includes medical, physiological, psychological and social as well as environmental factors [16, 18]. Whereas the ageing process can often explain physiological and psychological factors, environmental factors in terms of meal ambiance can be easily modulated. It appears that environmental stimuli are not changed during the ageing process; therefore, environmental factors should always be considered as part of a nutritional nursing plan for older people living in nursing homes [19]. Given that the population of older people is increasing worldwide, it is crucial that healthcare professionals and RNs in particular actively work to prevent malnutrition and identify ways to meet the diet and nutrition needs of this vulnerable population.

It is reasonable to suggest that if RNs highlight and promote the importance of older people's participation ('participation' and 'involvement' will be used synonymously in this paper) in their own nutritional nursing care, then the risk of malnutrition may decrease. Internationally and nationally there have been an obvious shift from the earlier hierarchical systems at the hospitals [20, 21] towards patients rights, which also encompass nursing.

One plausible explanation for this change of focus in care are likely to be the strong democratic movements during the twenty-first century [22]. Resulting in that patients now, and regardless of context, are viewed as active participants in their care and healthcare decisions [23]. This shift is not attributed to changes in professional values alone. Rather, the move towards patient empowerment and person-centredness, is according to Christensen and Hewitt-Taylor [20] most likely the result of "....changes in the dominant views of society and lack of confidence in healthcare professionals, not simply because the healthcare professionals have adapted their thinking to be more respectful of patients' rights ([20] p. 696)." In Sweden the patient's right to be informed and to be made part of their own care is nowadays regulated by the Patient Act [24] and the Health and Medical Services Act [25]. Older people's participation in all parts of their health care should therefore be considered as essential for healthcare professionals, particularly as a means to understand preferences and the optimisation of care [26]. Although previous research, conducted with a quantitative design, has shown that the involvement of older people has a positive effect on health outcomes, for example, in terms of health status, raising the energy intake [27] and satisfaction with care [28], older people are less often involved in their care than younger people [29, 30]. This despite studies that show older people want to be involved in their own care [31]. 'Participation' in care can mean to facilitate and encourage older people to share the responsibility of their own health and to support them in the decision-making process regarding their treatment and care [32] The involvement of older people in their own care is central for promoting person-centred nursing models, where RNs could play an important role in establishing this *modus operandi* in the care of older people.

Alharabi and colleagues [33] suggest that the lack of both understanding and confidence among healthcare professionals about involving older people in their nutritional care needs to be eliminated. The level of acceptance healthcare professionals has in regard to older people's participation in care, has been shown to be influenced by the professionals' need to maintain control and lack of time as well as the type of illnesses [34]. Further, ways to involve older people who reside in nursing homes in the food and meal activities appear to be limited [35, 36]. This may well be a factor that influences nutritional nursing care negatively in this population group. The majority of identified published nursing research seem to focus on the risk of malnutrition and its consequences either in the acute care setting or in the community alone, rather than older people's experiences of participation in their nutritional care at nursing homes. Thus, in-depth knowledge about RNs, and older people's experience of participation in nutritional care and the RN's experiences of this type of care in a nursing home context is therefore still sparse. To the best of our knowledge, very few studies exist exploring this phenomenon in a nursing home context while including both older people and RNs. Therefore, this study aimed to illuminate the experience of participation in nutritional care from the perspective of older people residing at nursing homes and RNs. A further aim was also to illuminate the latter's experience of nutritional care per se.

Methods

A qualitative, descriptive design [37] was used to understand the experiences of nurses and older people who participate in nursing care when assessed as 'at risk for malnutrition' or as 'malnourished' from the informant's point of view [38]. Data were collected through semi-structured interviews [37], and the subsequent analysis was inspired by Burnard's [39, 40] description of content analysis.

Study setting

This study took place in a city in the southern part of Sweden during spring 2016. In Sweden, the care of older people is primarily a public responsibility, and the provision of care and service for older people is mainly financed through taxes. The county councils are the regional providers of healthcare, but the municipalities are responsible for the care of older people living in their own homes or in nursing homes. The care is guided by RNs; however, the main providers of care and service in the municipalities are staff nurses and healthcare assistants. For the past 16 years in Sweden, the only way into the nursing profession has been through a degree programme, and since 2007, the only route has been via a bachelor's degree in Nursing Science, which involves 3 years of study at university. The university education aims to equip the Swedish nursing students with the knowledge, competencies and skills needed to take the lead of care. Particularly the competencies needed to assess, diagnose, intervene and evaluate, in relation to the same essential human needs that was highlighted in care already by Florence Nightingale in the nineteenth century. Eating and drinking i.e. nutrition is hence part of the fundamentals of care [9], and a required practice competency expectation for nursing care also in Sweden.

Nursing homes are homelike residential care facilities for older people with mainly one-bed rooms that provide around-the-clock care. Residents at nursing homes are quite frail, and eight out of ten are aged 80 years or older. In the nursing homes, staff nurses and healthcare assisstants are on duty around the clock to provide regular care as well as palliative care. A RN (or, at times, two RNs depending on the size of the nursing home) is on call and accessible during officetime between Monday to Friday. Most residents have a primary care physician who is employed by the county council and who works at the local healthcare centre usually located near the nursing home where the resident lives.

Sample and recruitment

In this study, 12 informants agreed to participate: The strategic sample [30] consisted of four older persons (65 +), of which three were female and one was male. Our sample also consisted of eight RNs working in six different special accommodations. Of the RNs, two were male and six were female.

The inclusion criteria for the older persons were that they should be age 65 or older, cognitively intact, and able to read, speak and understand Swedish. They must also reside in one of the municipality's nursing homes and have been assessed as 'at risk for malnutrition' or as 'malnourished' in accordance with the Mini Nutritional Assessment tool [41], which means they will have received a nursing diagnosis and intervention. Inclusion criteria for the RNs were that they should hold a permanent position at the nursing home, work at least 75% and be in charge of a ward not designated for older people suffering from cognitive decline.

Recruitment process

In the first step of the recruitment process, a sample of the city's boroughs was made and nine out of 10 boroughs were contacted. For obvious ethical reasons, the borough in which the second author (JN) was working where not included in our study. After having received permission from the relevant branch heads to contact the municipality services, the coordinator of care was contacted. The latter contacted the patients' responsible RNs in nine of the municipality's nursing homes via email to inform them about the study. They acted as recruiters alone, and were asked to forward an invitation about participation in the study to older people and RNs meeting the inclusion criteria. In addition, the email contained an information letter about the study for the RNs. Six of the nine nursing homes that were contacted agreed to take part in the study. One reason given by the nursing homes for not wishing to participate was a lack of time.

The RN in charge of each nursing home facilitated the recruitment of the older persons. In total, seven older persons were assessed as meeting the study's inclusion criteria and thus eligible for the study. Of these, four older persons with a mean age of 85.7 years (age range 74-90 years), residing in four different nursing homes, agreed to participate in the study (Table 1). Of the remaining three, one further individual initially agreed, but then withdrew at a later stage. Another became acutely ill, and the third withdrew due to feeling uninformed about malnutrition being the focus of the study.

Table 1 Characteristics – older persons

Code	Gender	Years in special accommodation	Body Mass Index [BMI]	Mini Nutritional Assessment [MNA scores]
A	Male	3	21.5	7 [malnourished]
B	Female	1	20.9	10 [risk of malnutrition]
C	Female	1	18.8	9 [risk of malnutrition]
D	Female	2	18	7 [malnourished]

The interviewer provided written and verbal information about the study both when arranging the time for the interviews and before each interview began. All older persons gave written and verbal consent to their participation in the study.

The interviewer approached 14 eligible RNs, of which eight RNs with a mean age of 44.1 years (age range 28-67 years) accepted to participate (Table 2). Reasons given for not wanting to participate were, once again, a lack of time. During a face-to-face meeting, they were once again provided with verbal and written information, and a time and place was arranged for the interview. All informants in this study ($n = 12$) were informed about confidentiality and their right to withdraw at any point without needing to give any explanation for doing so.

Semi-structured interviews

The semi-structured interview method was used to collect the data [30], and they were conducted by the second author (JN) during April 2016. The interviews began with one overarching question (Fig. 1), which became more specific as the interviews proceeded. The overarching interview question was tested, by the second author (JN), on two RNs and one older person ahead of the interviews to assure its understandability and its relevance for the study aim. This test did not lead to any changes. Data from this test were not included in our analysis. Whenever clarification was needed during the interviews, general probing was used (ibid). The interviews with the older people were conducted in their home and at a time and

Table 2 Characteristics – Registered nurses

Code	Gender	Work experience (years)	Educational level
E	Male	11	BSc Nursing
F	Female	3	BSc Nursing
G	Female	2	BSc Nursing
H	Female	4	BSc Nursing
I	Female	12	Diploma
J	Male	2	Diploma
K	Female	2	BSc Nursing
L	Female	43	Diploma

place of their choice, while the interviews with the RNs took place during working hours in a separate room at the informant's workplace – a place familiar to the informants and at a time that would maximise participation. The interviews lasted approximately 30–40 min and were tape recorded and transcribed before the analysis begun.

Content analysis

The transcribed texts were analysed by a method influenced by content analysis, as outlined by Burnard [39, 40], and focused on both the manifest and latent levels, as outlined by Graneheim and Lundman [42] The process involved four steps. In the first step, the transcribed texts were read to gain an overall understanding and parts of the texts that were found to respond to the aim of the study were highlighted. The highlighted parts were in the second step condensed without losing the central meaning. In the third step, codes were created and in the fourth and final step, the codes were once again read, compared and contrasted with the text to ensure trustworthiness [39, 40]. In the final step, sub-themes involving several similar codes were also created and interpreted to represent three predominant themes relating to older people's experience of being involved in their nutritional care as well as RN's experience of older person participation and their experience of nutritional care per se. The second author (JN) was the main lead in the above described process of analysis. Additionally, the research team independently read and analysed the text and met regularly (approximately 1 h once every second week for about 10 weeks) to discuss and reach a consensus in all the different steps of the analysis. To further ensure the trustworthiness of the analysis, quotes from the informants are reported in the results.

Results

Two of the themes, 'participation in nutritional care equals information' and 'nutritional care out of remit and competence' were interpreted to solely illuminate the RNs experience of older people's participation in nutritional care and their experience of nutritional care per se. Whilst the third and last theme, 'nutritional care – more than just choosing a flavour' were interpreted to mirror older peoples experience of participation in their nutritional care.

Participation in nutritional care equals information?

The theme, 'participation in nutritional care equals information', reflected how the RNs actually experienced older people's participation in nutritional care to be equal with supplying them with information. The theme also reflected an awareness among the RNs about that the low level of patient participation in nutritional care. Especially when the older persons were as at risk of malnourishment or already diagnosed by the RNs as malnourished needed

Overarching interview questions	
Older people	I am interested to hear about your experience of being involved in care, in particular, the care regarding you having been assessed as at risk for malnutrition or as malnourished.
Registered Nurses	I am interested to hear about not only your experience of nutritional care in general but also your experience of involving older people in their own care when they have been assessed as at risk for malnourishment or as malnourished?

Fig. 1 Overarching interview questions

to be developed further as a part of their nutritional care. Thus, the main nursing strategy used to involve the older persons in their nutritional care was to offer some brief information to them. However, the RNs recognised that the information they offered to the older persons could be of better quality. This was experienced by the RNs as especially true for not only the information concerning the implications of being at risk of malnutrition or diagnosed as malnourished, actions to prevent it, and actions to remedy it, but also the information about the anticipated development, goals and nursing interventions targeting nutrition. An RN expressed this sentiment in her interview:

If we would have been better in our information, and included... yeah, particularly the different options. If we really had taken the time to go through it and to check, as there actually are many interventions.... trying to find the cause and then treat the actual reason. Yeah, I do not think we do it to the extent we should. [RN/H]

On the other hand, whether one should involve older people in their nutritional care or not stood out as an antipode. Particularly as the RN's experiences also reflected that involving the older persons in his/her nutritional care was not at the top of the RN's agenda. It also appeared unimportant to the RNs to inform the older persons about the outcomes of assessments performed, the actions to possibly take, and/or any interventions targeting their nutritional issue. The theme appeared more to mirror nursing directives and strict orders to remedy nutritional problems than strategies to support participation in care as a tool to reach common possible solutions in regards to the older persons nutritional care. The directives and orders were interpreted to be purely based on the RN's experiences of what they thought was best for the older persons.

No, I do not do it [involve the older person] ... no. But if I see that they are losing weight, then I visit

them and tell them that I will order nutritional supplement drinks and that they should eat more. [RN/J]

Thus, this theme also reflected that, at times, the goal to involve older persons in their nutritional care departed from the common professional perspective of "I know what is best for you":

It becomes a bit of an "I know best" attitude in this. That you might feel [like], 'But I actually have this education and I do know this stuff, so therefore I choose this'. [RN/D]

Yeah. Thus, I think that one only thinks about it as any other treatment – that we think we know best about what works for them, and then we try that. [RN/K]

Involving older persons in their nutritional could be experiences as a challenge for some RNs. One particular challenge expressed as a barrier for participation in nutritional care became discernible when the older persons no longer experienced that their life was meaningful.

We try to involve them, but when they are at the point where they refuse [to engage] completely ... they see no future and nothing, and they have lost all interest – then it is difficult. It is really very difficult to motivate [them and get them to understand] why food [eating] would make them feel fitter. [RN/L]

Experiencing a constant lack of time was also a barrier and meant that sometimes other types of nursing care was prioritised as more important than nutritional care. This, along with an underestimation of the older persons' ability and willingness, were cited as reasons by the RNs to not involve older people in his/her nutritional care. One RN expresses this in plain terms:

> Ugh, this is maybe an issue that is not a top priority,
> so one, yeah … yeah, one simply doesn't have the time
> because we have other things to do here which one
> thinks is more important, but this is equally
> important. [RN/I]

Another experience by the RNs mirrored that the older persons did not always want to be involved in their nutritional care. Instead, the RNs experienced that they kicked the ball right back to the RNs corner. One RN expressed this as:

> It depends on how interested the patient is. Some
> patients don't want to know anything. If you start
> to talk about certain stuff, the reply is, "Yeah, yeah.
> You are handling it so well". [RN/G]

The theme also indicated that both how well-informed the RN is about the older person's general health and the RN's perception of how independent and capable the older person was, were factors in the RN's decision to involve the older person in their nutritional care or not.

> I am not sure if they are well-informed enough to
> participate, and that is of course on us to give them
> that information and maybe offer some more suggestions
> for action than to arrive in their room and say, "Now
> we are doing like this". I am bad at that [i.e. do the
> latter a lot]. [RN/H]

'Participation in nutritional care equals information' also illuminated certain insights concerning having missed out on an opportunity to engage and involve older persons in their own nutritional care. This was particularly mentioned as a lack of engagement in how the older persons experienced the mealtime ambience and the food served. One RN brought this up:

> I think that this is something we are not so very
> good at, I think. I think that we do not really
> consider that, actually. They [the older people]
> are all sitting there in the dining room. It is, yes …
> No, this is something one can work on much more,
> actually. [RN/E]

Furthermore, the theme reflected that involving older people in their nutritional care actually was viewed by some RNs as a natural and integral part of professional nursing – particularly if the RNs perceived that the older person's nutritional status were a vital factor for the older person's general condition of health, as exemplified in the following quotation:

> I usually inform that one has no energy, one cannot
> move around as much as one wishes. That the risk
> of attracting infections is bigger, and that one's pain
> threshold is lower if one is malnourished. On the
> whole, one can withstand much if one is normally
> nourished, so to speak. [RN/F]

The theme additionally echoed a wish to allocate more time for troubleshooting and for understanding the underlying cause of the older people's individual nutrition problems. The RNs felt that being able to depart from the root of the cause would facilitate older people's participation in their nutritional care. This could be expressed as:

> To inform them that there is a problem, what
> the alternatives could be to remedy it, and most
> importantly, why it is so important to not be
> malnourished – [to tell them] all the risks of
> being malnourished. [RN/K]

Nutritional care out of remit and competence?

In the theme, 'nutritional care out of remit and competence', RNs experience of nutritional care per se was reflected as contradictory in many ways. How each individual RN experienced nutritional care per se was interpreted as not only having an impact on their performance of the nutritional nursing care on offer. Their experiences also seemed to resolve to what degree the RNs engaged in involving the older person in her/his nutritional care. The texts mirrored some RNs awareness of the importance to work proactively with nutrition in general and other RNs obliviousness, where nutritional care was not given much thought or refection. Those RNs reflecting a greater awareness of, and proactive engagement in nutritional care also tended to indicate knowledge about the relationship between nutritional status, older people's health and their function expressed as:

> One [the older person] has no strength if one doesn't
> have enough food. One risks infections and sickness,
> and one has no resistance. Therefore, I put a strong
> emphasis on nourishment among old people. It
> should be frequent, small, calorie-dense portions
> and [served at] regular [times]: Three main meals
> and three in-between meals. One meal needs to be
> just before bedtime to avoid a long period of starvation
> at night, which will happen if one doesn't eat just before
> bedtime. [RN/F]

In contrast, the oblivious approach to nutritional care was reflected upon by this RN:

One tries to ask if they have any particular likings in regards to food. I do not ask them much more than that. I actually do not think that much about that part – nutrition – at all. You see... there is... nature has to have its cause. In general, one eats... you know, one has less appetite for food and drink when getting older, and yes, that is how I view it in the bigger picture. [RN/I]

The theme, 'nutritional care out of remit and competence', also reflected experiences of insecurity and certain challenges, especially when it concerned what nursing actions and/or interventions to take when the older person was at risk for malnutrition. Some self-critical voices were apparent:

It's most likely ignorance amongst the professionals, that is, by the nurse, um, yes. [RN/I]

Experiencing nutritional care as challenging could additionally mean that nutritional supplement drinks were the informants' first and main choice of nursing intervention. It was also here where more self-critical voices were illuminated, and one informant expressed that the task of giving nutritional supplement drinks meant a job done and ticked off the list:

When we have given complete nutritional supplement drinks, we believe we have done it all. One can tick it off and record it ... then one has done something. Is that not strange? [RN/K]

Another response which reflected this was made by another RN:

My initial thought is always complete nutritional supplement drinks ... We met with the dietician yesterday and talked about this, and then he said that these [nutritional supplement drinks] are actually the last way out/option. One should focus more on adjusting the meal environment or use simpler methods to find out what is causing the person in question to not eat. [RN/H]

Despite interpreting the above statement to mean that teaming up with other healthcare professionals could result in different perspectives on nutritional care, the text reflected a rather cool and distanced relationship to for example the dieticians:

At times, I contact them [the dieticians], yes. ...Yes, it can happen when there are problems with choking. It can happen when we do not [succeed with them] gaining weight despite us trying everything. ...They

might view it in a different way. ... You get clever tips, but it is absolutely not always – it is [rather] seldom. [RN/E]

Another distanced relationship in nutritional care was also experienced in regard to the General Practitioner (GP). The informants' overall experience was that not many "medical" actions could be done by the GP when an older person stops eating and drinking. Such issues had to be dealt with by the RNs, as this problem was situated within the domain of nursing. Here, another contradiction was reflected, as the texts mirrored both insecurity and challenges as well as experiences such as the RNs being much better equipped to handle nutrition involving older people and possessing more insight into how to deal with it despite being self-critical about the main nursing intervention i.e. nutritional supplement drinks.

I don't deal with the GP as much. If I would have some bigger issues with a patient, [then] I would contact the dietician, but not the GP. I don't really think they are much into this issue. [RN/F]

The theme 'nutritional care out of remit and competence' also reflected that the mealtime environment, mealtime ambiance and choice of what food served was not within the informant's remit in nutritional care. The main control and responsibility for these factors had instead been handed down to the healthcare assistants, and this handing down of actual responsibility was expressed by two of the informants:

I think it is mainly [that] one has put it on the healthcare assistants [because] they are there all the time. It is them handling it, so it has been put down to them. [RN/J]

I am trying to engage, but it is mainly the enrolled nurse. It is their environment in the kitchen and so [on]. But if I think something is wrong, I do try to point it out – that they need to think about this or maybe that. [RN/G].

Nutritional care more than just choosing a flavour?
In the final theme, 'nutritional care more than just choosing a flavour', the older persons' experiences of participation in their nutritional care reflected that no easy standard approach exists to achieve a satisfactory level of involvement in their care. Some of the experiences reflected by the RNs in the theme 'participation in nutritional care equals information' also mirrored the older persons' experiences. This was especially reflected amongst those older people who

experienced being uninformed about what could be done or which care could remedy their nutritional status. One older person states this plainly:

> No one tells you anything here. They do what they want ... that is how it is. [OP/D]

Additionally, the older persons' experience of not being involved or having the possibility to discuss things with the RNs about how the nutritional care was to be planned indicated frustration, and this came through in one plain-speaking older person's interview could be expressed as:

> One is not allowed to decide anything. [OP/C]

Other experiences were also recounted, as some of the older persons perceived that they had been informed about what malnutrition could mean when being older. They could describe how being malnourished affects their energy levels and is detrimental for their health. One informant expressed it in the following admission:

> It was okay. Yeah, one could say it was good [the information about being malnourished]. ... I needed to eat more. [OP/A]

In these cases, despite having been informed by the RN, the older persons perceived that they not had been involved in planning the treatment meant to target their malnourishment or risk of malnutrition. These older people experienced that they were passive receivers of the nutritional care and the information given.

> When malnourished, no, we did not [participate]. I got nutritional supplement drinks from the nurse. I got Actimel. [OP/A]

The theme 'nutritional care more than just choosing a flavour' also suggested that when having been assessed as at risk of or as malnourished the only nursing action for this was to instruct the older persons to drink supplemental nutrition drinks, and the older person's only involvement was to be allowed to "pick the flavour you like". The nutritional supplement drinks were given until the individual's weight was back up to a healthy level.

> For a while, I got these ... bottles. I got one three times a day, such bottle [nutritional supplement drinks]. But now, I am told by them that I don't need them anymore. [OP/B]

Having been slim and slender throughout life and consequently having a low BMI since youth meant that some older people experienced nutritional care and

weight gain as an upsetting ordeal. Emotions such as nervousness and anxiety about weight gain and a changed body image were expressed. This experience was corroborated by the RNs, who perceived that some older persons took on a highly passive role in regard to involvement and were not particularly adherent to the action plan purely based on anxiety about gaining too much weight.

> I am eating and gaining weight. Now I am scared to gain far too much weight. [OP/B]

In stark contrast to the one nursing intervention on offer (i.e. nutritional supplement drinks) was the older persons' views reflecting the possibility to decide his/her meals. On one hand, the older person would experience a boost in energy by the drinks, but on the other hand, they found them difficult, as they quickly felt full with them. If they were given a choice, the older people preferred normal food over drinking more than one nutritional supplement drink a day.

> They tell you that you can drink more in one day, but one can't. It is that much ... one cannot drink four or as much as possible. So, so that is how it is ... for me, there is a limit of one bottle [nutritional supplement drink] a day. And that is not enough to go up.... [in weight]. [OP/C]

The theme 'nutritional care more than just choosing a flavour' also entailed the older person's experiences of involvement in the mealtime environment and the setting of the daily food menu. They expressed a wish to be involved in both the shaping of the environment and the menu. One older person expressed her frustration:

> And I thought, 'It is only this time [that] it is a catastrophe. It is only this time ... and not tomorrow'. Oh, yes, I am put at the same place by the table every time [next to a resident she does not want to be near]. [They think,] 'She is so kind, and she is so tiny, so it doesn't matter, [so] we place her here'. [OP/C]

The food on offer at the nursing home was not experienced as highly rated, and when asked the direct question of whether the older persons experienced any possibility to become involved in the food that was served, two of the informants gave a reply indicating that the menu was not able to be changed:

> I get the menu, and then [I] have to eat [what's on it]. [OP/A]

Nothing [involving participation with food]. They only serve it. On the table in front of me. [OP/D]

The theme reflected that breakfast was the only meal where the older persons experienced that they could be involved. Breakfast food was presented on the table, and one could choose whatever they liked. The older persons perceived that they could ask for something else (i.e. extra outside ordinary mealtimes and the set menu), but otherwise their involvement was also limited here. The theme reflects the wish to be involved in the menu as well as the insight that if the food tasted a bit better, then they would automatically eat more. However, despite not experiencing any meaningful involvement in their nutrition, the food served or mealtime ambience, the older persons still felt that the staff tried to accommodate as many of their wishes as possible.

I would like to decide my food and [choose] food that is good. Good gravy. That the food is … when you get pork shops or pork shoulder. Then you get no gravy. They remove the best part. I would like to have my mum's great steaks [giggles]. I know I cannot get it. [OP/C]

Coffee and tea – one can have at any time you go down and say, "Now I fancy a cup of coffee" [then they say,] "I will arrange that for you". They are good in that sense: "Have all of you got [coffee or tea]?" [OP/C]

All meals were served at set times, but they could be slightly moved for the unique individual. This was perceived as some degree of being involved as well as being in control in some way. One older person explains:

We have our set mealtimes here: Breakfast at 8 o'clock, dinner at 12 o'clock, coffee at 2 o'clock, and supper at 5 o'clock. This is how it is every day. But if you are doing something, then they save your food and reheat it for you when you arrive. [OP/B]

Lastly, the theme reflects that the older persons would experience the need to accept what was laid out on the table, as they perceived that it would not be right to complain about the food being served. One of the older people explains:

If I don't want it, they can arrange something else. But I never do that. I am ashamed of doing that. They do all they can to prepare good food, and then how it comes out – that's another matter – but one has to try to eat it. [OP/A]

Discussion

The analysis indicate that RN's experience of older people's participation in nutritional care and their experiences of nutritional care per se could be understood in the light of two predominant themes: 'participation in nutritional care equals information' 'nutritional care out of remit and competence'. While the older peoples experience of their participation in their nutritional care could be understood in the light of the theme, 'nutritional care more than just choosing a flavour.'

The lack of engagement from the RNs regarding involving the older persons in their nutritional care stood out as noteworthy in the theme, 'participation in nutritional care equals information', particularly as the concept of *person-centred care* is cited as one of healthcare's main priorities today, but the concept is also one of the six core competencies [43] RNs are suggested to base care on. Our findings put forward that the RNs saw participation as analogous to simply informing the older persons about their nutritional status. When taking the time to reflect, the RNs experienced that the information they gave could have been better; however, a lack of time was cited one barrier for giving information. Our findings also revealed that RNs seemed to prefer to give directives and strict orders rather than engage the older person in a discussion about what could be the best ways to improve their nutritional status. However, our findings may not be unexpected, given that Longtin and colleagues [34] found that the staff's acceptance of patients' participation in care is affected by their need to preserve control and by a lack of time. Factors entrenched in the context of care such as a task-oriented practice (e.g. giving directives) is also known to obstruct participation [44]. Others [35, 36] have shown that the participation of older persons, particularly those residing in nursing homes like those of this study, are rarely, if at all, involved in activities relating to nutrition or nutritional care.

To involve older people in their own care and inform them adequately requires effective communication. However, research into participation in clinical practice found that although RNs speak about the importance of communication, they were only observed to have contact with the persons they cared for when they had a task to complete [44, 45]. This knowledge has implications, particularly in the Swedish context of nursing homes, as the daily care is delivered by healthcare assistants and not by the RNs. The latter are mainly called upon in unexpected care events; thus, this does not leave many natural interaction points between the RNs and the older persons. It is clearly important to acknowledge that adequate information [46] is vital in supporting people to participate in decision-making about their own care, especially as information is central for the patient's ability to make decisions about their care. In particular, when the information given is used as a tool to support the RN's agenda, it becomes ostensible rather than a factor that leads to true participation. We recommend that participation in care has to be more than simply informing the older person about directives and already planned actions. Collaboration and the sharing of power between the RN and the older persons appear just as important as offering them relevant information. Thus, our findings imply, despite that patient participation in care is regulated by law in Sweden, that nutritional care for older people residing in nursing homes may yet have some way to go before participation becomes a natural part of nutritional care in this context. There are no easy solutions to remedy this; however, a person-centred care approach should be central in the nutritional care of older people.

Involving older persons in their care appears to occur when RNs possess knowledge and awareness about the components of nutritional care as reflected in the theme 'nutritional care out of remit and competence' This stood out in stark contrast to some RNs views which suggested nature needs to have its place in old age. It also contrasts with certain RNs feelings of insecurity and frustration about nutritional nursing care and strategies for involvement. Despite the latter and that support was available both in the form of the GP and dietician, nutritional supplement drinks were shown to be the nurses' gold standard for those older people assessed at risk for malnutrition or as malnourished. It is clear that knowledge and competence support RNs in involving older persons in their care. However, the ease at which RNs confess to lack sufficient competence in nutritional care and how to involve the older persons in this care is unexpected, although others have also highlighted shortcomings in nutritional nursing care. For example, Alharabi and colleagues [33] suggest the need to remove the lack of understanding and confidence among healthcare professionals when it concerns how to involve older people in their nutritional care. Suominen and colleagues [1] further support this by putting forward that RNs need more in-depth knowledge about nutrition issues to raise their awareness about nutritional nursing care. This corroborates with our interpretation of the connection between RN's knowledge and awareness of nutrition and the RN's level of involving patients. Moreover, interprofessional collaboration in addition to the collaboration between RNs and older persons is required to establish appropriate and sustainable nutritional care.

Considering that one of the core competencies for RNs put forward by Cronenwett et al. [43] is that nursing care on offer should be evidence-based, it was rather unexpected that nutritional supplement drinks were the first line of nursing intervention in treating older people assessed at risk for malnutrition or as malnourished. Especially, considering the weak evidence about their actual effect on malnutrition i.e. effect in weight gain or

improved function among older people [47, 48]. It seems reasonable to draw the conclusion that nutritional care in this context seemingly still not rests on an evidence-based care. Taking this into account, it becomes difficult to whitewash or give alternative interpretations to the kind of nutritional nursing care reflected by statements such as "a job done and ticked off". Understanding and applying evidence-based nutritional knowledge are important ways to effectively assess dietary intake and provide appropriate guidance, counselling and treatment to older persons. This must be vital despite the fact that a recent systematic review [49] aiming to determine the effect of nursing interventions targeting fundamentals of care [9] such as nutritional care concluded that current evidence for nutritional nursing care interventions was sparse, of poor quality and unfit to provide evidence-based guidance to RNs in clinical practice. Consequently, educational efforts alone will not be enough to improve nutritional care as Richards et al. [49] highlights that nursing research additionally need to step up when it concerns effective nursing care interventions targeting fundamentals of care.

Although the RNs ultimately are responsible for care, thus expected to take on the role as the point-of-care leader, our findings indicated that some of the responsibilities for the older persons nutritional care depended upon the health care assistants. Leaving some of the RNs with the experience that some of the general nutritional care were out of their remit. On the other hand, RNs were quite determined that the GPs not were in a position to support nursing care in case of nutritional challenges i.e. older patients refusing to eat and drink as this belonged to the domain of nursing. It is not based on these findings reasonable to predict the reasons for these contradictory experiences. We know that RNs providing leadership at the point-of-care can have a positive impact on clinical practice but also introduce leadership behaviours of importance for all roles [50]. However, to be able to lead care demands competent and safe RNs and, our findings did at time, reflect experiences of both insecurity and lack of competency concerning nutritional care. Additionally, teamwork is known to improve patient planning, is clinically more efficient and supports a person-centred care [51]. Working in interprofessional teams in order to ensure continuity of care, patient safety and quality of care is also one of the six core competencies suggested for nurses to possess to meet health care standards [43] and would be a realistic approach to improve older peoples nutritional care in nursing homes.

Older persons' participation in their own nutritional care appears to be an ambiguous and tortuous path. In the theme, 'nutritional care more than just choosing a flavour', it is clear that, although the older people wished to be involved in both what was on the menu and in shaping the environment, their involvement was restricted to choosing what they wanted for breakfast and what flavour they wanted if they required a nutritional supplement drink. No easy standard approach exists to achieve a satisfactory level of involvement in their own care. The older people stated that communication often failed, and they were not able to be involved or have the possibility to discuss things over with the RNs about how their nutritional care was planned. Our findings are corroborated by others. Say and colleagues [26], conclude in their literature review that it is important to remember that participation may not be acceptable or appropriate for everyone. In a qualitative study by Nyborg and colleagues [52] the older people experienced difficulties when participating (i.e. their involvement in decisions and in their own care). The reason given by the older persons in the study was their deteriorating capability to do so. Additionally, an older person's desired level of participation in his/her care may be influenced by their generational values. This notion falls in line with Nyborg and colleagues [52], who state that today's participation ideology is based on individualism, which they suggest is likely to conflict with the current older generation's "commonly held values of solidarity and community" (p.1). Consequently, research [53] has shown that older people's gratitude for the health-care system and to healthcare staff at times overshadows not being informed or involved; that is, they reject their own needs and preferences. Another study by Penney and Wellard [54] found that participation in care was equated with being independent by the older persons. The later can be extra challenging for the RNs to handle when engaging in strategies promoting participation, as it is likely that older people residing in nursing homes already experience that their independence is restricted. Nursing that strives to involve older persons in their care and decisions about their care would therefore gain from departing from person-centred care models, particularly as is seems fair to assume that these kinds of nursing models automatically mean acceptance of the RNs to offer a care adapted to what degree the older person wishes to participate.

Study limitations – Strength and weaknesses
Our study design allowed an emphasis to be placed on the statements and interpretations of those being studied. However, its relatively small sample ($n = 12$) has implications for the trustworthiness of the findings. Our sampling technique ensured the possibility of capturing different views and perceptions, and although the sampling was strategically conducted [30], it was relatively homogenous in aspects like gender when it concerned the RNs. This implies that the result can be specific for female RNs within this context and that homogeneity can affect the transferability of the result. However, their heterogeneous ages, levels of education and amount of time in their position, in addition to including two RNs who are male,

may counterbalance this. It was a challenge to recruit older people, and the sample size ended up being restricted to four informants (three women and one man), as three informants chose to withdraw from the study prior to the interviews. Therefore, due to the small sample size and the homogeneity, generalisations must be made with caution. However, to the best of our knowledge, few studies regarding older people's experiences of involvement in nutritional care have been conducted, and thus, this study contributes with new knowledge to this field.

The amalgam of realities presented here may be regarded as the views of the informants, and as such, may be transferable to similar settings. Finally, the risk of subjectivity in the data interpretation always exists, as there is always more than one possible way to interpret a text. Our method of analysis – content analysis [35] – allows the possibility to justify the texts by structuring and presenting them using categories and themes. However, the risk of subjectivity always remains, as data interpretation can be influenced by the interpreter's life experience and ability [55]. To reduce this risk and to enhance the credibility of this study, the authors worked together throughout the phases of analysis to strengthen the interpretations, not by achieving consensus or arriving at identical formulations in interpretations but by supplementing and contesting each other's readings. By describing the analytical procedure used and presenting quotations from the interview texts, we have hopefully enabled the reader to consider the interpretation valid [56] and trustworthy. A qualitative study such as this is limited in regard to its transferability and its relevance to other types of settings; consequently, this should be taken into account when evaluating our findings.

Conclusion
Our findings are somewhat disheartening because today substantial existing knowledge confirms that it is important for healthcare professionals to strive towards true participation in care. However, we acknowledge that participation is a complex process which requires all factors to work together well before participation and decision-making become a natural part of essential care for older people. Although our findings suggest that RNs should be aware of the importance of involving older people in their care, they also indicate that, despite the knowledge that participation should be central to nursing, this has yet to become a reality despite its regulation by law. Therefore, educational strategies that support RNs in developing the competences needed to enable older people's participation in nursing care should be a priority, even during the first years of nurses' training. Furthermore, our findings indicate that a paternalistic attitude in care as well as asymmetry in the nurse-patient relationship are still common characteristics of modern clinical nursing practice in the care of older people. However, we envisage that this unsuccessful

approach in care will be phased out when new cohorts of older people such as baby boomers become the new consumers of health and social care.

Nursing care striving to involving older people in their own care, and those making the decisions need to be aware that different strategies may be needed to make participation a reality. Although our findings may need to be interpreted with caution, they reflect that getting involved in care was not always as high on the older persons' agenda as one might expect. Thus, developed strategies for participation need to take this into account. A person-centred approach to care could be one model of care to facilitate this. To be successful in this work, an interdisciplinary approach including both RNs, GPs and Health Care assistants is needed. To promote effective collaboration, it is important to assure that the roles of the team members is clear, but also that RNs are ready to take on the role as the point-of-care leader. Enhancement of collaboration by communicating roles and making work agreements should therefore be continuously on the agenda. It is also important find strategies to empower RNs to take the point-of-care leadership for the fundamentals of care and here especially for nutritional care. However, before doing this it seems that there is a need to raise competence and knowledge as our findings indicate both insecurity and lack of competence among RNs concerning nutritional care.

Finally, it appears important to conclude by suggesting that different strategies are needed for researchers to be able to explore more in-depth how participation can be achieved or experienced among older people, particularly those residing in nursing homes, as this is an extremely vulnerable group. For them to participate in and be able to decide about their care may be effective ways to support the older person's feelings of independence and well-being.

It is important to get a deeper understanding of what matters to patients and to RNs who are responsible for deliver nutritional care in an often complex and challenging environment, and more research in the field is needed. Nutritional care must be based on evidence and future research also need to focus on the effectiveness of fundamentals of care to support nursing knowledge in the deliverance of an evidence-based care.

Abbreviations
GP: General practitioner; RN: Registered nurses

Acknowledgements
We would like to thank the registered nurses and the older people who participated in this study and the Language Editing Group at Malmö University for support with language revision.

Funding
This research received no specific grant from any funding agency in the public, commercial, or not-for-profit sector.

Authors' contributions
JN and KSF were responsible for the study's inception and design. JN was responsible for the data acquisition and drafting the manuscript. JN, KSF and GB performed the data analysis. KSF and GB were responsible for the critical revision of the paper. KSF and GB added important intellectual content, while KSF supervised the study. All authors read and approved the final manuscript.

Ethics approval and consent to participate
This study was conducted in compliance with the established ethical guidelines of the Declaration of Helsinki. Although under the Swedish Ethical Review Act 2003:460 this study did not require ethical clearance, we applied for and received ethical guidance from the Ethical Advisory Board in Southern Sweden (No. HS2016/28). The researcher gave oral and written information and obtained written informed consent from all participants before the interviews. Participation was voluntary, and the participants had the right to withdraw at any time without further explanation. The participants gave consent for direct quotes from their interviews to be used in this paper. To ensure confidentiality, each quotation was assigned a pseudonym in the form of a capital letter. Data were stored securely and anonymously in compliance with the Data Protection Act.

Competing interests
The authors declare that they have no competing interest.

Author details
[1]Department of Care Science, Faculty of Health and Society, Malmö University, SE-205 06 Malmö, Sweden. [2]Malmö Town, Borough Administration West, SE-214 66 Malmö, Sweden.

References
1. Suominen MH, Sandelin E, Soini H, Pitkala KH. How well do nurses recognize malnutrition in elderly patients? Eur J Clin Nutr. 2009;63:292–6.
2. Adams N, Bowie A, Simmance N, Murray M, Crowe T. Recognition by medical and nursing professionals of malnutrition and risk of malnutrition in elderly hospitalized patients. Nutr Diet. 2008;65:144–50.
3. Carlsson M, Gustafson Y, Eriksson S, Haglin L. Body composition in Swedish old people aged 65–99 years, living in residential care facilities. Arch Gerontol Geriatr. 2009;49:98–107.
4. Kaiser MJ, Bauer JM, Rämsch C, Uter W, Guigoz Y, Cederholm T, Thomas DR, Anthony PS, Charlton KE, Maggio M, Tsai AC, Vellas B, Sieber CC. Frequency of malnutrition in older adults: a multinational perspective using the mini nutritional assessment. J Am Geriatr Soc. 2010;58:1734–8.
5. Chan M, Lim YP, Ernest A, Tan TL. Nutritional assessment in an Asian nursing home and its association with mortality. J Nutr Health Aging. 2010;14:23–8.
6. Verbrugghe M, Beeckman D, Van Hecke A, Vanderwee K, Van Herck K, Clays E, Bocquaert I, Derycke H, Geurden B, Verhaeghe S. Malnutrition and associated factors in nursing home residents: a cross-sectional, multi-Centre study. Clin Nutr. 2013;32:438–43.
7. Beattie E, O'Reilly M, Strange E, Franklin S, Isenring E. How much do residential aged care staff members know about the nutritional needs of residents? Int J Older People Nursing. 2013;9:54–64.
8. Bales C. What does it mean to be "at nutritional risk"? Seeking clarity on behalf of the elderly. Am J Clin Nutr. 2001;74:155–6.
9. Kitson AL, Muntlin Athlin A, Conroy T. Anything but basic: Nursing's challenge in meeting patients' fundamental care needs. J Nurs Scholarsh. 2014;46:331–9.
10. Bachrach-Lindström M, Jensen S, Lundin R, Christensson L. Attitudes of nursing staff working with older people towards nutritional nursing care. J Clin Nurs. 2007;16:2007–14.

11. Wentzel Persenius M, Hall-Lord ML, Bååth C, Wilde Larsson B. Assessment and documentation of patients' nutritional status: perceptions of registered nurses and their chief nurses. *J Clin Nurs. 2007;17:*2125–36.

12. Bjerrum M, Tewes M, Pedersen P. Nurses' self-reported knowledge about and attitude to nutrition – before and after a training programme. Scand J Caring Sci. 2012;26:81–9.

13. Christensson L, Unosson M, Ek AC. Individually adjusted meals for older people with protein-energy malnutrition: a single case study. J Clin Nurs. 2001;10:491–502.

14. Faxén-Irving G, Andren-Olsson B, af Geijerstam A, Basun H, Cederholm T. The effect of nutritional intervention in elderly subjects residing in group-living for the demented. Eur J Clin Nutr. 2002;56:221–7.

15. Jones J, Duffy M, Coull Y, Wilkinson H. Older people living in the community-nutritional needs, barriers and interventions: a literature review. Scott Gov Soc Res. 2009:1–78.

16. Chen CCH, Schilling LS, Lyder CH. A concept analysis of malnutrition in the elderly. J Advanced Nurs. 2001;36:131–42.

17. Chapman IM. Nutritional disorders in the elderly. Med Clin North Am. 2006;90:887–907.

18. Sauer AC, Alish CJ, Strausbaugh K, West K, Quatrara B. Nurses needed: identifying malnutrition in hospitalized older adults. NursingPlus Open. 2016;2:21–5.

19. Nijs K, de Graaf C, van Staveren WA, de Groot L. Malnutrition and mealtime ambiance in nursing homes. Jamda. 2009;10:226–9.

20. Christensen M, Hewitt-Taylor J. Empowerment in nursing: paternalism or maternalism? Br J Nurs. 2006;15:695–9.

21. Cody WK. Paternalism in nursing and healthcare: central issues and their relation to theory. Nurs Sci Q. 2003;16:288–96.

22. Gallant MH, Beaulieu MC, Carnevale FA. Partnership: an analysis of the concept within the nurse-client relationship. J Adv Nurs. 2002;40:149–57.

23. Sahlsten MJ, Larsson IE, Sjöström B, Lindencrona CS, Plos KA. Patient participation in nursing care: towards a concept clarification from a nurse perspective. J Clin Nurs. 2007;16:630–7.

24. The Patient Act (2014:821) Retrieved from https://www.riksdagen.se/sv/dokument-lagar/dokument/svensk-forfattningssamling/patientlag-2014821_sfs-2014-821 on 15 March 2018. Accessed 15 Mar 2018. In Swedish.

25. The Health and Medical Service Act (2017:30) Retrieved from https://www.riksdagen.se/sv/dokument-lagar/dokument/svensk-forfattningssamling/halso%2D-och-sjukvardslag_sfs-2017-30. Accessed 15 Mar 2018. In Swedish.

26. Say R, Murtagh M, Thomson R. Patients' preference for involvement in medical decision making: a narrative review. Patient Educ Couns. 2006;60:102–14.

27. Pedersen PU. Nutritional care: the effectiveness of actively involving older patients. J Clin Nurs. 2005;14:247–55.

28. Little P, Everitt H, Williamson I, Warner G, Moore M, Gould C, Payne S. Observational study of effect of patient centeredness and positive approach on outcomes of general practice consultations. BMJ. 2001;323:908–11.

29. Rosén P, Anell A, Hjortsberg C. Patient views on choice and participation in primary health care. Health Policy. 2001;55:121–8.

30. Levinson W, Kao A, Kuby A, Thisted RA. Not all patients want to participate in decision making: a national study of public preferences. J Gen Int Med. 2005;20:531–5.

31. Bastiaens H, Van Royen P, Pavlic DR, Raposo V, Baker R. Older people's preferences for involvement in their own care: a qualitative study in primary health care in 11 European countries. Patient Educ Couns. 2007;68:33–42.

32. Wetzels R, Harmsen M, Van Weel C, Grol R, Wensing M. Interventions for improving older patients' involvement in primary care episodes. Cochrane Database of Systematic Reviews 2007, Issue 1. Art. No.: CD004273.

33. Alharabi J, Carlström E, Ekman I, Jarneborn A, Olsson L-E. Experiences of person-centered care - patients' perceptions: qualitative study. BMC Nurs. 2014;13:28.

34. Longtin Y, Sax H, Leape LL, Sheridan SE, Donaldson L, Pittet D. Patient participation: current knowledge and applicability to patient safety. Mayo Clin Proc. 2010;85:53–62.

35. Winterburn S. Residents' choice of and control over food in care homes. Nurs Older People. 2009;21:34–7.

36. Abrahamsen Grøndahl V, Aagaard H. Older peolpe's involvement in activities related to meals in nursing homes. Int J Older People Nursing. 2016;11:204–13.

37. Polit D, Beck C. Essentials of nursing research: appraising evidence for nursing practice. 8th ed. Philadelphia: Wolters Kluwer Health/Lippincott Williams & Wilkins; 2013.

38. Kvale S, Brinkmann S. Interviews learning the craft of qualitative research interviewing. Thousand Oaks: Sage Publications; 2009.

39. Burnard P. A method of analysing interview transcripts in qualitative research. Nurse Educ Today. 1991;11:461–6.

40. Burnard P. Teaching the analysis of textual data: an experiential approach. Nurse Educ Today. 1996;16:278–81.

41. Vellas B, Guigoz Y, Garry PJ, Nourhashemi F, Bennahamm D, Langue S, Albarede JL. The mini nutritional assessment (MNA) and its use in grading the nutritional state of elderly patients. Nutr. 1999;15:116–22.

42. Graneheim UH, Lundman B. Qualitative content analysis in nursing research: concepts, procedures and measures to achieve trustworthiness. Nurse Educ Today. 2004;24:105–12.

43. Cronenwett L, Sherwood G, Barnsteiner J, Disch J, Johnson J, Mitchell P, Taylor Sullivan D, Warren J. Quality and safety education for nurses. Nurs Outlook. 2007;55:122–31.

44. Henderson S. Knowing the patient and the impact on patient participation: a grounded theory study. Int J Nurs Pract. 1997;3:111–8.

45. Wellard S, Lillibridge J, Beanland C, Lewis M. Consumer participation in acute care setting: an Australian experience. Int J Nurs Pract. 2003;9:255–60.

46. Thompson AG. The meaning of patient involvement and participation in health care consultations: a taxonomy. Soc Sci Med. 2007;64:1297–310.

47. Baldwin C, Kimber KL, Gibbs M, Weekes CE. Supportive interventions for enhancing dietary intake in malnourished or nutritionally at-risk adults. Cochrane Database Syst Rev. 2016;20(12):CD009840.

48. Milne AC, Potter J, Vivanti A, Avenell A. Protein and energy supplementation in elderly people at risk from malnutrition. Cochrane Database Syst Rev. 2009;15(2):CD003288.

49. Richards DA, Hilli A, Pentecost C, Goodwin VA, Frost J. Fundamental nursing care: a systematic review of the evidence on the effect of nursing care interventions for nutrition, elimination, mobility and hygiene. J Clin Nurs. 2017;00:1–11.

50. Abraham P. Developing nursing leaders: a program enhancing staff nurse leadership skills and professionalism. Nurs Adm Q. 2011;35:306–12.

51. Atwal A, Caldwell K. Nurses' perceptions of multidiscilplinary team work in acute healthcare. Int J Nurs Pract. 2006;12:359–65.

52. Nyborg I, Kvigne K, Danbolt LJ, Kirkevold M. Ambiguous participation in older hospitalized patients: gaining influence through active and passive approaches-a qualitative study. BMC Nurs. 2016;15:1–11.

53. Hvalvik S, Dale B. The transition from hospital to home: older people's experiences. Open J Nurs. 2015;05:622–31.

54. Penney W, Wellard S. Hearing what older consumers say about participation in their care. Int J Nurs Pract. 2007;13:61–8.

55. Wallace JB. Life stories. In: Gubrium JF, Sankar A, editors. Qualitative methods in aging research. London: Sage Publications; 1994.

56. Benner P. Quality of life: a phenomenological perspective on explanation, prediction, and understanding in nursing science. Adv Nurs Sci. 1994;8:1–14.

18

Accuracy of pulse oximetry in detection of oxygen saturation in patients admitted to the intensive care unit of heart surgery: comparison of finger, toe, forehead and earlobe probes

Sohila Seifi[1], Alireza Khatony[2*], Gholamreza Moradi[3], Alireza Abdi[2] and Farid Najafi[4]

Abstract

Background: Heart surgery patients are more at risk of poor peripheral perfusion, and peripheral capillary oxygen saturation (SpO2) measurement is regular care for continuous analysis of blood oxygen saturation in these patients. With regard to controversial studies on accuracy of the current pulse oximetry probes and lack of data related to patients undergoing heart surgery, the present study was conducted to determine accuracy of pulse oximetry probes of finger, toe, forehead and earlobe in detection of oxygen saturation in patients admitted to intensive care units for coronary artery bypass surgery.

Methods: In this clinical trial, 67 patients were recruited based on convenience sampling method among those admitted to intensive care units for coronary artery bypass surgery. The SpO2 value was measured using finger, toe, forehead and earlobe probes and then compared with the standard value of arterial oxygen saturation (SaO2). Data were entered into STATA-11 software and analyzed using descriptive, inferential and Bland-Altman statistical analyses.

Results: Highest and lowest correlational mean values of SpO2 and SaO2 were related to finger and earlobe probes, respectively. The highest and lowest agreement of SpO2 and SaO2 were related to forehead and earlobe probes.

Conclusion: The SpO2 of earlobe probes due to lesser mean difference, more limited confidence level and higher agreement ration with SaO2 resulted by arterial blood gas (ABG) analysis had higher accuracy. Thus, it is suggested to use earlobe probes in patients admitted to the intensive care unit for coronary artery bypass surgery.

Trial registration: Registration of this trial protocol has been approved in Iranian Registry of Clinical Trials at 2018–03–19 with reference IRCT20100913004736N22. "Retrospectively registered."

Keywords: Pulse oximetry, Critical care, Accuracy

Background

Pulse oximetry is a simple and non-invasive method used to examine oxygen saturation (SpO2) in various parts of body [1]. Using pulse oximetry is effective in accelerating the weaning from mechanical ventilation and extubation and reduces the frequency of bleeding for analysis of arterial blood gases (ABG), because for the

patients who just need checking for the O2 saturation, pulse oximetry could be a proper alternative [2, 3]. Convenient use, speed and high accuracy in detection of hypoxia and continuous monitoring of patients are other features of pulse oximetry [3–5]. This device detects the amount of oxyhemoglobin and deoxygenated hemoglobin in arterial blood and shows it as Oxyhemoglobin saturation (SpO2) [6] which is an indirect estimation of arterial oxygen saturation (SaO2) [7]. The normal amount of SpO2 in healthy individuals is 97% to 99% [8].

* Correspondence: Akhatony@kums.ac.ir
[2]Nursing department, Nursing and Midwifery School, Kermanshah University of Medical Sciences, Kermanshah, Iran
Full list of author information is available at the end of the article

If the SaO2 is 70% to 100%, the amount of SpO2 has high accuracy and is 2% different from the SaO2 amount obtained from ABG analysis [5]. Yet, in more critically ill patients, the amount of pulse oximetry error is reported as 7.2% [9]. Various factors can affect the accuracy of the device including the physiologic, environmental, technology failures and human error [1, 3, 7, 10–12].

There are contradictory and controversial results regarding the accurate detection of SpO2 by pulse oximeter obtained from the related studies [13–16]. Nessler et al. (2012) in their study concluded that among the patients under vasopressors, the forehead pulse oximeter sensor had higher accuracy in detection of SpO2 compared to transitional pulse oximetry of fingers [13]. The study of Bilan et al. (2006) indicated pulse oximetry by earlobe probe, had higher accuracy compared to pulse oximetry of finger and toe probes in detection of hypoxemia in children and babies. Further, it was shown that pulse oximetry of finger probes had the lowest agreement with SpO2 [14]. Korhan et al. (2011) suggested that in patients under physical restraints, the unfolded finger should be used to show the accurate value of SpO2 [15]. Wilson et al. (2010), in a retrospective cohort study, reported the difference of 2.7% between SpO2 and SaO2 in emergency patients with severe sepsis and septic shock and suggested using ABG where there is a need for more accurate detection of SaO2 [1]; the authors suggested doing more investigations due to the limitations of the study such as insufficient sample size.

Sugino et al. (2004) compared the pulse oximetry of forehead and finger probes in patients under general anesthesia. For this purpose, eighteen patients were induced by Propofol and time of lowest, time to recovery and lag time of beginning of SpO2 were measured for finger and forehead probes. The results showed that there are no differences between pulse oximetry of forehead and finger in terms of the mentioned times in a general anesthesia, and the authors suggested, the forehead probe can be a proper replacement when it is not possible to use finger probe [16]. Common methods such as forehead and finger probes have higher reliability in detection of peripheral oxygen saturation in patients with normal condition. However, these methods are not effective in critically ill patients hospitalized in intensive care unit with changes in vital signs because they have some limitations such as having edema in attached sites, and difficulties to matched control group [17, 18].

Considering the limitations and advantages of pulse oximetry in various parts of the body, the importance of accurate detection of hypoxemia and lack of studies about the proper method of pulse oximetry in patients admitted to intensive care units for coronary artery bypass surgery, the present study was conducted to determine the accuracy of pulse oximetry probes of finger, toe, forehead and earlobe in detection of oxygen saturation in the patients admitted to the intensive care unit for coronary artery bypass surgery.

Methods

In this clinical trial, the study population was the patients admitted to the intensive care unit of Imam Ali (AS) Hospital affiliated to Kermanshah University of Medical Sciences (KUMS) for coronary artery bypass surgery. Study sample included 67 patients estimated based on the mean difference of 0.15 between measured SpO2 of finger, toe and forehead probes in the study by Yunt et al. (2011) [12], test power of 90% and probability error of first type as 5%.

These patients were selected based on convenience sampling and the inclusion criteria included having arterial line, oral temperature above 35 °C, Hemoglobin greater than 9 g/dl, mean arterial pressure of higher than 60 mmHg, PaO2 between 70% to 100% and pCO_2 less than 45 mmHg, lack of underlying problems such as blood disorders (for example anemia, methemoglobinemia, carboxyhemoglobinemia), left ventricular failure, peripheral vascular disease, and acute and chronic renal failure, not having nail polish and finger clubbing, no history of smoking, and lack of ulcers, burns, edema and dressing in probe placement. Patients whose mean arterial pressure reached less than 60 mmHg or needed suction, received medicines affecting vessel diameter and had change position, were excluded from the study.

Instrument

The portable probes of finger, toe and the forehead reflectance and earlobe pulse oximeter of Novametrx, Max-Fast, Nellcor Puritan Bennett INC, Pleasanton, Calif made in USA were used regarding all the patients for measurement of SpO2 values, respectively. In addition, four similar portable monitoring OXYPLETH 520A devices made in USA were used. The ABG reader XHOP SPLUL device made in USA was used in order to measure the ABG. Tympanic thermometer Jinus (series stat profile PHOX) was also used for measuring the temperature. In order to determine the reliability of ABG device which is considered as the standard of the study, two sample of arterial blood of 2 cm^3 were taken from one of the patients. One of the samples was sent to the laboratory and the second sample was put in refrigerator after bleeding. The second sample was send to the laboratory in a time interval of two minutes following the first sample. Results of the study showed that there was an error of 0.11 between the SaO2 of both samples which showed the high reliability of the device.

Three blood samples of 2 cm^3 were taken from one of the patients in order to determine the reliability of the ABG device. One of the samples was analyzed using the ABG reader device of the study and the other two

Table 1 Comparing the correlation and agreement of SpO2 of four probes with standardized SaO2

Statistical index	Correlation			Agreement	
Probe type	r	p	CI	Rho	CI 95%
Finger	0.76	< 0.001	−1.02-2.08	0.68	−0.80- 0.57
Toe	0.60	< 0.001	−1.69- 2.28	0.58	−0.74- 0.43
Earlobe	0.77	< 0.001	−1.54- 1.83	0.76	−0.87- 0.67
Forehead	0.73	< 0.001	−1.07- 3.58	0.50	−0.62- 0.38

samples were analyzed using another ABG reader device. Results of the study showed that there was a correlation of 0.93 between the SaO2 obtained from three ABG reader devices which indicated high correlation and reliability of the device. Four monitoring devices were of a same type and calibrated before the study. Tympanic thermometer was also calibrated prior to be used.

Data collection

In order to collect the data, permission to conduct the study was issued by the Ethical Committee of KUMS. Then the required permissions were taken from Deputy of Research and Technology of KUMS and provided to the officials of the Imam Ali Hospital. Then, the researcher referred to the intensive care unit of the hospital every day and invited the patients having inclusion criteria. For this purpose, first of all the research purpose was explained to the patients and if they wished to be included in the study, they were asked to sign a written informed consent. The patients were assured about the anonymity and confidentiality of personal information. First of all, a blood sample 2 cm^3 was taken from each patients through artery catheter by the researcher. Then the samples were put inside an ice container and immediately sent to the laboratory next to the ICU. Hb (Hemoglobin) and temperature of the patients were also recorded in the ABG test. Tympanic thermometer was used in order to measure the patients' temperature. Further, the ratio and duration of SpO2 was also measured at the same time using the finger, toe, earlobe and forehead probes. It should also be mentioned that the same probes were used for all the patients.

Devices were calibrated prior to using the pulse oximetry. All the patients were in supine position and while the bed was 30 degrees above body surface area. A cover

was put around the probes in order to prevent the intervention of environmental light with the performance of each four pulse oximetry probes. Moreover, unnecessary actions such as changing the position, suction, and medication were avoided while using probes to prevent any change in hemodynamic condition of the patients. SpO2 value showed on the monitor in finger, toe, earlobe and forehead probes were measured and recorded at the same time per 60 s for 5 min in time intervals of 0, 1,2,3,4 and 5 min. Finally, the mean SpO2 was calculated for each probe. The SpO2 values of each probe and also the SaO2 values were recorded on the information sheet.

Data analysis

Data were analyzed using STATA-11 software. Independent t-test, Pearson correlation coefficient and Rho coefficient were used to compare the SpO2 and SaO2 of four probes. Bland- Altman analysis was used to compare the accuracy of each pulse oximetry probes. Lesser mean difference and higher agreement indicated higher accuracy of the probe. Kappa coefficient was used in order to divide the agreement ratio with the range of 0–1. Closer amounts indicate higher agreement [19].

Results

Of the 67 patients, 56.7% (n = 38) were female and 43.3% (n = 29) were male. The mean and standard deviation of patients' age were 57.22 ± 13.71 years. The mean and standard deviation of sample Hb was estimated as 13.21 ± 2.01 g/dl. The mean PaO2 in 43.3% of the sample was about 70–70.9 mmHg. The mean and standard deviation of the samples' temperature were and 36.8 ± 0.6 °C and 58. 2% of the sample had the temperature of 36–36.9 °C. The mean and standard deviation of PaCO2 were 35.03 ± 5. 57 mmHg and this values for PaO2 were 96.81 ± 1.20%.

Table 2 agreement and mean difference of Finger, Toe, Earlobe and Forehead pulse oximeters comparing to Standard SaO2

Statistical index / SpO2 probe	Mean	SD	Mean difference SaO2-SpO2	p-Value for t-test of mean difference	CI 95% for agreement
Forehead	95.55	1.75	1.25 ± 1.18	< 0.001	0.38–0.62
Earlobe	96.67	1.34	0.14 ± 0.86	0.019	0.67–0.87
Finger	96.28	1.06	0.53 ± 0.79	< 0.001	0.57–0.80
Toe	96.52	1.06	0.29 ± 1.01	0.22	0.43–0.74

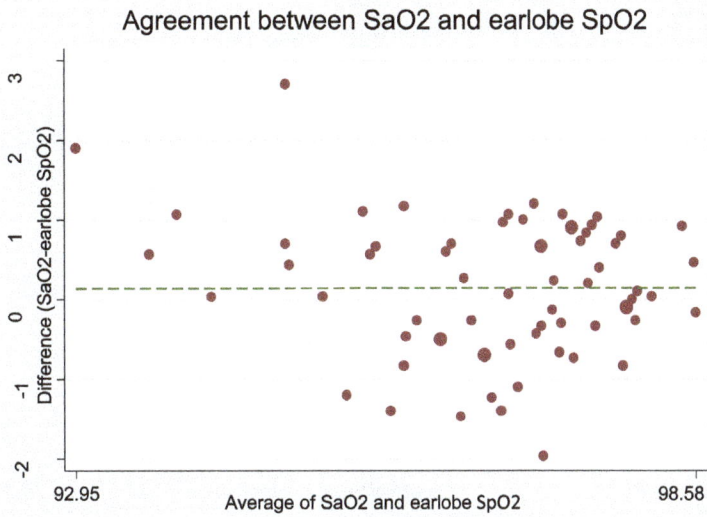

Fig. 1 Bland-Altman plot of earlobe for measuring SpO2

Based on the Pearson correlation test, the highest and lowest correlation between the mean SpO2 and mean SaO2 were related to earlobe probe ($r = 0.77$, $P < 0.001$) and toe probe ($r = 0.60$, $P < 0.001$). The highest and lowest clinical agreement with standard SaO2 were related to earlobe probes (0.76) and forehead probes (0. 50), respectively. The confidence level (CI) calculated for clinical agreement in earlobe probe was less than other probes (Table 1).

The lowest mean difference of SpO2 or SaO2 was related to earlobe probe (0.14 ± 0.86) and the highest difference ratio was related to forehead probe (1.25 ± 1.18) (Table 2).

Figures 1, 2, 3 and 4 show the Bland-Altman plot of comparing the clinical agreement between SaO2 or SpO2 values of earlobe, toe, forehead and finger probes where the earlobe probe with the agreement of 0.76 and confidence interval of 1.54–1.83 had the highest agreement with SaO2.

Discussion

In this study, the earlobe probes had the highest clinical agreement with SaO2 and higher accuracy due to less mean difference and limited confidence interval following by the finger, toe and forehead probes. Results of the study by Bilan et al. (2010) indicated pulse oximetry of

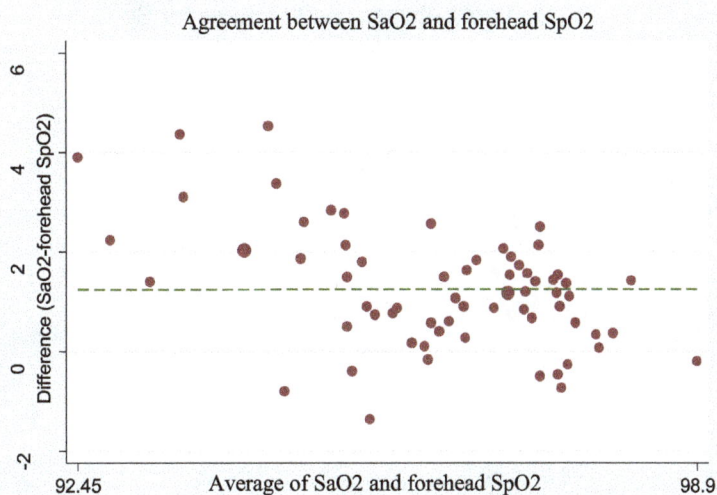

Fig. 2 Bland-Altman plot of forehead for measuring SpO2

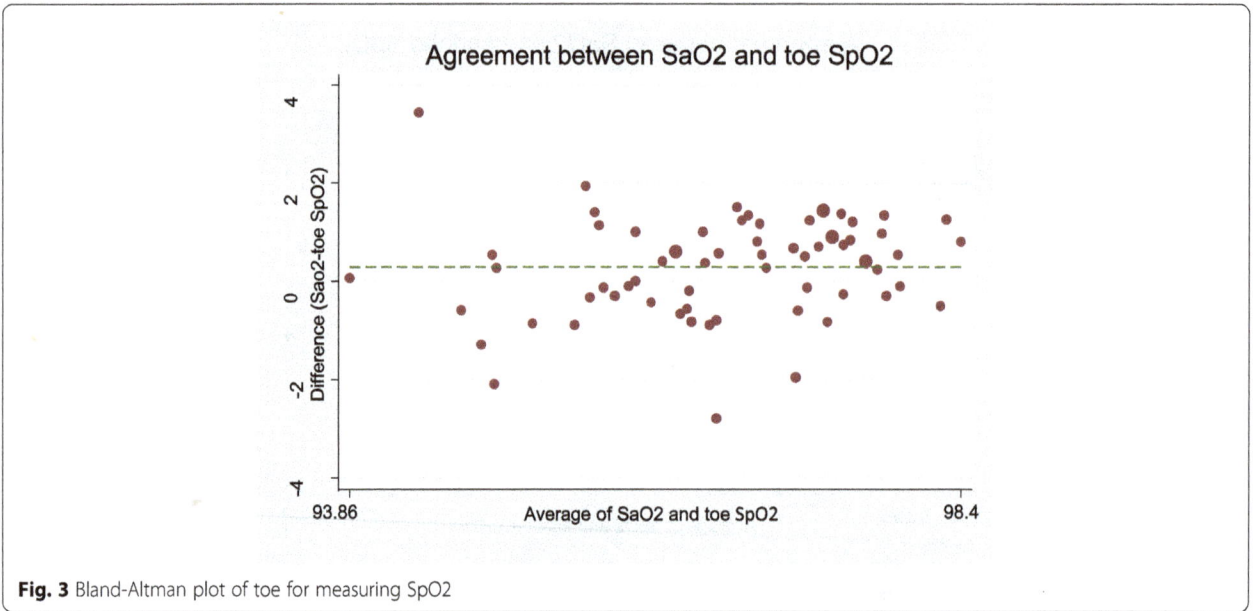

Fig. 3 Bland-Altman plot of toe for measuring SpO2

earlobe probe had higher accuracy compared to pulse oximetry of finger and toe probes in detection of hypoxemia in children and babies. Further, it was shown that pulse oximetry of finger probe had the lowest agreement with SaO2 [4]. However, Vax et al. (2009) compared the ear and forehead probes in patients under coronary surgery and reported that forehead probe had higher clinical agreement compared to ear probe [20]. Benz et al. (1991) also examined the accuracy of Biox 3700 pulse oximeter in patients receiving medicines affecting vessel diameter and reported that the ear probe of patients receiving medicines affecting vessel diameter was not reliable for monitoring SaO2 [21]. It seems that measuring the oxygen saturation using pulse oximeter can be influenced by the patient's condition; in this regard, Eberhard et al. (2002) stated that earlobe probe was the proper method in patients under anesthesia due to high speed of detecting SaO2 [22]. Lindholm et al. (2007) also argued that earlobe probe was the more proper method compared to finger probe due to more sensitivity to peripheral hypoxia in detection of SaO2 in patients with apnea [23]. Simon et al. (2003) also showed that ear probe was a more proper approach compared to finger probe in hypothermia [24].

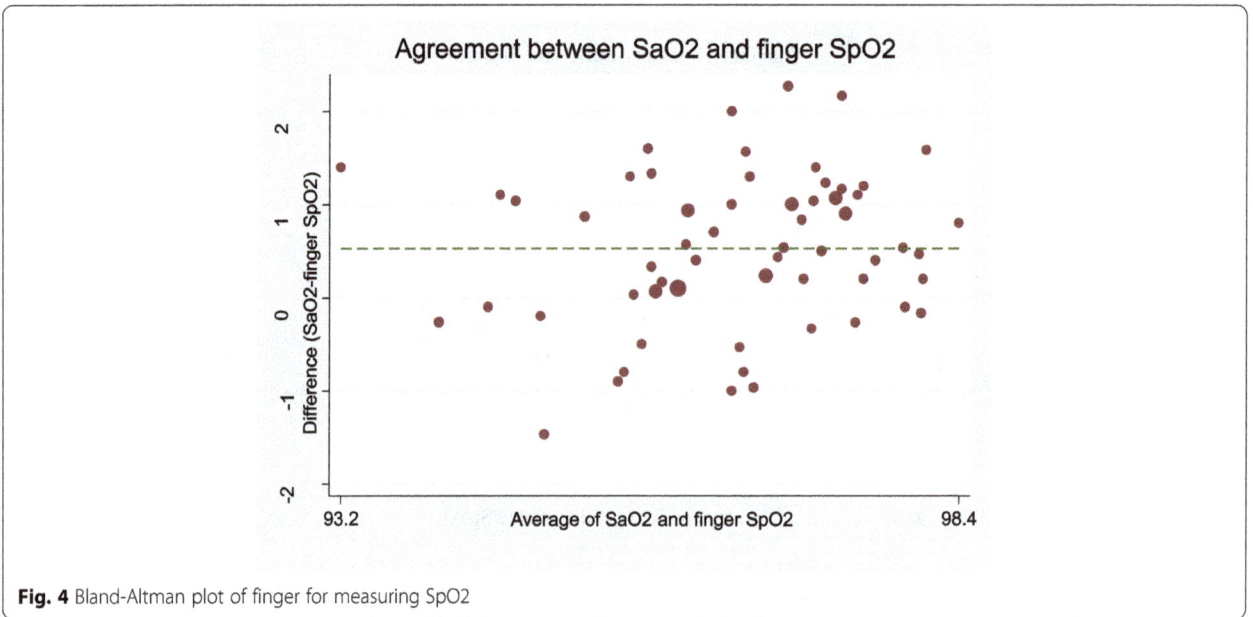

Fig. 4 Bland-Altman plot of finger for measuring SpO2

However, other studies had different results based on patients' condition [7, 25–27]. In this regard, Fernandez et al. (2007), in a method-comparison study, assessed the agreement between SpO2 values by digit-based and forehead pulse oximeters in low cardiac index patients, they suggested using forehead probe in these patients since the peripheral blood flow and body temperature are decreased [25]. Schallom et al. also claimed that in critically ill patients under surgery or with trauma exposed to the risk of peripheral hypoperfusion, the SpO2 ratio by forehead probe was more accurate than finger probe [26]. Das et al. (2010) also believe that there is no proper method for the placement of pulse oximeter sensor in children with cyanotic heart disease due to their specific condition to show the accurate value of SpO2. However, foot sensor can be the more appropriate one in this regard [7]. Sedaghat Yazdi et al. (2008) examined the effect of placement on the accuracy and reliability of the pulse oximeter sensor in children with cyanotic heart disease and found that if the SaO2 $\leq$ 90%, the foot sensor had the worst accuracy and reliability. Further, regardless of SaO2 amount, there was no difference between finger and toe sensor in terms of accuracy and reliability [27].

Although the accuracy of pulse oximetry is reduced in patients with severe and rapid O_2 desaturation, low blood pressure, body temperature, dyshemoglobinemia and reduced blood perfusion conditions [28], the earlobe pulse oximetry had more accurate and reliable performance regarding these changes [22, 23, 29]. Haynes (2007) claimed that earlobe probe can be considered as the proper method of finger pulse oximetry since in finger probe, the body movement is limited and the risk of reduced tissue perfusion is increased [18]. Thus, regarding the importance of continuous monitoring and maintaining hemodynamic stability in patients under heart surgery [29] and considering the results of our study, the earlobe probe can be used as the proper method for examining the oxygen saturation in patients under heart surgery.

In this study, the environmental light could intervene with the performance of each four pulse oximetry probes. However, a cover was put around the probes in order to prevent the intervention of environmental light with the performance of each four pulse oximetry probes. Non-random sampling was used for this study which could affect the generalizability of the findings. Thus, it is suggested to replicate the study using random sampling in various patients. The study was conducted on the patients admitted to the intensive care unit for cardiac surgery and it is suggested to conduct the similar study on the patients admitted to emergency and operating rooms.

Conclusion

Results of the study indicated that earlobe probe had higher accuracy in showing the SpO$_2$ among patients admitted to the intensive care unit for heart surgery compared to finger, toe and forehead probes and the obtained SpO$_2$ value of earlobe probe approximated to the SaO$_2$ obtained from ABG test. Thus, earlobe probe can be used in intensive care units to measure the peripheral oxygen saturation.

Abbreviations

ABG: Arterial Blood Gases; C: Centigrade; Hg: hemoglobin; KUMS: Kermanshah University of Medical Sciences; Sao2: Saturation of Oxygen (arterial blood); Spo2: Spot Oxygen Saturation

Acknowledgements

This work was perform in partial fulfillment of the requirements for MSc. degree of soheila seifi, in faculty of nursing and midwifery, Kermanshah University of Medical Sciences, Kermanshah, Iran. This article was drawn from a research project (No. 90099) sponsored by deputy of research and technology of KUMS. We appreciate Clinical research development Unit of Imam Reza Hospital and patients who contributed to the study.

Funding

This study was drawn from a research project (No. 90099) sponsored by deputy of research and technology of KUMS. The cost of the payment is spent on the design and implementation of the study.

Authors' contributions

SS, AK, GM, FN and AA contributed in designing the study, SS, AK and GM collected the data, and analyzed by FN and AA. The final report and article were written by SS, AK, FN, and AA and they were read and approved by all the authors.

Competing interests

The authors declare there are no competing interests.

Author details

[1]Students Research Committee, Kermanshah University of Medical Sciences, Kermanshah, Iran. [2]Nursing department, Nursing and Midwifery School, Kermanshah University of Medical Sciences, Kermanshah, Iran. [3]Department of anesthesiology, Medicine School, Kermanshah University of Medical Sciences, Kermanshah, Iran. [4]Research Center for Environmental Determinants of Health (RCEDH), School of Public Health, Kermanshah University of Medical Sciences, Kermanshah, Iran.

References:
1. Wilson BJ, Cowan HJ, Lord JA, Zuege DJ, Zygun DA. The accuracy of pulse oximetry in emergency department patients with severe sepsis and septic shock: a retrospective cohort study. BMC emergency medicine. 2010;10(1):1.
2. Niknafs P, Norouzi E, Bijari BB, Baneshi MR. Can we replace arterial blood gas analysis by pulse oximetry in neonates with respiratory distress syndrome, who are treated according to INSURE protocol? Iranian journal of medical sciences. 2015;40(3):264.

3. Berkenbosch JW, Tobias JD. Comparison of a new forehead reflectance pulse oximeter sensor with a conventional digit sensor in pediatric patients. Respir Care. 2006;51(7):726–31.

4. Bilan N, Behbahan AG, Abdinia B, Mahallei M. Validity of pulse oximetry in detection of hypoxaemia in children: comparison of ear, thumb and toe probe placements/Validité de l'oxymétrie de pouls pour détecter l'hypoxémie chez l'enfant: comparaison du placement de la sonde au niveau de l'oreille, du pouce et de l'orteil. East Mediterr Health J. 2010;16(2):218.

5. Pluddemann A, Thompson M, Heneghan C, Price C. Pulse oximetry in primary care: primary care diagnostic technology update. Br J Gen Pract. 2011;61(586):358–9.

6. Ruskin KJ, Wagner JL. Pulse oximetry: basic principles and applications in aerospace medicine. Aviat Space Environ Med. 2008;79(4):444.

7. Das J, Aggarwal A, Aggarwal NK. Pulse oximeter accuracy and precision at five different sensor locations in infants and children with cyanotic heart disease. Indian journal of anaesthesia. 2010;54(6):531.

8. Schutz SL. Oxygen saturation monitoring by pulse oximetry. AACN procedure manual for crit care. 2001;4:77–82.

9. Durbin CG Jr, Rostow SK. More reliable oximetry reduces the frequency of arterial blood gas analyses and hastens oxygen weaning after cardiac surgery: a prospective, randomized trial of the clinical impact of a new technology. Crit Care Med. 2002;30(8):1735–40.

10. Blaylock V, Brinkman M, Carver S, McLain P, Matteson S, Newland P, et al. Comparison of finger and forehead oximetry sensors in postanesthesia care patients. J Perianesth Nurs. 2008;23(6):379–86.

11. Hodgson CL, Tuxen DV, Holland AE, Keating JL. Comparison of forehead max-fast pulse oximetry sensor with finger sensor at high positive end-expiratory pressure in adult patients with acute respiratory distress syndrome. Anaesth Intensive Care. 2009;37(6):953.

12. GIHI Y, Korhan EA, Khorshid L. Comparison of oxygen saturation values and measurement times by pulse oximetry in various parts of the body. Appl Nurs Res. 2011;24(4):e39–43.

13. Nesseler N, Frnel JV, Launey Y, Morcet J, Malldant Y, Seguin P. Pulse oximetry and high-dose vasopressors: a comparison between forehead reflectance and finger transmission sensors. Intensive Care Med. 2012;38(10):1718–22.

14. Bilan N, ABDI NB, Mahallei M. Validity of pulse oximetry of earlobe, toe and finger in the detection of pediatric hypoxemia. 2006.

15. Korhan EA, Yont GH, Khorshid L. Comparison of oxygen saturation values obtained from fingers on physically restrained or unrestrained sides of the body. Clinical Nurse Specialist. 2011;25(2):71–4.

16. Sugino S, Kanaya N, Mizuuchi M, Nakayama M, Namiki A. Forehead is as sensitive as finger pulse oximetry during general anesthesia. Can J Anesth. 2004;51(5):432–6.

17. Cheng EY, Hopwood MB, Kay J. Forehead pulse oximetry compared with finger pulse oximetry and arterial blood gas measurement. J Clin Monit. 1988;4(3):223–6.

18. Haynes JM. The ear as an alternative site for a pulse oximeter finger clip sensor. Respir Care. 2007;52(6):727–9.

19. Viera AJ, Garrett JM. Understanding interobserver agreement: the kappa statistic. Fam Med. 2005;37(5):360–3.

20. Wax DB, Rubin P, Neustein S. A comparison of transmittance and reflectance pulse oximetry during vascular surgery. Anesth Analg. 2009;109(6):1847–9.

21. Ibanez J, Velasco J, Raurich JM. The accuracy of the biox 3700 pulse oximeter in patients receiving vasoactive therapy. Intensive Care Med. 1991;17(8):484–6.

22. Eberhard P, Gisiger PA, Gardaz JP, Spahn DR. Combining transcutaneous blood gas measurement and pulse oximetry. Anesth Analg. 2002;94(1 Suppl):S76–80.

23. Lindholm P, Blogg SL, Gennser M. Pulse oximetry to detect hypoxemia during apnea: comparison of finger and ear probes. Aviat Space Environ Med. 2007;78(8):770–3.

24. Simon SB, Clark RA. (Mis) using pulse oximetry: a review of pulse oximetry use in acute care medical wards. Clin Eff Nurs. 2002;6(3):106–10.

25. Fernandez M, Burns K, Calhoun B, George S, Martin B, Weaver C. Evaluation of a new pulse oximeter sensor. Am J Crit Care. 2007;16(2):146–52.

26. Schallom L, Sona C, McSweeney M, Mazuski J. Comparison of forehead and digit oximetry in surgical/trauma patients at risk for decreased peripheral perfusion. Heart & Lung: The Journal of Acute and Critical Care. 2007;36(3):188–94.

27. Sedaghat-Yazdi F, Torres A Jr, Fortuna R, Geiss DM. Pulse oximeter accuracy and precision affected by sensor location in cyanotic children. Pediatr Crit Care Med. 2008;9(4):393–7.

28. Jensen LA, Onyskiw JE, Prasad NGN. Meta-analysis of arterial oxygen saturation monitoring by pulse oximetry in adults. Heart & Lung: The Journal of Acute and Critical Care. 1998;27(6):387–408.

29. Westphal GA, Silva E, Gonçalves AR, Caldeira Filho M, Poli-de-Figueiredo LF. Pulse oximetry wave variation as a noninvasive tool to assess volume status in cardiac surgery. Clinics. 2009 Apr;64(4):337–43.

19

Modelling job support, job fit, job role and job satisfaction for school of nursing sessional academic staff

Leanne S. Cowin[*] and Robyn Moroney

Abstract

Background: Sessional academic staff are an important part of nursing education. Increases in casualisation of the academic workforce continue and satisfaction with the job role is an important bench mark for quality curricula delivery and influences recruitment and retention. This study examined relations between four job constructs - organisation fit, organisation support, staff role and job satisfaction for Sessional Academic Staff at a School of Nursing by creating two path analysis models.

Methods: A cross-sectional correlational survey design was utilised. Participants who were currently working as sessional or casual teaching staff members were invited to complete an online anonymous survey. The data represents a convenience sample of Sessional Academic Staff in 2016 at a large school of Nursing and Midwifery in Australia. After psychometric evaluation of each of the job construct measures in this study we utilised Structural Equation Modelling to better understand the relations of the variables.

Results: The measures used in this study were found to be both valid and reliable for this sample. Job support and job fit are positively linked to job satisfaction. Although the hypothesised model did not meet model fit standards, a new 'nested' model made substantive sense.

Conclusion: This small study explored a new scale for measuring academic job role, and demonstrated how it promotes the constructs of job fit and job supports. All four job constructs are important in providing job satisfaction – an outcome that in turn supports staffing stability, retention, and motivation.

Keywords: Sessional staff, Job satisfaction, Organisational fit, Job support, Job role, Nursing education

Background

The importance of Sessional Academic Staff in teaching and learning at universities throughout Australia continues to increase [1]. The term Sessional Staff includes casual, associate, adjunct or part-time, ancillary or auxiliary academic staff aiming to capture the transient or temporary state of employment. There are now more sessional staff employed in Australian Universities than full time academics [2]. Attracting and retaining dedicated teaching staff is now crucial to the functioning of some Schools of Nursing in Australia and the provision of a quality curriculum [3]. Nurses of the future are dependent on sessional as well as full time academic staff.

The quality of teaching at tertiary level has never been more important to student outcomes and workforce contributions [4]. High quality teaching, according to Queensland University of Technology [5], should capture students into a learning partnership whereby personal and professional development is inspired, fostered, and ultimately practised as new graduates. Such teaching provides rigorous feedback and evaluation within the learning environment with the support of sessional academic teaching staff being critical to the success of the graduate, particularly in health care professions [6]. However, despite higher numbers of Sessional Staff (SS), less support is available now and it is provided by fewer staff members [6].

Recent liberal directions of universities throughout Australia have involved policies such as 'uncapped

* Correspondence: l.cowin@westernsydney.edu.au
School of Nursing & Midwifery, Western Sydney University, Locked Bag 1797, Penrith Soutah DC, NSW 2751, Australia

enrolment' whereby University programs such as the Bachelor of Nursing are able to recruit as many students as they wish [7]. Previously, student numbers were capped and according to the 'Group of Eight' [8], universities are calling for a recapping of placements within courses including nursing due to spiralling costs and student quality issues. The 'Group of Eight' consists of Australia's eight leading research Universities [8]. Ever increasing numbers of students have not been matched by staffing and resources [7] leading to greater stress than ever before on academic staff [9]. As stated by Harvey, 'the main failure of university expansion is the unwillingness to fund it' [10].

The need for further SS continues to grow as the numbers of full time nursing academics dwindle. Shortages of full time academic staff persists in countries such as the USA and Canada [11], and causes identified for the growing shortages include distressingly high workloads, aging academics, perceived lack of teaching support and inflexible work life [12, 13]. In 2003, the Australian Universities Teaching Committee found that the tertiary education sector had managed the 'casualisation' of the teaching workforce 'quite poorly' in terms of training and support ([14]p. i). More than a decade on, it remains unclear whether the SS member receives the support, training, resources, and satisfaction they need to continue working in a part time capacity [2]. Over the past 20 years, the numbers of SS have increased to more than the number of tenured staff [2, 14]. SS are employed as lecturers, tutors, and lab demonstrators on a casual or sessional basis. While SS bring 'flexibility, diversity and financial savings' ([14] p. i), job satisfaction, support and training remain problematic and retention becomes a critical employment issue. Sessional staff (SS) are people employed on a part time basis for a short period to deliver and assess curricula to university students [13]. McCormack [15], describe this group as teachers employed on a casual, contractual or sessional basis.

Within nursing education, a tension exists between clinical currency and teaching expertise [16]. Do nursing academics, who divide their time between the clinical field and the university environment, provide superior and more relevant nursing education, or do they have more teaching difficulties because of this dual focus? Currently, there are signs of a rise in teaching expertise and a decrease in dual roles of teaching and clinical work as the need for SS increases. This is in contrast to previously held notions of the SS member being unqualified in adult education [17], and being commonly engaged in clinical practice [18]. Evidence from recent workforce assessment reveals some Australian universities are extensively 'casualised' and many tasks attributable to the academic role such as journal reviewing, editing, student feedback, and committee attendance are not possible in the timeframe available [19].

Enjoyment of work is an important construct in any workplace but it is probably most important for those people who work casually. If SS are not satisfied with their work, the option of employment elsewhere is potentially much easier than for the full time permanent academic [2]. Indeed, much of the attraction of sessional work centres on a sense of flexibility with work choices [20]. For the organisation to attract the best academics job satisfaction is vital and that assessing and making adjustments to increase job satisfaction is critical [21].

Research into job satisfaction continues to be popular in all organisational studies primarily because of the strong empirical evidence supporting causal relationships between satisfaction with work and retention [22, 23]. Coates et al. [24] found that Australian academics have among the lowest levels of satisfaction in the world. In addition, the connection between satisfaction and performance quality and effectiveness is also important and has significant financial and productivity implications [23]. The workplace of SS varies substantially from that of the fulltime academic in management and work setting. For example, access to office space may be limited or even non-existent. Access to the teaching team may also be varied. Accessing other SS may be easier than accessing fulltime academics. The role of the SS is fraught with issues relating to work flexibility, multiple campus sites, financial reimbursement, and team communication [15].

Aims

The purpose of this study was to create and test a path analysis model containing the variables of job satisfaction, organisational support, organisational fit, and sessional staff role. In a previous quality improvement project from 2014, the SS raised the subjects of job satisfaction, job fit, job support, and job role as important themes. These four topics were reviewed in the research literature, specifically those with valid and reliable tools. Where possible the shortest tools were sought due to potential sample size limitations and survey length issues. Theoretical support for this model is gained from the well supported notion that increased job satisfaction promotes retention and intrinsic rewards [25, 26], (see extensive literature based on these 'work and motivation' theorists). It is hypothesised that: Organisational support, organisational fit, and sessional staff role will positively and significantly contribute to job satisfaction. In this model, job satisfaction is treated as the dependent variable.

Methods
Sample
This study was conducted in the School of Nursing and Midwifery at a large multi-campus university in

Australia. In 2015–6 approximately 85 fulltime teaching academics and 150 regular SS taught or marked assignments. All SS were emailed an invitation to participate in this study and the invitation was displayed on the SS electronic resource site. The email and advertisement directed potential participants to the survey site www.Qualtrics.com at the end of the second semester for the year – November-December 2015 and again in early 2016. Sixty-six sessional staff attempted the survey in second semester 2015 and 67 in first semester 2016 thereby providing 133 completed surveys for cross sectional analysis. As different subjects are conducted in the semesters, different SS were accessed in each semester thereby allowing us to treat participants as one homogenous group. The online survey precluded missing data, contained a brief outline of the study, a series of short answer questions, and the four scales utilised in this study. The qualitative data gathered will be reported elsewhere.

Measures

Global Job Satisfaction is measured using a six item tool by Pond and Geyer [27] (see Additional file 1). The items assess affective 'facet free' responses, and although Quinn and Sheppard originally posited a 5 item scale in 1974 ($\alpha = 0.88$, M = 3.75), it is the 6 item version by Pond and Geyer in1991 [27] that has been utilised in this study. Psychometrics from the 1991 Pond and Geyer study indicate a mean score of 2.76 (SD 0.92) and an alpha of 0.89 in a sample of 70 non-unionised textile workers. In a more recent study by Gutierrez, Candela and Carver [28] the researchers, using the Pond and Geyer version, reported a mean score for global job satisfaction as 4.18 (SD 0.65) and an alpha of 0.93 in a sample of 570 nursing academics in the USA.

Support for SS is measured using the *Perceived Organisational Support Scale* (POSS) by Eisenberger et al. [29]. Originally, this measure contained 36 items, and was designed to explore employees' beliefs of how much the organisation they worked for valued their work and their well-being. In 2012 Gutierrez et al. [28] also utilised nine relevant items from the Eisenberger et al. [29] scale for their sample of 570 nursing academics and demonstrated a mean score of 5.20 (SD1.16) by utilising a 7-point Likert scale (1 = strongly disagree, 7 = strongly agree) however, no alpha score is reported. Tourangeau et al. [11]also utilised the POSS nine item 7-point scale for their study of 650 nursing academics, reporting a mean score of 4.09 (SD 1.38). The authors [11] reported an alpha score of 0.93.

For the current study, it was agreed by the research team that only six items of Guitierrez et al., [28]and Tourangeau et al., [11] nine item POSS related to SS. The use of the original phrase – 'The Organisation', would

be altered to - The School of Nursing & Midwifery (*see* Table 1).

Organisational suitability was measured using the 3 item '*Perceived-Person Organization Fit*' scale (PPOF) by Cable and Judge [30]. The internal consistency estimate for the 3-item scale was 0.68 based on a study of 320 job seekers utilising 3 points in time (Time 1 N = 320, Time 2 N = 96, and Time 3 N = 68). In the Gutierrez et al. 2012 study of 1453 nursing academics, a sample of 570 demonstrated a mean score of 3.96 (SD 0.60) and an alpha score of 0.90.

The *Sessional Staff Role Scale* ([15] p. 56) (Table 2) is a 12 item checklist for SS. The checklist was not initially designed to be a measure of the role of the SS member however, each item can be assessed using a Likert type scale and the assumption is that the higher the score rated by the participant the greater the agreement there is with the particular item. Further analysis may be required as this is the first time the Sessional Staff Role Scale has been used to assess understanding of the role of a sessional academic in teaching and learning.

Ethical considerations

Approval for this study was obtained from the Western Sydney University Human Research Ethics Committee project number H11352 and the study was conducted according to ethical requirements. As data was collected using an online survey consent to participate was assumed by completion of survey. No names or identifying details were collected.

Analysis

The psychometric details of each measure were examined using SPSS (IBM SPSS version 24 2016), for the participant's response to job satisfaction, person-organisation fit (job fit), perceived organisational support (job support) and the sessional staff role scale (job role). Path analysis is an extension of multiple regression where the estimates of significance are demonstrable between the variables. This includes direction of effects and can provide some measure of causal modeling. The advantage of using Structural Equation Modelling (SEM) here is that it combines 'path and factor analytic techniques in the one predictive model' ([31] p. 2126). The use of the term model is as a descriptor of the relations amongst the variables as a statistical statement and the term path diagram is a pictorial representation of this model. Path analysis; where job satisfaction is treated as the endogenous (dependent) variable and job fit, job support, and job role are exogenous variables, is graphically created by the use of AMOS (IBM SPSS version 24 2016). Maximum likelihood estimation is utilised for normally distributed data such as ours as it is more 'forgiving' of a smaller sample [32].

Table 1 Perceived Organisational Support Scale (POSS) by Eisenberger et al. (1986)

Item number	Item wording
27	The School of Nursing & Midwifery takes pride in my accomplishments at work.
9	The School of Nursing & Midwifery really cares about my well-being.
1	The School of Nursing & Midwifery values my contributions to its well-being.
4	The School of Nursing & Midwifery strongly considers my goals and values.
23[a]	The School of Nursing & Midwifery shows little concern for me.
20	The School of Nursing & Midwifery is willing to help me if I need a special favour.

[a]- reverse scored

Results

Psychometric testing of scales

The results begin with descriptive analyses of the measures used with this sample followed by path analysis and model restructure. Reliability assessment of the *Global Job Satisfaction Scale* [27] using Cronbach's Alpha resulted in a score of 0.82 for the six items and all items were correlated at the 0.05 level (see Table 3). A Confirmatory Factor Analysis (CFA) of the total group ($N = 133$) utilising AMOS revealed a good model fit of >

Table 2 Sessional Staff Role items

	Item
1.	I identify my own professional development needs
2.	I actively engage in formal and/or informal professional development in learning and teaching
3.	I am familiar with, and keep up to date with, policies and procedures that affect my work
4.	I am aware of institutional student support such as academic skills programs, counselling, and disability services.
5.	I receive ongoing formal and informal feedback from the unit coordinator, peers and students
6.	I am aware of my roles and responsibilities as a sessional staff member
7.	I critically reflect (with myself and/or with others) on students' learning, my teaching, and my professional development as a teacher
8.	I provide ongoing feedback to my department and unit coordinator
9.	I participate in, or contribute to, institutional/department/unit events and activities
10.	I am aware of opportunities in my school/university to gain recognition and reward for my contribution to quality teaching and learning.
11.	I am aware of departmental websites, learning management systems, discussion fora, and email
12.	I maintain regular and timely communication with my unit coordinator, department, and human resources.

0.90 (GFI of 0.97, RMSEA 0.07, chi-sq of 15.84 (df 9), and $p = 0.07$).

An initial Exploratory Factor Analysis (EFA) utilising Principal Axis factoring (PAF) was performed on the six item *Perceived Organisational Support Scale* by Eisenberger et al. (1986 *see* Table 3) as the item group were uniquely selected from the larger original scale of 36 items. This resulted in a one factor model with factor loadings ranging from 0.65 to 0.95, and which accounted for 67.49% of variance. A CFA revealed a good model fit (GFI of 0.97, RMSEA 0.05, chi-sq of 12.53 (df 9), and $p = 0.16$).

The three item *Perceived-Person Organisation Fit* by Cable and Judge 1996 *(see* Table 3) model is not identifiable using CFA as the degrees of freedom are 0 and the probability level cannot be computed [33]. An EFA was examined instead, again utilising PAF and this resulted in a one factor model with good factor loadings ranging from 0.75 to 0.94, and which accounted for a high 81.87% of variance.

The 12-item *Sessional Staff Role Scale* by Harvey and Fredericks 2015 *(see* Table 3) has no previous data to compare. This is a new measure arising from a 'checklist' created by Harvey and Fredericks in response to three areas – 1) assessing – achieving and sustaining good practice (items 1–7), 2) participating in the life of the institution/faculty (items 8–10), and 3) communicating with others regarding teaching (items 11 & 12). The authors were agreeable to the use of these items as a potential pilot test. A correlation matrix revealed all items were weakly to moderately related. The 12 items do not provide an adequate model fit (GFI < 0.81). However, as the authors had initially constructed their item list in three subscales. Items 1 to 7 (Achieving and sustain good practice) did provide a better model fit (GFI 0.92, RMSEA = 0.11 (Chi^2 = 37.69, DF = 14, $p = 0.001$)).

Using items 8–12 did not provide an adequate model fit however, and item 12 was highly correlated with item 8 (> 0.8). as this was the first time the Sessional Staff Role Scale was used in a survey a decision was made to use the 11-item model for the measurement of Job Role. This includes the first 11 items in Table 2. A CFA with a one factor solution is gained from the 11 item model (VE = 49.85%).

Path analysis model

The goal of inference from this data was to determine if organisational support, organisational fit, and job role positively and significantly contributed to global job satisfaction. To this end a regression analysis was initially conducted and confirmatory models were created and interpreted. While the regression is a useful sequential method of estimating the relations amongst the

Table 3 Descriptive statistics and correlation estimates (N = 133)

Variable	Scale α	M(SD)	1	2	3	4
1. Global Job Satisfaction	0.82	4.50 (0.44)	–			
2. Perceived Organisational Support Scale	0.92	3.71 (0.71)	.403**	–		
3. Perceived-person organisation fit	0.89	3.76 (0.69)	.474**	.478**	–	
4. Sessional Staff Role Scale (revised)	0.82	4.01 (4.02)	.182*	.401**	.458**	–

Note: * $p < 0.05$; ** $p < 0.01$

variables, it does not take into account measurement error and covariance [32].

The size of path coefficients (see Table 4) in the output path diagram demonstrate that Job Fit (as measured by PPOF) followed by Job Support (as measured by POSS) data have greater effects on Global Job Satisfaction. Parameter estimations for a path analysis are conducted using SEM. However, the model is such a poor fit to the data here the model is unacceptable using these parameters (Fig. 1).

Nested model

The three variables of Job Role, Job Fit and Job Support did not demonstrate an acceptable model despite statistically significant pathways. Therefore, an alternative model was tested and described (see Model 2 below). In this model, the Job Role variable is set to mediate through the Job Fit and Job Support variables. This is based on the premise that if a person is attempting to determine if they fit well with the organisation and have the forms of supports tailored to their work, then knowing what their role is would be a mediating factor rather than as an independent effect on Global Job Satisfaction as seen in the inadequate Model 1. Consequently, in this alternative model, Job Role should not be modelled as a main effect as it is in the first model. Job Role creates and supports Job Fit and Job Support in this hypothesis as a smaller model occurring within a larger model. This alternate approach creates a 'nested' model [34] and demonstrates good model fit indices and is thereby superior to the first model (Fig. 2).

Table 4 Regression Results using a Stepwise process (N = 133)

Model		Unstandardised Coefficients		Standardised Coefficients
		B	Std. Error	Beta
1				
	Job Support	.207	.065	.344[b]
	Job Fit	.458	.140	.404[a]
	Job Role11	−.025	.068	−.045

Note: dependent variable is Global Job Satisfaction
[a]significant at 1% level
[b]significant at 0.1% level

Discussion

In this study we hypothesised that organisational support, organisational fit and SS role will positively and significantly contribute to the job satisfaction of sessional academic staff. Through the use of SEM this has been demonstrated, albeit in an alternative model to that first proposed. Three of the four measures used in this study demonstrated good psychometric qualities with the fourth one (Job Role) requiring some adjustment.

Global job satisfaction

The results of the sample revealed a statistically significant (0.02) mean score for satisfaction (4.50) when compared with the Gutierrez et al. score of 4.18 [28]. This was an important finding for us as recent literature on the current academic workplace portrays it as a stress ridden role with a somewhat gloomy outlook [35]. Baker [36] found that an increase in satisfaction was linked to retention of SS. However, job satisfaction is a dynamic and flexible construct [22] and as stated by Hagedorn 'no single conceptual model can completely and accurately portray the construct' ([23] p.6).

The global approach to a job satisfaction scale aimed to capture a 'worker's general affective reaction to the job without reference to any specific job facets' ([37] p.50). There are many reliable and valid global job satisfaction measures but as Quinn and Sheppard pointed out nearly 50 years ago – many are occupation specific or 'homogeneous', or simply too long and complicated [37].

Our SS may or may not be registered nurses as a small number of the staff who teach science based subjects are science experts - not nurses. Use of an occupation specific tool such as the McCloskey Muller Satisfaction Scale (MMSS) [38] would be inappropriate in this study. There is also a perception that sessional teaching may be the beginning step needed for a full time academic career [39], and that boundaries of work and responsibilities may be blurred in an eager effort to appeal at job interviews. It is argued here however, that job satisfaction would be impacted by such plans and the results of this small study do not support this.

Staff selection is fraught with many contextual issues such as experiential and qualification issues. The contribution of Job Fit to Job Satisfaction (0.36 Fig. 2)

Path model of total effects on Job Satisfaction N= 133

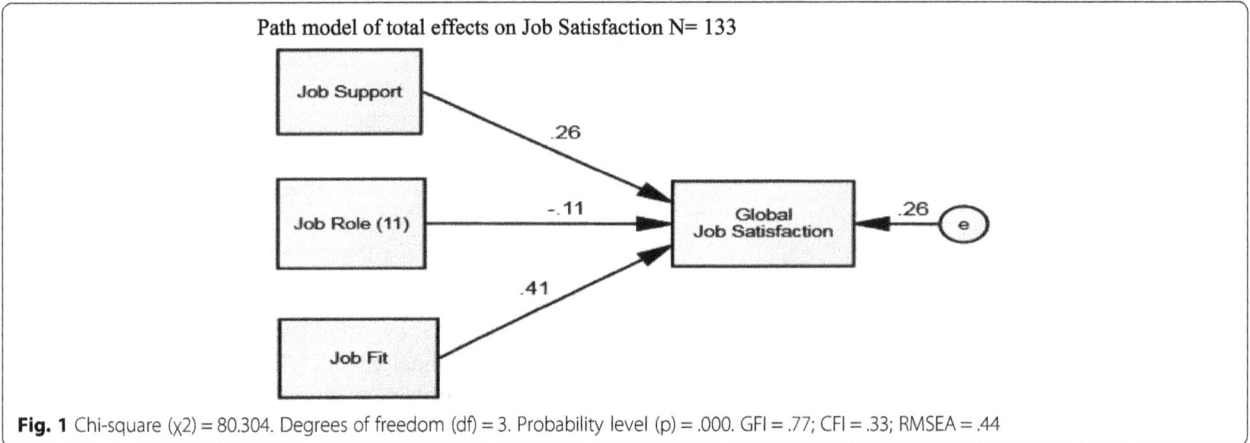

Fig. 1 Chi-square (χ2) = 80.304. Degrees of freedom (df) = 3. Probability level (p) = .000. GFI = .77; CFI = .33; RMSEA = .44

demonstrates good selection processes and commitment to the job by the SS. In this study, more than half of the sample have an ongoing SS role each year- some in the first half of the calendar year, and others in the second half according to when their subjects are conducted. However, many new SS are assessed and employed each year. Job fit is important to job satisfaction. The question posed is - how much of job fit is achieved by the individual and how much is created through good employment selection and institutional processes?

Job support (POSS) demonstrated good psychometric properties and similar results in the path analysis to job fit. The question of whether a SS person feels supported in fulfilling their employment is essential to the management and organisation of SS. In this study, support is significantly related to job satisfaction. Needleman et al. [40] also found that support is critical to job satisfaction amongst tenured staff. This can be interpreted as 'support increases satisfaction'. The implication of this finding is that, – in order to retain SS - an investment in support management is required. Institutional support however, is less well explored than educational delivery [40]. Mentorship and team collegiality are aspects of

institutional structures that can provide support to the SS and thereby increase job satisfaction.

Research indicates that if support (be it perceived or actual) is not available to the new and even the seasoned academic staff person, the flow-on effect leads to lowered job satisfaction and lowered performance [40]. Baker also supports this stating that 'high levels of empowerment and low levels of burnout were significant predictors of work satisfaction, with empowerment being the stronger predictor' ([40] p. 413).

Recognition, inclusion, engagement and collegiality are some of the forms of supports needed for an inclusive workplace according to Rea [19]. The author claims that limitations of sessional work can cause financial as well as professional hardship. Rea states that 'inequities and gross exploitation cannot be kept hidden as the dirty secret of the contemporary academic profession' which lends a great deal of weight to the need for highly visible and structural support for SS ([19] p.13).

The staff role scale was the least successful tool used in this study. The 12 statements utilised performed poorly in CFA assessment, although the use of an 11 item model was found to work well within the model. Understanding the role of the SS is crucial to providing

Nested model of Job Role to Organisational Fit and Job Support N= 133

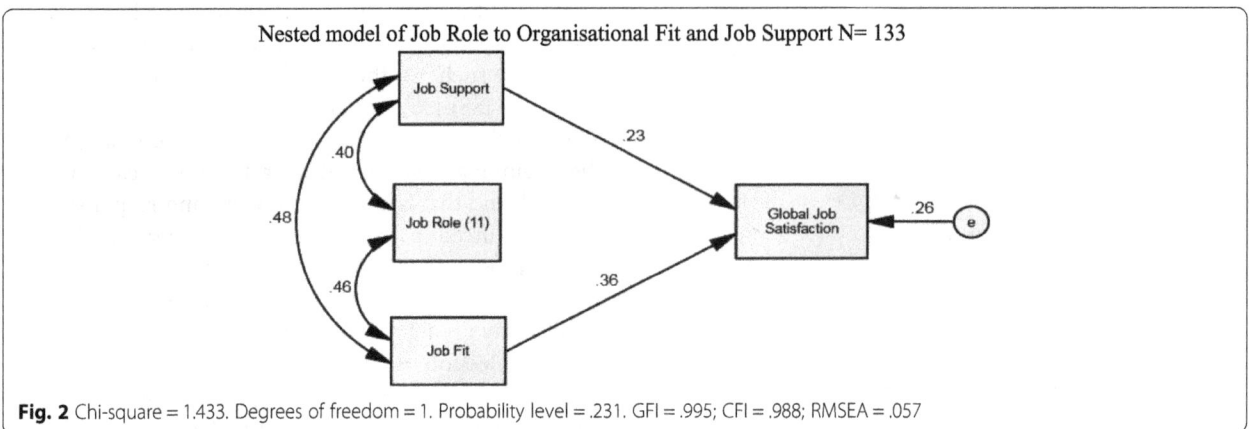

Fig. 2 Chi-square = 1.433. Degrees of freedom = 1. Probability level = .231. GFI = .995; CFI = .988; RMSEA = .057

quality teaching and learning but the future may create entirely different blended and online learning environments. The role of SS will continue to change. Budget restrictions may target both ongoing and sessional nursing academics forcing some classroom education into on-line delivery thereby saving the organisation money or raise the costs of nursing studies [41].

Model

The results of modelling role, job fit and job support on job satisfaction were statistically significant for job fit and job support and non-significant for job role in the first model (see Fig. 1). The model did not demonstrate a good fit with the data producing unacceptable fit indices. What is not in this model may well be of greater importance to job satisfaction of SS. However, it is important for good SS management to explore the importance of support and job fit (right person right job) when numbers of casual staff now exceed those of permanent staff.

An alternate model examined the 'mediation' of Job Role through Job Fit and Job Support and demonstrated a good fit with the data as supported by high fit indices (see Fig. 2). Path analysis is used to refine the causal hypothesis. The path coefficient for job role is very small, so it made sense for us to eliminate the pathway. The new, 'nested' model, which has the same variables but fewer pathways, provided a more sensible outcome and good model fit. The strength of this model indicates a strong mediating effect of Job Role with Job fit and Job Support. This is based on the premise that if a person is attempting to determine if they fit well with the organisation then knowing what their role is likely to be would be is a strong intervening consideration.

Limitations

One of the strengths of this small study was the use of valid and reliable measures to explore potential effects on job satisfaction. However, results are limited by the sample size, sample type, and what is left out of the modelling such as career progression planning and workplace location, which may also have a significant impact on job satisfaction for SS. Correlations are between variables in this specific data set and cannot be generalised beyond this population.

Causality requires longitudinal data and as this was cross-sectional data, causal inference cannot be drawn. One issue of the small sample size is that all results should be read with caution if not rejected outright as SEM is particularly sensitive to sample size and those with $N <$ 200 are 'undesirable' [31]. As Green states though – when variables are reliable, the model is simple, and the effects are strong, it may be acceptable if not rigorous practice to utilise a sample size such as ours. Green also points out

Bentler and Chou's [42] recommendation of applying at least 5 cases to each model parameter (5:1 ratio). As there are 10 model parameters our sample meets this criteria.

Future directions

This study indicates that job satisfaction for SS is predicated on having the right person for the job as well as adequate supports [43] for the academic role. In her study of casual teachers, Bamberry ([44] p. 49) claims 'casual employment can erode the job quality of otherwise decent work within professional occupations' yet this study does not demonstrate support for this claim. Further research could include use of these measures on full time staff as a group for comparison.

More than half of the curricula is delivered here by SS and according to Crimmins et al. [45] this trend is likely to increase in the future. Support for and selection of SS are important mediators of job satisfaction whereas SS role did not contribute to this small model with this sample. Job satisfaction relates to retention, which completes a round circle back to stability of staff. Replication of this study would be useful to address the current limitation of causality and incorporate Hierarchical Linear Modelling analyses for the issue of nested models, hierarchical structures, and for longitudinal data.

Conclusion

An investigation into the relationships of support, job fit and job role on the global job satisfaction of SS staff has yielded important information that can be especially useful in recruiting and retaining valuable academic staff. Investments at all levels in universities must now be made to create a seamless team of full time, part time, and sessional academics or the system will fail our newest professionals. As the full-time academic disappears from our universities and sessional academics become the new normal, there are new imperatives in terms of maintaining high quality learning and learning outcomes. Knowing what the job role entails feeds into job fit and job supports, which are important in providing job satisfaction – an outcome that supports staffing stability, retention, and motivation.

Abbreviations
GJS: Global job satisfaction; M: Mean; POSS: Perceived organisational support scale; PPOF: Perceived-person organization fit; SD: Standard deviation; SEM: Structural equation modelling; SS: Sessional staff

Acknowledgements
The authors would like to acknowledge Drs Peter Jonason and Renu Narchal for their consultation and assistance with statistical analyses – nested

models. The authors would also like to thank all Sessional Staff who completed this survey and thereby contributed to this paper.

Authors' contributions

LSC– survey construction, ethics application, online survey set up and monitoring, data analysis, manuscript construction, reading and approval of the final manuscript. RM– conceptual directions, survey construction editing, data analysis, manuscript editing, reading and approval of the final manuscript. Both authors read and approved the final manuscript.

Competing interests

The authors declare that they have no competing interests.

References

1. Australian Learning and Teaching Council [ALTC]. The RED resource – The contribution of sessional teachers to higher education. Australian Learning and Teaching Council. 2008. http://www.cadad.edu.au. Accessed Dec 2017.
2. Andrews S, Bare L, Bentley P, Goedegebuure L, Pugsley C, Rance B. "Contingent academic employment in Australian universities." LH Martin Institute. 2016. http://www.lhmartininstitute.edu.au/documents/publications/2016-contingent-academic-employment-in-australian-universities-updatedapr16.pdf Accessed Dec 2017.
3. Welk DS, Thomas PL. Considering a career change to a nursing faculty position? Key interview questions to ask and why. J Contin Educ Nurs. 2016; 40(4):165–70.
4. Knott G, Crane L, Heslop I, Glass BD. Training and support of sessional staff to improve quality of teaching and learning at universities. Am J Pharm Educ. 2015;79(5):1–8.
5. Queensland University of Technology. Annual Report 2003 Volume One. 2003. https://cms.qut.edu.au/__data/assets/pdf_file/0005/72095/annual-report-2003.pdf Accessed Dec 2017.
6. Lekkas D, Winning TA. Using quality enhancement processes to achieve sustainable development and support for sessional staff. Int J Acad Dev. 2017; https://doi.org/10.1080/1360144X.2016.1261357.
7. French S, James R. Australian higher education. In: Collins CS, Lee MN, Hawkins J, Neubauer DE, editors. The Palgrave handbook of Asia Pacific higher education. USA: Palgrave Macmillan; 2016. Chapter 38.
8. Group of Eight Australia. Priority Directions. 2016. https://go8.edu.au/article/go8-media-release-group-eight-priority-directions-time-action-not-activity Accessed Dec 2017.
9. Roughton SE. Nursing faculty characteristics and perceptions predicting intent to leave. Nurs Educ Perspect. 2013;34(4):217–25.
10. Harvey A. Uncapping of university places achieved what it set out to do. So why is it dubbed a policy failure? In: The Conversation. 2016. https://theconversation.com Accessed Dec 2017.
11. Tourangeau A, Saari M, Patterson E., Ferron EM, Thomson KW, MacMillan K. (2014). Work, work environments and other factors influencing nurse faculty intention to remain employed: A cross-sectional study. Nurse Educ Today 2014;34:940–947. doi.org/https://doi.org/10.1016/j.nedt.2013.10.010.
12. Yedidia MJ, Chou J, Brownlee S, Flynn L, Tanner C. Association of faculty perceptions of work–life with emotional exhaustion and intent to leave academic nursing: report on a national survey of nurse faculty. J Nurs Educ. 2014;53(10):569 79.
13. Klopper CJ, Power BM. The casual approach to teacher education: what effect does casualisation have for Australian university teaching? Aust J Teach Educ. 2014;39(4):101–14. https://doi.org/10.14221/ajte.2014v39n4.1
14. University of Queensland and Queensland University of Technology Training, support and management of sessional teaching staff. Final Report: Australian Universities Teaching Committee (AUTC). Canberra: Australian Universities Teaching Committee; 2003.
15. Harvey M, Fredericks V. Quality learning and teaching with sessional staff. Higher education Research and Development Society of Australasia (HERDSA) 2015. ISBN: 9780908557974.
16. Andrew S, Halcomb E, Jackson D, Peters K, Salamonson Y. Sessional teachers in a BN program: bridging the divide or widening the gap? Nurse Educ Today. 2010;30:453–7. https://doi.org/10.1016/j.nedt.2009.10.004.
17. Coombe K, Clancy S. Reconceptualizing the teaching team in universities: working with sessional staff. Int J Acad Dev. 2002;7(2):159–66.
18. Gappa J, Leslie D. The invisible faculty: improving the status of part-timers in higher education. San Francisco: Jossey-Bass; 1993.
19. Rea J. Stop being so casual. NTEU National President, Advocate 2016;23:2: 13–14. http://www.unicasual.org.au/article/Stop-being-so-casual-%28Advocate-23-02%29-18735 Accessed Dec 2017.
20. Candela L, Gutierrez AP, Keating S. What predicts nurse faculty members' intent to stay in the academic organization? A structural equation model of a national survey of nursing faculty. Nurse Educ Today. 2015;35:580–9. https://doi.org/10.1016/j.nedt.2014.12.018
21. Beigi M, Shirmohammadi M, Kim S. Living the academic life: a model for work-family conflict. Work. 2016;53:459–68. https://doi.org/10.3233/WOR-152173.
22. Judge TA, Weiss HM, Kammeyer-Mueller JD, Hulin CL. Job attitudes, job satisfaction, and job affect: a century of continuity and of change. J Appl Psychol. 2017;102(3):356–74. https://doi.org/10.1037/apl0000181
23. Hagedorn LS. Conceptualizing faculty job satisfaction: components, theories, and outcomes. New Dir Inst Res. 2000;(105):5–21.
24. Coates H, Dobson IR, Geodegebuure L, Meek L. Australia's casual approach to its academic teaching workforce. People and Place. 2009;17(4):47–54.
25. Herzberg F, Mausner B, Snyderman BB. The motivation to work. 2nd ed. New York: John Wiley; 1959.
26. Spector PE. Job satisfaction: application, assessment, causes and consequences. Thousand Oaks, CA: SAGE. 1997.
27. Pond SB III, Geyer PD. Differences in the relation between job satisfaction and perceived work alternatives among older and younger blue-collar workers. J Vocat Behav. 1991;39:251–62.
28. Gutierrez AP, Candela LL, Carver L. The structural relationships between organizational commitment, global job satisfaction, developmental experiences, work values, organizational support, and person-organization fit among nursing faculty. J Adv Nurs. 2012;68(7):1601–14. https://doi.org/10.1111/j.1365-2648.2012.05990.x.
29. Eisenberger R, Huntington R, Hutchison S, Sowa D. Perceived organizational support. J Appl Psychol. 1986;71(3):500–7.
30. Cable DM, Judge TA. Person-organization fit, job choice decisions, and organizational entry. Organ Behav Hum Decis Process. 1996;67(3):294–311.
31. Green T. A methodological review of structural equation modelling in higher education research. Stud High Educ. 2016;41(12):2125–55. https://doi.org/10.1080/03075079.2015.1021670.
32. Kline RB. Principles and practice of Struct Equ Model. 4th ed. New York: Guilford Publications; 2016.
33. Bollen KA. Structural equations with latent variables. 1st ed. New York: John Wiley & Sons; 1986.
34. Cox DR, Donnelly C. Principles of applied statistics. Cambridge, UK: Cambridge University Press; 2011.
35. Crimmins G. The spaces and places that women casual academics (often fail to) inhabit. High Educ Res Dev. 2016;35(1):45–57. https://doi.org/10.1080/07294360.2015.1121211.
36. Baker SL. Nurse educator orientation: professional development that promotes retention. J Contin Educ Nurs. 2010;41(9):413–7.
37. Quinn RP, Shepard LJ. The 1972–73 Quality of Employment Survey. Survey Research Center of the Institute for Social Research. Ann Arbor, Michigan: The University of Michigan; 1974.

38. Lee SE, Dahinten SV, Macphee M. Psychometric evaluation of the McCloskey/Mueller satisfaction scale. Jpn J Nurs Sci. 2016;13:487–95. https://doi.org/10.1111/jjns.12128.

39. Baranay I. The academic underclass. Griffith REVIEW Edition 11 – Getting Smart: The battle for ideas in Education. Australia: Griffith University; 2006.

40. Needleman J, Bowman CC, Wyte-Lake T, Dobalian A. Faculty recruitment and engagement in academic-practice partnerships. Nurs Educ Perspect. 2014;35(6):372–9. https://doi.org/10.5480/13-1234.

41. Yucha C, Smyer T, Strano-Perry S. Sustaining nursing programs in the face of budget cuts and faculty shortages. J Prof Nurs. 2014;30(1):5–9. https://doi.org/10.1016/j.profnurs.2013.07.002. Accessed Dec 2017

42. Bentler PM, Chou CP. Practical Issues in Structural Equation Modeling. Sociol Methods Res. 1987;16:78–117. https://doi.org/10.1177/0049124187016001004.

43. Neves P, Eisenberger R. Perceived organizational support and risk taking. J Manag Psychol. 2014;29(2):187–205. doi.org/10.1108/JMP-07-2011-0021

44. Bamberry L. As disposable as the next tissue out of the box . . .: Casual teaching and job quality in new South Wales public school education. J Ind Relat. 2011;5(31):49–64. https://doi.org/10.1177/0022185610390296.

45. Crimmins G, Nash G, Oprescu F, Alla K, Brock G, Hickson-Jamieson B, Noakes C. Can a systematic assessment moderation process assure the quality and integrity of assessment practice while supporting the professional development of casual academics? Assessment & Evaluation in Higher Education - on-line, 2015. https://doi.org/10.1080/02602938.2015.1017754 Accessed Dec 2017.

20

Understanding why child welfare clinic attendance and growth of children in the nutrition surveillance programme is below target: lessons learnt from a mixed methods study in Ghana

Faith Agbozo[1,2]* (iD), Esi Colecraft[3], Albrecht Jahn[2] and Timothy Guetterman[4]

Abstract

Background: Growth monitoring and promotion (GMP) programmes promote not only child health but serve as a service delivery strategy to enhance coverage for other crucial nutrition-specific interventions. This study compared community-based and facility-based GMP programme with respect to attendance rates, children's nutritional status, caregivers' satisfaction with services received and perceptions of service providers and users on factors influencing utilization.

Methods: Explanatory sequential mixed methods study conducted in Ga West municipality, Ghana. It comprised 12-month secondary data analysis using growth monitoring registers of 220 infants aged 0–3 months enrolled in two community-based (CB = 104) and two facility-based (FB = 116) child welfare clinics; cross-sectional survey (exit interview) of 232 caregiver-child pairs accessing CB ($n = 104$) and FB services ($n = 116$); and in-depth interviews with 10 health workers and 15 mothers. Quantitative data were analyzed through Fisher's exact, unpaired t-tests, and logistic regression at 95% confidence interval (CI) using SPSS version 20. Qualitative data were analyzed by thematic content analysis using ATLAS.ti 7.0.

Results: Mean annual attendance to both programmes was similar with an average of six visits per year. Only 13.6% of caregiver-child pairs attained more than nine visits in the 12-months period. At least 60% of children in both programs had improved weight-for-age z-scores (WAZ) scores during participation. Predictors for improved WAZ were being underweight at baseline (AOR:11.1, 95%CI:4.0–31.0), annual attendance of at least six visits (AOR:2.2, 95%CI:1.1–4.1) and meeting the Ghana Health Service target of nine visits (AOR:4.65, 95%CI:1.4–15.1). Compared to 31.5% CB users, significant proportion of FB caregivers (57.4%) were visited at home. Half were dissatisfied with services received (CB:55.6% vs. FB:62.0%, $p = 0.437$) citing long waiting times, negative staff attitude and extortions of money. Regarding perceptions on factors hindering service utilization, emerged themes included extremes of maternal age, high parity, postpartum socio-cultural beliefs and practices, financial commitments, undue delays, unprofessional staff behaviours, high premium on vaccination and general misconceptions about the programme.

(Continued on next page)

* Correspondence: faagbozo@uhas.edu.gh
[1]Department of Family and Community Health, School of Public Health, University of Health and Allied Sciences, PMG, 31 Ho, Ghana
[2]Institute of Public Health, University of Heidelberg Medical Faculty, Heidelberg, Germany
Full list of author information is available at the end of the article

(Continued from previous page)

Conclusion: The association of increased attendance with improved growth reaffirms the need to strengthen primary healthcare systems to improve service delivery; sensitize caregivers on contribution of growth monitoring and promotion to early child development; and increase contacts through home visits.

Keywords: Quantitative and qualitative research, Research methodology, Nutritional surveillance, Service utilization, Growth monitoring and promotion, Community health nursing, Child health

Background

Promoting child health during the window of opportunity period, that is the first thousand days starting from conception to a child's second birthday, is crucial for survival [1]. Globally, child mortality has reduced significantly [2] from 91 deaths per 1000 live birth in 1990 to 43 in 2015 [3]. Implementation of evidenced-based cost-effective nutrition-specific and nutrition-sensitive interventions that address the immediate and underlying causes of malnutrition have contributed to this progress.

One such strategy is the growth monitoring and promotion (GMP) programme. This essential preventive health intervention uses multi-sectoral approach to routinely assess child growth. It is implemented through the health and nutrition sectors, and serves as delivery channel to achieve coverage for other nutrition-specific interventions [4]. Growth monitoring promotes early child development and is associated with long term health, economic, and social benefits [5].

This programme is widely implemented in many low resource settings at the primary healthcare level as a nutritional surveillance activity linked with health promotion [6]. The intervention involves monthly weight measurement and charting, and using the information to counsel caregivers. It creates awareness about child growth and care practices with the aim of increasing demand for other health services. The long-term goal is to serve as a focal activity in an integrated child health system where caregivers are empowered to take actions to foster growth-enabling environments for children [6].

Central to the GMP programme in Ghana are three core activities: child weighing and charting of the weight-for-age Z-scores; identification of growth faltering; and counselling of caregivers on age-appropriate infant and young child feeding. Typically, GMP services are delivered in combination with other child health services such as vaccinations, vitamin A supplementation, free distribution of insecticide-treated bed nets, birth registration, education on infection prevention and family planning motivation. GMP services are provided at child welfare clinics (CWC) predominantly by community health nurses (CHN). The clinics are run as facility-based, community-based and outreach clinics. Details of the GMP programme is documented

elsewhere [7]. The facility-based CWC are static clinics situated within health facilities whereas the community-based CWC are typically mobile and outreach clinics where clinic days are scheduled.

Over the past five decades of monitoring growth in Ghana, the main challenges that have confronted the programme are unavailability of and inaccessibility to weighing centres, high participant drop outs and slow progress in reducing malnutrition rates [8]. To tackle these challenges, trained volunteers called community child growth promoters were integrated into the programme in selected community-based clinics in 2005. Their primary task includes child weighing, identification of growth faltering, vitamin A supplementation, child-centred counselling on infant and young child feeding and conducting home visitations.

Adequate participation in the programme enables caregivers to track changes in their children's weight enabling them to associate child's weight to overall health status [9]. It rises awareness on importance of growth charts [10] and its interpretation [11]. Moreover, optimum participation contributes to early identification of growth faltering [12], increases vaccinations coverage [13] and provides avenues for education on nutrition and health [14].

Although caregivers in Ghana are increasingly becoming aware of the importance of regular growth monitoring, [15], in the past, participation was low. Some reasons cited by caregivers in the 1990s for the low participation and high drop-out rates were advancing age of child, unavailability of and inaccessibility to the service, financial constraints, transportation difficulties, unsuitable schedules, uncomfortable venues and long waiting times [16]. In addition, service providers have cited poor knowledge of caregivers on importance of immunization, excessive workload on under-staffed health workers, and poorly motivated service providers [17] which have persisted for decades [18]. The Ghana Health Service has also attributed the irregular attendance mainly to lack of maternal interest after completion of most vaccinations [19]. Nonetheless, these challenges are not limited to Ghana. Other factors such as misconceptions about childhood malnutrition, inadequate skills of health providers, ineffective supervision and shortage of logistics have emerged in Ethiopia [15] and Zambia [9].

Evidence suggest that GMP is most effective when coverage and utilization is high [13]. As part of the nutritional surveillance system in Ghana, caregivers are encouraged to send their children aged 0–24 months old to CWCs on monthly basis to receive GMP services. In this present study, we evaluated effectiveness of the GMP programme in two community-based and two facility-based child welfare clinics in terms of two key performance indicators: utilization and undernutrition rates. We also sought to identify the factors that motivated caregivers to meet appointment schedules and their level of satisfaction with services received. Finally, we explored the perception of service providers and users on barriers to adequate participation.

Methods

Study location

The study was conducted in four child welfare clinics (CWCs) located in the Ga West municipality of the Greater-Accra region, Ghana. All communities within the municipality were classified into rural and urban geographic zones. Within each zone, one health facility-based and one community-based CWC was randomly selected.

Mixed methods design

The explanatory sequential mixed methods design was used [20]. The research started with a quantitative part where the investigators assessed the levels of participation of caregiver-infant pairs enrolled on the GMP programme offered at two community-based and two facility-based CWC in 2011. The resultant change in anthropometric indices of the infants was assessed during their first and last attendance within the 12-months retrospective follow up period. Findings from the study informed the design of a qualitative follow-up in 2015. The aim was to gain in-depth understanding from service providers (community health nurses and community child growth promoters) and users (caregivers) regarding their perspectives on the attendance trends observed in the quantitative

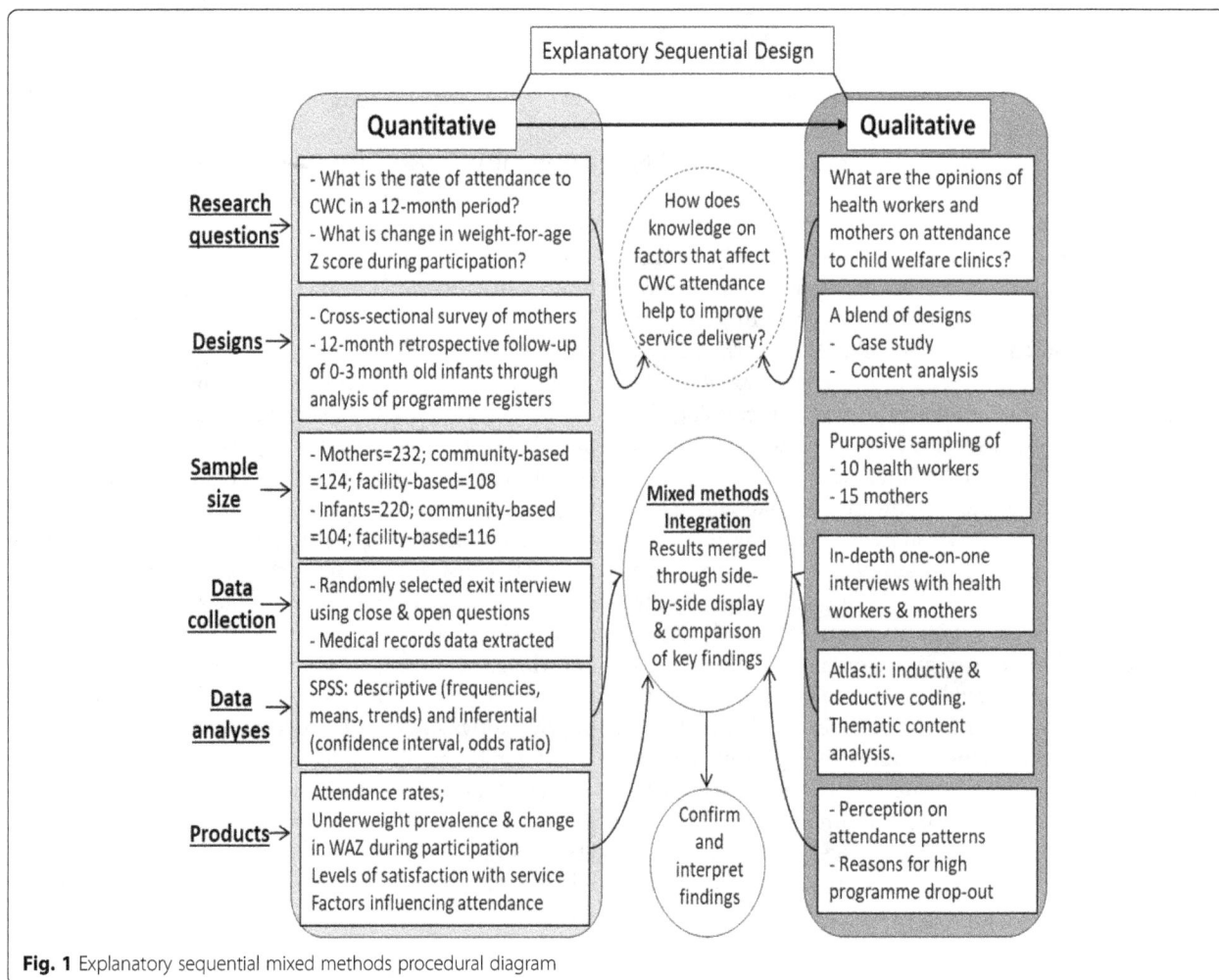

Fig. 1 Explanatory sequential mixed methods procedural diagram

phase of the study. The step-by-step mixed methodology employed in conducting the study is shown in Fig. 1.

Quantitative study

The quantitative part was an observational study with components of cross-sectional survey and retrospective follow-up using secondary data. The study design, data collection and analysis procedures are embedded in the mixed methods procedural diagram presented in Fig. 1.

Retrospective follow-up through secondary data extraction

In the closed-cohort retrospective follow-up, secondary data were extracted from the medical records over a 12-month period spanning from January to December 2011. Information on age and sex of participants, monthly attendance rates and body weight measurements were documented. The inclusion criterion was infants aged 0 to 3 months. This age bracket was chosen because of the increased likelihood of this group participating in the programme for a relatively longer period. Infants enrolled after January 2011 were excluded.

Based on the inclusion criteria, data on 220 registered infants aged 0 to 3 months was extracted from the registers of the facility-based ($n = 116$) and community-based ($n = 104$) programmes. To determine whether the sample size of 220 was sufficiently powered to generate results generalizable to the study population, post-hoc statistical power was tested. First, the standardized difference (effect size) for the two groups was calculated with the aid of a formula provided by Whitley and Ball. The 0.37 standardized difference obtained was then applied on the Altman nomogram at 0.05 alpha level. This yielded a statistical power of 83%; an indication that the sample size had the probability of detecting an effect when it actually existed [21].

A score of one was awarded for each monthly attendance and zero for non-attendance, with the maximum possible score of 12. Data on the extraction forms was entered into SPSS (version 20). Average annual visits as well as proportion of infants who attended the CWC at least six times (≥50%) or met the Ghana Health Service recommended visits of nine times (≥75%) within the 12-months period were compared using independent sample t-test and Fisher's exact test statistic respectively. Body weight measurements were converted to weight-for-age z-scores (WAZ) using WHO AnthroPlus software (version 3.2.2). The resulting z-scores were used to determine the proportions of underweight children (WAZ < – 2 standard deviation) at baseline and at the last CWC visit within the 12-months follow-up period. Change in WAZ between first and last attendance was computed for each child and categorized as a binary variable, to indicate whether the child's WAZ improved or deteriorated during participation. Using improvement or deterioration in WAZ as the dependent variable, a backward stepwise binary logistic regression model was built to determine the adjusted odds ratios (AOR) for improved WAZ during participation. The independent variables were type of programme, age and nutritional status of the child at enrollment, child's sex and attendance levels.

Cross-sectional survey

A cross-sectional survey was conducted to assess the level of satisfaction of caregivers whose children received child welfare services in the community-based and facility-based GMP programmes. The target population was caregiver-child pairs who registered on the GMP programme between January and March 2012. To be eligible for inclusion, caregiver-infant pairs should have attended the clinic at least three times. The sample size was estimated based on a total population of 492 registered infants enrolled in the programme in the study sites at the end of December 2011. A 95% confidence level, 5% margin of error and reliability coefficient of 1.96 [22] generated a sample size of 232. This was proportionately distributed among caregivers enrolled in the community-based ($n = 124$) and facility-based ($n = 108$) programmes. A pre-tested semi-structured questionnaire with close and open-ended questions was used. The questionnaire was purposefully designed to achieve the objectives of the study. Face-to-face interviews were conducted with 232 caregivers who had received child welfare services and were exiting the clinic. Selection of caregivers to partake in the exit interviews was done randomly using the systematic sampling technique. Every fifth caregiver who assessed services and was about to leave the clinic was invited for interviewing. Brief information on socio-demography, home visitation by community health workers, and caregivers' perceptions on the factors that motivated them to attend the clinic as scheduled were elicited. A three-point scale (satisfied, neutral and dissatisfied) was used to evaluate caregivers' levels of satisfaction with the services received. From the pre-testing, this scale was found to be more reliable due to its robustness in clearly discriminating responses coupled with better comprehension among participants with low education. Data obtained were entered into SPSS (version 20) software and analyzed descriptively. Differences between the community-based and the facility-based programmes were determined using Fisher's exact test and unpaired t-test reported with the corresponding 95% confidence intervals (CI) at $p < 0.05$.

Qualitative study

A blend of case study and content analysis designs were used for the qualitative part (Fig. 1). The aim was to gain holistic understanding of the experiences of mothers who received child welfare services from facility-based and community-based CWC. The GMP programme was considered as the case whereas the content analysis provided knowledge of the phenomenon of receiving child welfare services. The case study design has been credited for its usefulness in the health sciences to evaluate programmes and interventions [23]. The qualitative content analysis facilitates a subjective interpretation of the content of text data because codes are systematically classified to identify themes [24].

Qualitative data collection and analysis

Ten categories of health workers and 15 mothers were purposively-selected for the qualitative follow-up. Aided by a topic guide, face-to-face in-depth interviews were conducted from July to September 2014 to explore the experiences and opinions of service providers and clients on the low patterns of attendance to the facility and community-based GMP clinics. Each interview lasted for about 45 min. Saturation was achieved after these 25 interviews necessitating termination of the qualitative data collection. The interview questions had five major domains. We delved into caregivers' motives for taking their children to the GMP clinic, benefits derived from the programme, factors that contributed to regular or irregular attendance, effect of sporadic turnout and how participation would be improved. For instance, we asked a question on the characteristics of irregular attendees and measures to motivating caregivers to attend as scheduled.

The interview sessions were audio-recorded and afterward transcribed verbatim. The transcriptions were exported into the computer-assisted Atlas.ti software (version 7.0) for thematic content analysis. Before commencement of data analysis, a list of pre-determined codes was prepared deductively. These a priori codes were derived based on the research questions, literature on factors that influence participation in community health promotion programmes, and knowledge of the GMP programme in Ghana. Any text that could not be categorized with the initial coding scheme were given a new code. Inductive codes (in-vivo) were then generated from the textual data as result of the new ideas and concepts that emerged during analysis of the data. The lists of codes were reviewed for recurring themes. After relevant themes were mapped out from the codes, related themes were categorized into families and the thematic analysis process was completed. Important themes with accompanying quotes were extracted and summarized. Analysis was computer

assisted in that the software managed the coding process and reporting.

Mixed methods integration

The quantitative and qualitative analyses were done independent of each other. After statistical analysis of the numerical data and qualitative analysis of the textual data, key results were integrated through merging at the interpretation and reporting level. The essence of the merging was to link the quantitative to the qualitative data in order to explain findings from the latter [25]. Through comparison and visual presentation of key findings, new insights were unveiled. According to Fetters et al. [25], when similar conclusions are obtained from merged numeric and textual data, confirmation of findings provides greater credibility to the results. Presentation of quantitative and qualitative data was by side-by-side joint tabular display. Inferences and interpretations were drawn from the merged findings.

Results

Attendance levels and change in weight-for-age z-score

Table 1 shows attendance levels and weight-for-age z-scores (WAZ) of children in the facility- and community-based programme registers. In January when the assessment began, 32.7% ($n = 72$) of the infants were 1 mo old, 14.5% ($n = 32$) were 2 mos old, and the remainder (52.7%) were 3 mos old. Mean annual attendance was six visits (SD = 2.9). This was similar in the facility-based (5.95 ± 2.77) and community-based (6.05 ± 3.06) programmes. Overall, 46.8% ($n = 103$) of the infants received CWC services at least six times but only 13.6% ($n = 30$) met the recommended nine or more visits in the 12-months period. At baseline, mean weight of the children was 5.04 kg (SD = 1.36). Participants in the community-based programme were significantly heavier than their facility-based counterparts (5.29 ± 1.43 vs. 4.85 ± 1.28 kg). Consequently, significantly more children (19.8%) in the facility-based community-based programme were underweight compared to 8.7% in the community-based programme (Table 1). At the end of the one-year follow-up period, the overall mean weight increased to 8.87 kg (SD = 1.18). Uunderweight prevalence in the community-based cohort increased by 3%-points to 11.5% while decreasing by 4%-point to (15.5%) in the facility-based cohort ($p = 0.436$). Cumulatively, underweight levels during the 12-months period was 16.5%. Between the first and last month of attendance within the 12-months, there was about 70% increase in WAZ among both groups of children (Table 2).

With regards to monthly attendance patterns, in the first month, attendance was 75%. This decreased until it tapered to the lowest rate of 16% in December 2011. Five participants (2.3%) never missed a session. The

Table 1 Comparison of anthropometric characteristics at baseline and after the 12-months observation period

Characteristics	Baseline					12th month				
	Community-based (n = 104)		Facility-based (n = 116)		P value	Community-based (n = 104)		Facility-based (n = 116)		P value
	Mean±SD n (%)	95% CI	Mean±SD n (%)	95% CI		Mean±SD n (%)	95% CI	Mean±SD n (%)	95% CI	
Age (months) [a]	2.25±0.86	2.08–2.24	2.16±0.95	1.98–2.33	0.439	13.25±0.86	13.08–13.42	13.17±0.97	13.00–13.36	0.532
Weight (kg) [a]	5.29±1.43	4.80–6.10	4.85±1.28	4.38–5.30	0.035	8.97±1.95	8.55–9.24	8.79±1.35	8.26–9.15	0.547
WAZ [a]	− 0.60±1.04	−0.81 - -0.40	− 0.94±1.44	−1.21 - -0.71	0.049	− 0.27±1.32	−0.56 - 0.02	− 0.62±1.65	−0.94 - -0.33	0.081
Underweight (%) [b]	9(8.7)	3.8–14.4	23(19.8)	12.9–26.7	0.022	12(11.5)	5.8–18.3	18(15.5)	9.5–22.4	0.436

[a]unpaired t test
[b]Fisher's exact test

highest number of four visits was recorded by 15.5% (n = 34) of the participants. The overall drop-out rate was 59.5%; 58.7% in the community-based and 57.3% in the facility-based clinics. Due to the sporadic monthly attendance rates, underweight proportions within the 12-months period did not follow any peculiar trend. Underweight was highest in February (24%) and lowest in June (11%). Comparison of attendance levels, mean weight, weight-for-age z-scores and underweight prevalence in the community- and facility-based programmes is shown in Fig. 2.

Determinants for improved WAZ during programme participation

Overall, between first and last attendance, WAZ of 69.1% children (n = 152, 95% CI = 63.2–75.0) improved while 30.9% (n = 68, 95% CI:25.0–36.8) either deteriorated (28.2%) or remained unchanged (2.7%). Infants who were underweight at baseline were eleven times more likely (95% CI:3.95–31.03, p < 0.0001) to increase their WAZ during participation compared to normal weight infants (Table 3). Also, females were two times more likely (95% CI:1.07–3.62, p = 0.029) to improve their WAZ compared to males. Children who recorded six visits (95% CI:1.14–4.07, p = 0.018)

or met the recommended nine annual visits (95% CI:1.44–15.06, p = 0.010) were two and five times more likely to respectively increase their WAZ during participation. Neither enrolment in community-based or facility-based programme nor age of the child significantly affected the change in WAZ.

Caregivers' level of satisfaction with GMP services

Socio-demographic characteristics of the 232 caregivers who participated in the cross-sectional survey have been extensively described in a previous publication [7]. Mean age of the caregivers was 26 years (±5.6 SD) ranging from 15 to 45 years. Eighty-five percent (n = 197) lived with a partner while the remainder were single parents. One third of the mothers (37.5%, n = 87) were educated to the junior high school level (equivalent to the eighth grade) and 16.8% (n = 39) to the secondary high school/technical level (equivalent to the twelfth grade). One-fifth (17.2%, n = 40) had no formal education whereas only one participant had tertiary education. Almost 80% were engaged in some form of income generating venture. The mean parity among the women was three children and the average household size was five members. Mean age of the

Table 2 Attendance levels and change in weight-for-age z-score during first and last appearance on the programme in the 12-months period

Characteristics	Community-based (n = 104)		Facility-based (n = 116)		P value
	Mean ± SD n (%)	95% CI	Mean ± SD n (%)	95% CI	
Average annual visits [a]	5.95 ± 2.77	5.42–6.47	6.05 ± 3.06	5.48–6.62	0.800
Attend ≥6 times (%) [b]	48 (46.2)	36.5–55.8	55 (47.4)	38.8–56.0	0.893
Attend ≥9 times (%) [b]	13 (12.5)	5.8–18.3	17 (14.7%)	8.6–21.6	0.697
Average annual WAZ [b]	− 0.48 ± 1.02	−0.68 - -0.29	− 0.86 ± 1.54	− 1.14 - 0.57	0.035
Change in WAZ (%) [b]					0.772
Improved	70.2% (73)	61.5–77.9	68.1% (79)	59.5–75.9	
Deteriorated	29.8% (31)	22.1–38.5	31.9% (37)	24.1–40.5	

[a]unpaired t test
[b]Fisher's exact test

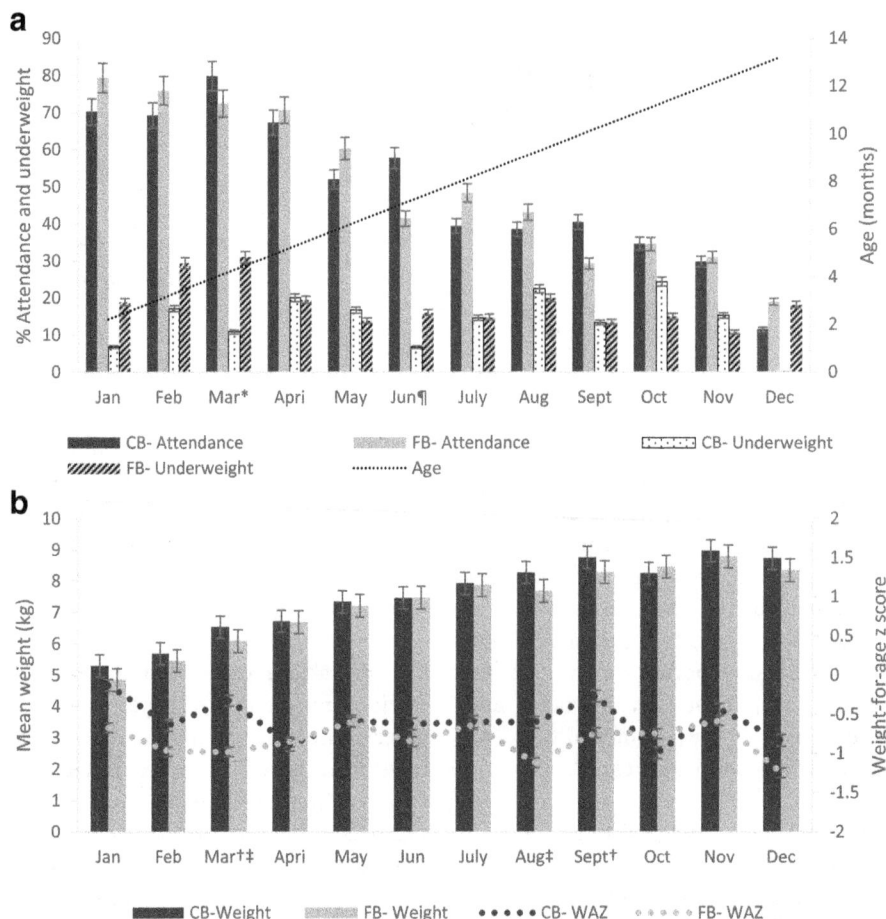

Fig. 2 Monthly attendance and underweight prevalence per month (**a**), and the mean weight and weight-for-age z scores (**b**) in the community-based (CB) and facility-based (FB) programmes. A superscript on the month implies $p < 0.05$. Statistically significant difference for ¶attendance; *underweight; †weight-for-age z-score; and ‡mean weight

Table 3 Binary logistic regression model showing factors that predicted an increase in weight-for-age z-score between the first and last attendance on the programme

Variables	n	%	Adjusted regression model		
			AOR	95% CI	P value
Programme (Facility-based)	116	47.3	Ref		
Community-based	104	52.7	1.27	0.70–2.33	0.434
Age at registration (> 4 weeks)	148	67.3	Ref		
Neonatal (≤4 weeks)	72	32.7	0.75	0.39–1.44	0.382
Sex (male)	110	50.0	Ref		
Female	110	50.0	1.97	1.07–3.62	0.029
Underweight at baseline (No)	188	85.5	Ref		
Yes	32	14.5	11.07	3.95–31.03	< 0.0001
Annual attendance (< 6 visits)	117	53.2	Ref		
≥ 6 visits	103	46.8	2.15	1.14–4.07	0.018
Attendance (< 9 annual visits)	190	86.4	Ref		
≥ 9 annual visits	30	13.6	4.65	1.44–15.06	0.010

Hosmer-Lemeshow goodness-of-fit test, Chi-square = 10.192, $p = 0.252$. Cox and Snell $R^2 = 0.155$, Nagelkerke $R^2 = 0.210$

Table 4 Caregivers' experiences with the community- and facility-based child growth monitoring and promotion programmes

Variables	Community-based (n = 124)		Facility-based (n = 108)		P value
	n (%)	95% CI	n (%)	95% CI	
Enrollment time					0.047
At birth	33 (26.6)	18.5–35.5	29 (26.9)	18.5–35.2	
Two weeks after birth	36 (29.0)	21.8–37.9	43 (39.8)	29.6–50.0	
1 month after birth	31 (25.0)	17.7–33.1	28 (25.9)	18.5–35.2	
After neonatal period	24 (19.4)	12.9–25.8	8 (7.4)	2.8–13.0	
Visited at home	39 (31.5)	23.4–39.5	57.4 (62)	48.1–66.7	< 0.0001
Motivation for participation					0.004
Know child's growth	58 (46.8)	38.7–56.5	39 (36.1)	26.9–45.4	
Receive vaccinations	38 (30.6)	22.6–38.7	19 (17.6)	11.1–25.0	
Treat minor ailments	22 (17.7)	11.3–25.0	38 (35.2)	25.9–43.5	
Nutrition education	4 (3.2)	0.8–6.5	8.3 (9)	3.7–13.9	
None	2 (1.6)	0–4.0	3 (2.8)	0.0–6.5	
Satisfied with services					0.437
Yes	43 (34.7)	25.8–42.7	29 (26.9)	5.6–16.7	
Neutral	12 (9.7)	4.8–15.3	12 (11.1)	18.5–35.2	
No	69 (55.6)	46.8–64.5	97 (62.0)	52.8–70.4	
Reasons for satisfaction					0.774
Knowledge on child's growth	31 (70.5)	56.8–81.8	19 (65.5)	48.3–82.8	
Educated on child care	8 (18.2)	6.8–29.5	5 (17.2)	3.4–31.0	
Free complementary services	5 (11.4)	2.3–20.5	5 (17.2)	3.4–31.0	
Reasons for dissatisfaction					0.051
Long waiting times	43 (62.3)	52.2–73.9	53 (77.9)	67.6–86.8	
Unfriendly staff attitude	15 (21.7)	13.0–31.9	12 (17.6)	8.8–27.9	
Extortion of money	11 (15.9)	7.3–24.6	3 (4.4)	0–10.3	

children sent to the CWC was eight months (7.9 ± 5.0 months). Although majority of caregivers registered their infants before within the neonatal period, it was significantly higher in the facility-based group (93% vs. 81%). Also, 57% of the caregivers who used the facility-based services reported being visited at home at least once by a community health worker, compared to 32% in the community-based programme ($p < 0.0001$). In both groups, caregivers mentioned knowledge on their child's growth status and vaccinations as the most important motivating factors for regular attendance. Overall, 35% expressed satisfaction with the services received citing education on child care and the free complementary services such as birth registration and distribution of insecticide-treated bed nets. However, over half of the caregivers expressed dissatisfaction citing long waiting times, unfriendly staff attitude and service fees charged by some staff particularly the community volunteers. Breakdown of the responses in the community- and facility-based CWC is presented in Table 4.

Characteristics of participants in the qualitative study
In-depth interviews were conducted with ten health workers who ran the GMP programme or supervised its implementation and 15 clients who accessed the service. The aim was to explore perceptions on the trends in attendance observed in the quantitative study.

Four out of the ten health workers were stationed at the district as core members of the District Health Management Team and the remainder worked at the primary healthcare level. The district health team comprised two Public Health Nurses, one nutrition officer and one disease control officer. The public health nurses had over 15 years work experience and played supervisory roles as nurse-managers. The nutrition and disease control officers provided logistics and technical support for the programme. Four were low cadre community health nurses (CHN) with on average, ten years post-qualification experience. One was selected from each of the four study facilities. The remaining two interviewees were the trained community child growth promoters who supported the CHNs and served as liaison with the community.

The mothers' age ranged from 21 to 46 years, and the age of their accompanying children ranged from 4 to 18 months. Six mothers were uniparous and the remaining nine were multiparous with the highest parity being six children. Two had no formal education whereas three had primary education. Five completed junior (eighth grade) and senior high schools (twelfth grade). In terms of occupation, three were unemployed, eight were traders and four were self-employed artisan. Seven used community-based and eight used facility-based CWC.

Perception of service providers/users on reasons for low attendance to CWC

The process of coding and thematic analysis of the transcribed data led to the generation of about 50 initial codes. By summarizing and synthesizing the codes, it was reorganized into 16 non-hierarchical codes from which seven themes were developed. The themes elucidated why attendance to child welfare clinics were often below set targets and the drop-out rate was high. The seven themes are described below.

Extremes of maternal age and high parity

It was deduced that teenage mothers and women above the age of 40 years who were grand multiparous mothers (with more than five children) failed to attend the clinics as scheduled. While the teenagers were scolded for "doing what was the reserve of their mothers", the older and multiparous mothers were condemned for not adopting a family planning method to avert the pregnancy, despite numerous sensitization campaigns. This 43 years old mother of five children expressed her sentiment:

> "Without considering the presence of other mothers, the nurse asked me why I gave birth at my age when I already had five children while they (the nurses) were preaching family planning every time. I felt so embarrassed".

Socio-cultural beliefs and practices during early postpartum

Both the health workers and the mothers mentioned conformity to certain entrenched postpartum cultural practices as a reason for irregular CWC attendance. In certain cultures, women with newborn babies were required to remain in-doors till the umbilical cord of the newborn fell off; the circumcision wound of the baby boy completely healed or until the baby was 'out-doored' and/or the naming ceremony performed. Another reason that strongly emanated was the

practice of mothers-newborn pairs adorning in all white attractive outfits as a way of expressing joy and gratitude to God for safe delivery. Mothers who were unable to purchase new set of clothing and apparels for adornment were reluctant to go to public places. A public health nurse at the district health directorate and a mother confirmed this assertion:

> "....as tradition demands, newly delivered mothers wear white clothes as a way of openly expressing their happiness for safe delivery. If the mothers cannot afford to buy new clothes, especially teenage and single mothers, they are likely to remain at home. We keep telling them that the health of the infant is more important than their looks".

> "My mother told me to stay indoors for some time to keep evil eyes off my baby. She said the baby is too young to be exposed. It was very difficult convincing her to come for today's weighing" (Mother age 22 years).

Financial commitments

Financial commitments towards transportation, purchasing items sold at the clinic and sometimes paying service charges was a major concern. Mothers lamented about constant persuasion from the health workers to purchase stuff they sold at the clinic. These items ranged from weighing pants, 'weanimix' (complementary food produced from cereal-legume-peanut blend), cosmetics, diapers to medications especially analgesics for fever, teething and colicky pain.

> "The nurses sell ...... If they ask you to buy sometime and you say you don't have money, they will say you are not concerned about your baby's health" (Mother age 28 years).

Unemployed and single mothers complained of lack of money for transportation, and to buy new apparels/clothing to look socially acceptable at the clinic. A single mother aged 21 years with a seven-month old infant epitomized this by saying: "the day I have money, I come". In few cases, mothers accused the community volunteers of demanding payment for service provision.

> "Some of the workers (community volunteers) ask us to pay money. But I know that weighing is free of charge. I didn't pay any money for my previous children. If you don't pay, they will refuse to give you your child's weighing card. That's why I don't like coming here" (Mother age 33 years).

The community volunteers admitted this allegation but attributed it to irregular remuneration by the District Health Directorate.

"The district is supposed to pay us every month. But we are hardly remembered. That is why we resolved to charge one Ghana cedi per client .... yes, it is compulsory for them to pay" (Community Volunteer).

Implications of long waiting times

The mothers complained of undue delays and late commencement of activities at the clinic. This situation they bemoaned restricted them from trading on clinic days leading to loss of income. Another opportunity cost cited was inability to perform household responsibilities. Thirty-six and 29-year old mothers confirmed this concern:

"Anytime I bring my child for weighing, I'm not able to go and sell my wares". I spend most part of the day at weighing". "When my children return from school, there's no one at home to take care of them. They just keep loitering until I return".

The service providers on the other hand argued that the siting of clinics within wide catchment zones contributed to overcrowding at the sessions and stagnated workflow. Nonetheless, they reiterated that inadequate personnel and heavy work schedules were the primary reasons for the delays and not just the limited availability and accessibility to the service.

"We hear mothers complain about spending long hours at the clinic. But while most of these centres are understaffed, how can the work move fast? .... Sometimes, the community health nurses have to pick-up vaccines at the directorate in the morning of the clinic. Unfortunately, we lack enough vehicles to convey them (the nurses) to their respective clinics, so they get there late". (Public Health Nurse).

Unprofessional behaviours and attitudes

A major concern was inflexibility in scheduling appointments. The mothers believed their non-involvement in deciding on the visit date added to the dwindling attendance. Also, they expressed concern about the unprofessional behaviours exhibited by some staff which demoralized them from being consistent with schedules. Behaviours such as public scolding, lack of rapport, impatience to listen and lack of confidentiality especially during counselling sessions were specified. These communication lapses resulted in difficulty understanding the counselling messages. In instances of inadequate child growth, mothers lamented about inability to reach clear consensus on agreed actions to implement at home.

"Some of the nurses are unfriendly. If your child is not growing well, they will shout at you as if it is your fault. They won't even allow you to explain yourself". (29-year mother) .

High priority on immunization

The health workers seemingly focused on meeting immunization targets to the neglect of other vital components of the programme such as growth assessment and counselling on infant and young child feeding. Optimizing the use of the vaccines was vital. They clarified that once a vial of vaccine was opened; it ought to be used within a limited time. Low turn-up therefore implied vaccine wastage. However, they thought that the lack of knowledge by caregivers and their families on the usefulness of GMP played a role. On the other hand, the mothers patronized the child welfare services primarily because of the immunizations given to the infants, without which they were reluctant to attend.

"The role of immunization in reducing childhood illnesses has contributed to mothers not attending the sessions as most of them have never seen a child with poliomyelitis, serious measles, whooping cough, and so on before. Hence they do not believe these diseases are real and therefore have to vaccinate against it". (Disease Control Officer)

"For most mothers, their main reason for sending their children to child welfare clinics is to receive vaccinations. When reports are collated, we notice that attendance is highest among participants that receive immunizations. This is making our surveillance on growth faltering difficult". (Nutrition Officer)

"I just ignore coming if I know my baby is not due for injection.... because they only weigh the baby and give you the next date to come.... nothing more" (Mother age 35 years).

Misconceptions about the programme

According to the health workers, sections of the public held some misconceptions that prevented them from optimally utilizing the service. Allegations such as hoarding and using items meant for mother-infant pairs,

Table 5 Side-by-side display of key quantitative and qualitative findings and implications for practice

Attribute	Quantitative findings	Qualitative findings	Implications
Attendance to the growth monitoring and promotion programme	- Mean annual attendance 6.0 ± 2.9 - Proportion meeting ≥6 visits: 46.8% - Proportion meeting the recommended ≥9 visits: 13.6% - Overall drop-out rate: 59.5%	Attendance based on maternal age, parity, postpartum socio-cultural practices, financial constraints, irregular staff remuneration, delays, unprofessional staff behaviours, high premium on vaccinations & general misconceptions about GMP programme	Increase home visitations and target the following mothers: teenagers, single parents, women above 40 years, and those with parity above four children
Change in weight-for-age z-score during participation and the determining factors	WAZ of 69.1% of the children improved. Determinants: - Underweight at baseline (AOR:11.1, 95% CI:4.0–31.0) - ≥6 annual visits (AOR:2.2, 95% CI:1.1–4.1) ≥9 annual visits (AOR:4.7, 95% CI:1.4–15.1)	Deterioration in growth attributed to drop-out rates from the GMP programme, inadequate counselling, ineffective staff-client rapport, communication lapses, emphasis on achieving meeting vaccinations to the neglect of the other components of the programme	- Sensitization on contribution of routine growth monitoring and promotion to early child development and the dangers associated with unidentified growth faltering
Motivation to attend and level of satisfaction with service delivery	- Motivators for attendance were knowledge of child's growth status and child vaccination. - 31% (95% CI: 25–37) of mothers satisfied - 59% (95% CI: 52–65) of mothers dissatisfied with service delivery	Satisfied as result of awareness of child's growth and education provided on child care. Dissatisfaction resulted from: long waiting times; late start of clinic; uncomfortable clinic area, monies collected as services charges and negative staff attitude	- Primary healthcare systems should be strengthened to improve service delivery by increasing availability and accessibility to the service; staff supervision, training and monitoring

extortions of money from clients, and making unwarranted financial gains through sale of items were mentioned.

> "As was done in the past, some mothers expect to be given tokens as such weanimix, weighing pants and medicines free of charge. We need to tell them (mothers) that the situation has changed".
> (Community Health Nurse)

Integration of mixed methods results
Presented in Table 5 are key findings obtained from the quantitative and qualitative studies and its implications for preventive child health practice.

Discussion
The aim of the quantitative study was to evaluate the trends in utilization of facility-based and community-based preventive child welfare services, change in weight-for-age z-scores of participants and caregivers' level of satisfaction with the services received. Findings informed a qualitative follow-up study to explore viewpoints of mothers and health workers on why attendance to the clinics was below targets.

Average annual visit was six with overall drop-out rate of 60%. Reports from the Family Health Division of the Ghana Health Service shows that although children age 0–11 months continue to record the highest registration, trends in CWC service utilization has been sub-optimum compared to the 12–23 months and 24–59 months age groups [26]. The target for children age 0–11 months achieving nine visits per year has never been realized at the national level. For instance, from 2013 to 2015, average annual visits were 4.9, 5.7 and 5.5 respectively [26]. These number of annual visit are similar to the 5.95 and 6.05 mean annual attendance recorded in the community- and facility-based clinics. It is therefore not surprising that only 13.6% children met the nine-visit target which is an improvement over the national trend.

The drop-out rate of 59.5% is lower compared to the 74.1% observed in the Lusaka district of Zambia after a 3 month prospective follow-up [9]. Cross-sectional surveys conducted in both rural and urban Ghana show that on monthly basis, 30% of caregivers miss CWC sessions [18, 27]. These findings concur to our closed-cohort retrospective follow-up using secondary data. We observed that in the first month of the follow-up, clients who missed the sessions were about 30%.

The Ghana Health Service has linked drops in attendance to completion of majority of immunization and supplementations schedules. The health workers we interviewed acknowledged this situation. Widespread investments towards meeting immunization targets in Ghana is also accountable [28]. From the exit interviews, caregivers mentioned knowledge of child's growth status as the most beneficial service received. But from the in-depth interviews, vaccinations ranked highest as the most important motivator for meeting schedules. Ashworth has observed that in preventive programmes, provision of medications including vaccinations are more valued than preventive services such as nutrition counselling [4].

Aside socio-demographic factors [29], long waiting times [30] transportation difficulties, inconvenient scheduling dates [18], poor client-staff relationship [31], and poorly motivated service providers [9] have been identified to reduce child welfare service utilization. However, other interesting findings emerged. These include public scolding of teenage and grand multiparous mothers, socio-cultural beliefs and practices that restricted early postpartum mothers-newborn pairs from going to public places and paying for an otherwise free service.

Utilization of preventive and promotion child health services in most developing countries vary widely depending on the mode of operation. Utilization of community-based programmes is usually higher than the traditional facility-based clinics. For example, in Honduras, monthly attendance rate among caregivers participating in the community-based growth promotion programme was significantly higher compared to those enrolled in the traditional health facility-based programme (60% vs. 40%) [32]. Average attendance in the Ugandan community-based programme was even higher (72%) [33]. In Rwanda, attendance was 53% in 2004 and increased to 78% in 2008 [34]. In our study however, caregiver-child pairs enrolled in the facility-based clinics tended to utilize the service more often.

Reasons for higher attendance to the facility-based clinics are evident from both the quantitative and qualitative studies. The community health nurses who run the facility-based clinics conduct more home visitation than their volunteer counterparts in the community-based clinics. In Ghana, home visitation is an effective mechanism to follow-up on defaulters, reinforce educational and counselling messages, observe practices in the natural environment, provide support, and link families to primary healthcare systems. It emerged from the in-depth interviews that due to infrequent remuneration, the free GMP programme was delivered at a fee by the volunteers, thereby deterring mothers from attending regularly. Meanwhile, frequent health worker-child contact is associated with better health outcomes [4]. This could explain why the proportion of underweight children increased among the community-based participants during the 12-months period. Despite this, more community-based clients were satisfied with the quality of services provided. Compliant of unprofessional behaviours were mainly against the community health

nurses who run the facility-based clinics. This could contribute to the higher satisfaction expressed by the community-based clinic users. But this 31% satisfaction level is low compared to the 88% of primary healthcare users who expressed satisfaction in urban Nigeria [35].

Although WAZ of 30% participants deteriorated during the 12-months period, in Zambia, WAZ of all children ($n = 698$) deteriorated [9]. We found that more CWC visits and being underweight at enrolment were associated with improved WAZ. Unfortunately, children at high risk of malnutrition tend to attend CWC less often [13]. As noted from the qualitative study, the practice of scolding mothers whose children were faltering growth demotivated them from using the service.

Strengths and limitations

This study has affirmed the potential effects of routine growth monitoring on improving the nutritional status of regular attendees and underweight children. This study is unique because of the innovation of applying mixed methods design to child development in primary healthcare systems research in Ghana. Methodology-wise, the combination of diverse designs both in the quantitative (cross-sectional survey and retrospective study using secondary data) and qualitative (case study and content analysis designs) research has enriched the findings as it has provided a holistic synopsis of the extent of child welfare service utilization and the factors mitigate patronage. Also, blending the conventional and directed approach as part of the content analysis design harnessed the strength of this qualitative methodology. The researchers did not only gain direct information from the caregivers without imposing preconceived theoretical perspectives but also expanded existing literature on the phenomenon of CWC utilisation. Instead of underweight rates, change in WAZ was used to build the regression model. WAZ corrects for age and eliminates the effect of change in age over time. Therefore, marginal changes in body weight and WAZ during participation were detected.

Nevertheless, the investigators acknowledge that the study is limited to one district in Ghana. To establish cause and effect, a prospective study would have been ideal. It is possible that the association of number of CWC visits predicting change in WAZ may actually be due to other unobserved differences in the mothers. That could not be determined in this observational study. It is worth noting that secondary data is not devoid of problems such as incomplete and multiple entries. Finally, background of the field investigator as a registered nurse and GMP service user could influence interpretations made.

Conclusion

This study has shown that higher contact is associated with improved growth. For growth monitoring and promotion programmes to achieve the needed impact, intensity of contact with service providers is crucial. Strategies to enhance contact such as home visitation should be targeted at groups of people identified from both the quantitative and qualitative studies to be prone to sporadic attendance. These include malnourished children; early postpartum mother-child pairs; teenage, single and grand multiparous mothers; and children who have completed their vaccinations. To increase adherence to appointment schedules, health workers could consider consulting with caregivers to agree on suitable appointment dates. Parents and families need to be sensitized on the role of growth monitoring in promoting child health even after completion of vaccinations. Since the complementary role of community volunteers in increasing availability and accessibility of GMP services is indispensable, [36], issues relating to their remuneration require critical review by policy makers.

Abbreviations

AOR: Adjusted odds ratio; CB : Community-based; CHN: Community health nurses; CI: Confidence interval; CWC : Child welfare clinic; FB : Facility-based; GMP : Growth monitoring and promotion; SD: Standard deviation; WAZ : Weight-for-age z-scores

Acknowledgements

We thank Kafui Doh for his extensive support with data collection and entry.

Authors' contributions

FA and EC conceptualized and designed the study. FA conducted the field work, analyzed the data and wrote the first draft. All authors critically revised the manuscript for important intellectual content. TG provided direction particularly on the methodological content and JA aligned the manuscript in the context of primary healthcare systems research. All authors approved the final submitted version.

Authors' information

FA (MPhil Nutrition), a Registered Nurse, is presently a doctoral student at the Institute of Public Health, University of Heidelberg, Germany. EC (Dr Public Health) is a Lecturer of Nutrition at the University of Ghana. AJ (PhD Tropical Medicine), an Obstetrics and Gynaecology specialist and a Professor of Public Health, is the group leader of the Research Group on Global Health Policies and Systems at the Institute of Public Health, University of Heidelberg, Germany. TG (PhD Educational Psychology) is an applied research methodologist and Assistant Professor at University of Michigan Medical School, USA.

Ethics approval and consent to participate

The study protocol was approved by the Institutional Review Board of the Noguchi Memorial Institute for Medical Research, University of Ghana (NMIMR-IRB CPN 040/11–12). The literate participants provided written informed consent. Where illiterate, the information sheet was read out to the participant in a local language of choice, in the presence of a witness, usually a relative/friend. Participants who verbalized their willingness to participate thumb-printed the consent form as evidence. In addition, participants with whom the in-depth interviews were conducted granted permission for verbatim quoting of excerpts of their interviews in any publication.

Parental consent was not obtained for teenage mothers because they were considered as emancipated adults.

Competing interests

The authors declare that they have no competing interests.

Author details

[1]Department of Family and Community Health, School of Public Health, University of Health and Allied Sciences, PMG, 31 Ho, Ghana. [2]Institute of Public Health, University of Heidelberg Medical Faculty, Heidelberg, Germany. [3]Department of Nutrition and Food Science, University of Ghana, Legon, Accra, Ghana. [4]Department of Family Medicine, University of Michigan Medical School, Ann Arbor, MI, USA.

References

1. Shekar M, Kakietek J, D'Alimonte M, Walters D, Rogers H, Eberwein J, et al. Investing in nutrition: the Foundation for Development: an investment framework to reach the global nutrition targets. Washington, DC: World Bank, results for development, Bill and Melinda Gates Foundation, CIFF, Thousand days; 2016.
2. Bhutta ZA, Das JK, Rizvi A, Gaffey MF, Walker N, Horton S, et al. Evidence-based interventions for improvement of maternal and child nutrition: what can be done and at what cost? Lancet. 2013;382(9890):452–77.
3. WHO. Monitoring of the achievement of the health-related Millennium Development Goals. Report by the Secretariat. Geneva: Switzerland: World Health Organization; 2016. Contract No.: EB138/13
4. Ashworth A, Shrimpton R, Jamil K. Growth monitoring and promotion: review of evidence of impact. Matern Child Nutr. 2008;4(s1):86–117.
5. Daelmans B, Black MM, Lombardi J, Lucas J, Richter L, Silver K, et al. Effective interventions and strategies for improving early child development. Br Med J. 2015;351:h4029. https://doi.org/10.1136/bmj.h4029.
6. Griffiths M, Del Rosso J. Growth monitoring and the promotion of healthy young child growth. In: Evidence of effectiveness and potential to prevent malnutrition. Washington, DC 20008: The Manoff Group; 2007.
7. Agbozo F, Colecraft E, Ellahi B. Impact of type of child growth intervention program on caregivers' child feeding knowledge and practices: a comparative study in Ga west municipality, Ghana. Food Sci Nutr. 2016;4(4):562–72. https://doi.org/10.1002/fsn3.318.
8. Ghana Health Service. Nutrition and Malaria Control for Child Survival Project. Sub-project Manual. Accra, Ghana: Ghana Health Service and Ministry of Health; 2008.
9. Charlton K, Kawana B, Hendricks M. An assessment of the effectiveness of growth monitoring and promotion practices in the Lusaka district of Zambia. Nutrition. 2009;25(10):1035–46. https://doi.org/10.1016/j.nut.2009.03.008.
10. Nyavani SM, Xikombiso GM, Fhumudzani ML. Caregivers' interpretation of the growth chart and feeding practices of children under five years: a case of Greater Tzaneen municipality, South Africa. Journal of food and Nutr Res. 2016;4(6):369–76. http://pubs.sciepub.com/jfnr/4/6/5
11. Roberfroid D, Pelto GH, Kolsteren P. Plot and see! Maternal comprehension of growth charts worldwide. Tropical Med Int Health. 2007;12(9):1074–86.
12. de Onis M, Wijnhoven TM, Onyango AW. Worldwide practices in child growth monitoring. J Pediatr. 2004;144(4):461–5.
13. Ashworth A, Shrimpton R, Jamil K. Growth monitoring and promotion: review of evidence of impact. Matern Child Nutr. 2008;4(s1):86–117. https://doi.org/10.1111/j.1740-8709.2007.00125.x.
14. Dewey KG, Adu-Afarwuah S. Systematic review of the efficacy and effectiveness of complementary feeding interventions in developing countries. Maternal Child Nutr. 2008;4(s1):24–85.
15. Bilal SM, Moser A, Blanco R, Spigt M, Dinant GJ. Practices and challenges of growth monitoring and promotion in Ethiopia: a qualitative study. J Health Popul Nutr. 2014;32:441.

16. Owusu WB, Lartey A. Growth monitoring: experience from Ghana education. 1992;48:23.0.

17. Bosu WK, Ahelegbe D, Edum-Fotwe E, Kobina AB, Kobina Turkson P. Factors influencing attendance to immunization sessions for children in a rural district of Ghana. Acta Trop. 1997;68:259–67. https://doi.org/10.1016/S0001-706X(97)00094-6.

18. Laar M, Marquis G, Lartey A, Gray-Donald K. Growth Monitoring and Promotion in rural Ghana: lack of motivation or tools? FASEB J. 2015; 29(1Suppl):31–4. https://www.fasebj.org/doi/abs/10.1096/fasebj.29.1_supplement.31.4.

19. Ghana Health Service. 2014 Family Health Annu Rep. Accra, Ghana: Ghana Health Service and Ministry of Health, Division FH; 2014.

20. Creswell JW. Research design: Qualitative, quantitative, and mixed methods approaches. United States of America: Library of Congress Cataloging-in-Publication Data; 2009.

21. Cohen J. Statistical power analysis for the behavioral sciences. 2nd ed. Hillsdale, NJ: Lawrence Erlbaum Associates; 1988.

22. Whitley E, Ball J. Statistics review 4: sample size calculations. Crit Care. 2002;6:1.

23. Stake R. The art of case study research. Thousand Oaks: SAGE Publications Inc; 1995.

24. Hsieh H-F, Shannon SE. Three approaches to qualitative content analysis. Qual Health Res. 2005;15:1277–88.

25. Fetters MD, Curry LA, Creswell JW. Achieving integration in mixed methods designs—principles and practices. Health Serv Res. 2013;48:2134–56. https://doi.org/10.1111/1475-6773.12117.

26. Ghana Health Service. Family health Annu Rep. Accra, Ghana: Ghana Health Service, Division FH; 2015.

27. Gyampoh S, Otoo GE, Aryeetey RNO. Child feeding knowledge and practices among women participating in growth monitoring and promotion in Accra, Ghana. BMC Pregnancy and Childbirth. 2014;14(1):180. https://doi.org/10.1186/1471-2393-14-180.

28. LaFond A, Kanagat N, Steinglass R, Fields R, Sequeira J, Mookherji S. Drivers of routine immunization coverage improvement in Africa: findings from district-level case studies. Health policy and planning. 2014;30(3):298-308. https://doi.org/10.1093/heapol/czu011.

29. Cameron E, Heath G, Redwood S, Greenfield S, Cummins C, Kelly D, et al. Health care professionals' views of paediatric outpatient non-attendance: implications for general practice. Fam Pract. 2014;31(1):111-17. https://doi.org/10.1093/fampra/cmt063.

30. Turkson P. Perceived quality of healthcare delivery in a rural district of Ghana. Ghana Med J. 2009;43(2):65-70.

31. Martin C, Perfect T, Mantle G. Non-attendance in primary care: the views of patients and practices on its causes, impact and solutions. Fam Pract. 2005; 22:638–43.

32. Van Roekel K, Plowman B, Griffiths M, Vivas V, de Alvarado J, Matute M. BASICS II Midterm evaluation of the AIN program in Honduras. Arlington, Virginia; U.S A: United States Agency for International Development; 2002. Contract No.: Contract No. HRN-C-00-99-00007-00

33. Muyeti RS, Miller del Rosso J. Uganda Community Based Growth promotion: Program review. Uganda. In: Uganda program for human and holistic development (UPHOLD), The Manoff group and USAID: JSI Res Training Inst Inc, 2008; 2007.

34. Ngirabega J, Leonard W, Munyanshongore C, Dramaix-Wilmet M. Utilization of community based growth monitoring services by eligible children in rural Rwanda. Rwanda Medical Journal. 2010;68:40–7.

35. Sule S, Olawuyi O, Afolabi O, Onajole A, Ogunowo B. Caregivers knowledge and utilization of child health services in an Urban District of Lagos, Nigeria. West African J Med. 2013;32:163–72.

36. Afulani PA, Awoonor-Williams JK, Opoku EC, Asunka J. Using community health workers in community-based growth promotion: what stakeholders think. Health Educ Res. 2012;27:1005–17.

21

Systematic development of CHEMO-SUPPORT, a nursing intervention to support adult patients with cancer in dealing with chemotherapy-related symptoms at home

Annemarie Coolbrandt[1,2]* (iD), Hans Wildiers[3], Bert Aertgeerts[4], Bernadette Dierckx de Casterlé[2], Theo van Achterberg[2] and Koen Milisen[2]

Abstract

Background: Given the great symptom burden associated with chemotherapy on the one hand and generally poor self-management of symptoms by cancer patients on the other hand, our aim was to develop a nursing intervention to reduce symptom burden in adult cancer patients treated with chemotherapy and to support them in dealing with their various symptoms at home.

Methods: Development of the intervention was guided by the Intervention Mapping Approach and included following steps: needs assessment, formulation of proximal programme objectives, selection of methods and strategies, production of programme components, and planning for implementation and evaluation of the intervention. A panel of multidisciplinary healthcare professionals ($n = 12$) and a panel of patients and family caregivers ($n = 7$) were actively involved developing the intervention at each stage.

Results: For the intervention, four patient performance objectives relating to self-management were advanced. Self-efficacy and outcome expectations were selected as key determinants of dealing with chemotherapy-related symptoms. As methods for supporting patients, motivational interviewing and tailoring were found to fit best with the change objectives and determinants. Existing patient information materials were re-designed after panel input to reinforce the new intervention approach.

Conclusion: The intervention mapping approach, including active involvement of the intervention providers and receivers, informed the design of this nursing intervention with two or more contacts. Further evaluation is needed to gain insight into the potential effects, feasibility and mechanisms of this complex intervention.

Keywords: Chemotherapy, Symptoms, Nursing, Intervention, Complex intervention, Intervention-mapping approach, Self-management

Background

Chemotherapy is associated with multiple, often distressing, side effects. The negative impact of these on quality of life is widely recognized [1, 2]. Typically, these side effects are experienced at home, in the absence of professional assistance [3]. Consequently, chemotherapy that includes ambulatory treatments forces patients to actively self-manage their symptoms. However, few patients seem to be able to do so adequately [4]. Performance of symptom self-management strategies is generally poor [5–8]. Also, patients sub-optimally report their symptoms to healthcare professionals [9, 10]. Patients report lacking knowledge and experience [11], and report high levels of unmet needs in relation to self-care support [12]. Evidence suggests that greater symptom burden is associated with poorer self-care [8, 13].

* Correspondence: annemarie.coolbrandt@uzleuven.be
[1]Department of Oncology Nursing, University Hospitals Leuven, Herestraat 49, 3000 Leuven, Belgium
[2]Department of Public Health and Primary Care, Academic Centre for Nursing and Midwifery, KU Leuven, Leuven, Belgium
Full list of author information is available at the end of the article

The burden of chemotherapy-related symptoms and (often unmet) patient needs related to their self-management has catalysed the development of several new nursing interventions to address these issues [12, 14–16]. Many have focused on managing a single symptom, such as oral mucositis or fatigue, but it is likely that meaningful improvement in quality of life can only be achieved by interventions that focus on multiple symptoms that cancer patients face [17]. Some interventions targeting multiple symptoms have indeed produced a positive impact on symptom burden [18, 19]. However, a recent systematic review revealed that these interventions have produced inconsistent results [20]. Combined with variable degrees of efficacy, many of these intervention studies face reproducibility limitations. Some studies contain little description of the studied interventions, their core components and intervention development [17, 21, 22]. The usual care that was employed for comparison is generally poorly described [20]. Intermediate outcomes, contributing to a better understanding of the effect mechanism of the intervention, are evaluated and reported in only one study [23]. Also, qualitative data on the intervention is presented in only one case [24–27]. Consequently, many questions remain unanswered: How were outcomes reached? Which intervention components produced measurable effects and by what mechanism(s)? Also, what factors promoted or hindered their results? [28, 29].

While the systematic development of complex interventions using the best available evidence and appropriate theory is becoming increasingly encouraged and acknowledged [30–32], such approaches are rarely applied or reported in interventions targeting chemotherapy-related symptom burden [20]. The Intervention-Mapping Approach (IM) is a conceptual framework for systematically developing healthcare programmes [33–35]. It has been used to further advance theory and evidence-based health promotion programmes in many health domains, such as smoking cessation, preventing HIV transmission, sun protection, asthma management, etc. [34] The framework assists programme developers in making and documenting decisions for influencing change in behaviour and improving health, while making use of available evidence and theory and collaborating with future intervention providers and receivers. Using IM in intervention development is presumed to improve the potential effects of healthcare programmes [34].

This paper describes a step-by-step overview of the development of a nursing intervention aimed at reducing chemotherapy-related symptom burden. We call it CHEMO-SUPPORT. In the development process, we used the best available evidence and theory and employed the IM Approach. The second aim of this paper is to fully describe the actual intervention, as it will be implemented and studied. We used the Template for Intervention Description and Replication (TIDieR) checklist to describe our intervention. The TIDieR is presented as an extension of the CONSORT 2010 statement and the SPIRIT 2013 statement with the aim of improving the completeness of reporting and ultimately the replicability of interventions [36].

Methods

We followed the Intervention Mapping Approach of Bartholomew et al. [34] to guide development of the intervention. Table 1 summarizes the 6 steps and their specific objectives. It also provides an overview of the methods used and the results obtained at each step.

Two groups of individuals were involved throughout development of the intervention. A panel of multidisciplinary health professionals from several different centres comprised one group. This panel included 3 oncologists and 4 nurses from 3 different hospitals (1 academic and 2 non-academic); 1 general practitioner; 3 home care nurses from different primary care organisations; and 1 psychologist, with expertise in self-management of chronic disease.

The other panel of individuals included patients and caregivers. Five of them were patients who had been treated with chemotherapy, and 2 were family caregivers (spouses in both cases). They represented patients/caregivers from 3 different hospitals (1 academic and 2 non-academic). Patients were recruited with the help of nurses and doctors from the hospitals, or through self-help groups. One participating caregiver also came from a self-help group, other caregivers from a group session for partners of people with cancer.

The cancer diagnoses associated with the seven participants comprising the patient and caregiver group spanned a mix of diagnoses (haematological cancer, digestive tract cancer, breast cancer, brain tumour, and gynaecological cancer). Three patients were women and 2 were men, 1 caregiver was a man, and the remaining one was a woman. The mean age in this panel was 54 years. Patients' age ranged from 18 to 69 years. This mix was important to achieve a diversity of perspectives [34] and to produce an intervention that is employable and generalizable to patients with cancer regardless of their demographical or clinical variables.

All panel members participated in five meetings for which they were compensated. Anonymity, confidentiality, non-binding and well-informed participation were closely guarded as ethical principles of the panel members' involvement.

Every panel meeting had its specific objectives according to the stage in the IM process, e.g. validating the needs assessment and getting consensus about the program objective. Relevant evidence was collected in preparation for

Table 1 Overview of the step-by-step process of Intervention Mapping with methods used and results produced at each step

	Methods	Results
Step 1 Needs assessment: Objectives: establishing participatory planning groups, conducting the needs assessment, specifying desired programme goals	♦ Literature review of symptom self-management in patients with cancer ♦ Qualitative study on dealing with chemotherapy-related symptoms at home [3] ♦ One discussion session with professional panel and one with patients and caregivers panel	♦ Needs structured in PRECEDE-model (Fig. 1) ♦ Reported and observed behavioral problems: patients' poor/inadequate self-management, poor communication and reporting of chemotherapy-related symptoms ♦ Desired program goals: improving self-management and communication/reporting of chemotherapy-related symptoms
Step 2 Matrices of proximal programme objectives Objectives: stating behavioral and environmental outcomes of the intervention, defining clear performance objectives (POs), creating matrices of change objectives by crossing POs with determinants	♦ Outline of matrices of proximal programme objectives by project leader ♦ Review of theory and outline of potential determinants ♦ One discussion session with professional panel and two discussion sessions with patients and caregivers panel	♦ Consensus on four patient performance objectives (POs): *Preventing, monitoring, reporting and managing chemotherapy-related symptoms at home* ♦ Consensus reached on vital determinants: *Self-efficacy and outcome expectations of patients* ♦ Matrices of proximal programme objectives for future program receivers (patients) (example in Table 2) ♦ Definition of nursing objectives to support patients' performance objectives
Step 3 Selecting theoretical methods and practical strategies Objectives: generating programme ideas, identifying and selecting theoretical methods, selecting or designing practical applications	♦ Study of methods and theories [16, 18, 19] ♦ Evaluation of the ideas on methods and strategies yielded in the earlier panel meetings ♦ Systematic review of complex nursing interventions aimed at reducing chemotherapy-related symptom burden [10] ♦ One discussion session with professional panel and one with patients and caregivers panel ♦ One discussion session with nursing panel	♦ Consensus on principal methods of the intervention: tailoring and motivational interviewing ♦ General outline of the intervention (Fig. 2): Brief motivational intervention, advanced on the basis of estimated individual need ♦ Formulation of additional project objective for the purpose of the intervention: revision of written patient information and advices
Step 4 Producing programme components Objectives: determining preferences for programme design, creating programme scope and sequence, preparing design, reviewing, developing and pretesting programme materials	Intervention manual development: ♦ Formulating nursing approach at every patient contact in the program ♦ Discussion with project team, nursing panel, 2 onco-psychologists New written patient information development: ♦ Web survey eliciting patient feedback (*n* = 102, characteristics see Table 3) on information and advice for 19 chemotherapy-related symptoms (question format see Table 1) ♦ First revision and second patient feedback round (*n* = 21) ♦ Feedback and discussion with healthcare professionals (*n* = 17)	Final intervention manual produced New booklet produced "Dealing with side effects from chemotherapy at home", outlining the 4 recommended self-management behaviours and presenting information and (professional and fellow patient) advice on 19 side effects
Step 5 Planning for adoption, implementation and sustainability Objectives: identifying potential adopters, stating outcomes for programme use, specifying determinants and creating matrices (defining determinants and change objectives) for programme adoption, implementation and sustainability	Planning for the implementation of the intervention in an intervention study: ♦ Planning selection strategy and criteria for the intervention providers in the study ♦ Translating nurse POs into training programme for the intervention nurses ♦ Outlining communication strategy for clinical nurses and other healthcare professionals	♦ Selection of 6 intervention nurses ♦ 2-day long training programme for the intervention nurses ♦ Meetings (*n* = 9) with clinical nurses (*n* = 114) ♦ Meetings with doctors and paramedics
Step 6 Planning for intervention evaluation Objectives: describing programme outcomes, writing evaluation questions, developing indicators and measues, specifying evaluation design	Together with the project team: ♦ Translating health and quality of life targets, POs and determinants into study outcomes ♦ Choosing appropriate methods and study design	♦ Protocol of a mixed-methods study ♦ Qualitative approach to explore patient experience with the intervention: satisfaction with intervention, open questions and semi-structured interviews ♦ Quantitative approach to study intervention effect: experimental before-after study with sequential design *Primary outcome: Symptom distress* *Secondary outcomes:* *Symptom severity* *Self-efficacy* *Outcome expectations* *Self-care*

panel meetings and additional literature was searched after collaborative consultation at the meetings, when necessary. The project leader (A.C.) applied different techniques to facilitate interpersonal communication, idea generation and consensus: e.g. responding to a paper or presentation of evidence, brainstorming, nominal group technique.

Step 1: Needs assessment

The needs assessment component comprised a qualitative study of how adult chemotherapy patients deal with side effects at home [13], a literature review of how cancer patients manage their symptoms, the development of a needs assessment model and an independent discussion with each panel. Panel discussions were conducted in order to discuss the model and to gain insights into the relative importance of behavioural and environmental factors and their determinants.

Step 2: Matrices of proximal programme objectives

Two independent meetings with the panels formulated the most relevant behavioural outcomes and necessary performance objectives (POs). The latter described what intervention receivers and performers "need to do in order to accomplish improvement in health outcomes" ([16], p. 239). These meetings also yielded a preliminary set of determinants. An additional meeting was held with the intended programme recipients (i.e., the patient and caregiver panel) to further discuss and prioritise the determinants for each PO.

Step 3: Selecting methods and strategies

In selecting theoretical methods and practical strategies appropriate for the intervention, the panels took into account the evidence on methods and theories linked with the change objectives and determinants recommended by the panel members [34, 37, 38], methods and strategies used by other nursing interventions aimed at reducing chemotherapy-related symptom burden [20] and methods and strategies suggested by the panel members during previous patient/caregiver and professional meetings. A provisional draft of the intervention was discussed with both panels to further refine the new nursing intervention. An auxiliary nursing panel was organised to query oncology nurses (the future intervention providers) for their opinions on the perceived relevance and feasibility of the intervention.

Step 4: Producing programme components

The first component that needed to be developed was a detailed scenario or plan of action for executing the nursing intervention. We call this the intervention manual. The intervention manual described every relevant patient contact, from start of the intervention to programme termination.

A second objective prioritized at this stage was to re-orient the currently used patient information tools to fit the new intervention. Some members of the patient/caregiver panel proposed that this was necessary so that patient information could better support and empower the determinants of the programme receivers' POs, i.e., self-efficacy and outcome expectations. An online survey was set-up to obtain patient testimonies and feedback. Its aim was to produce improved phrasing and to complete the symptom description and self-care advice in order to better reflect the patients' perspective and experience. Additionally, quotes that well supported, illustrated, or supplemented the professional advice were extracted. The survey overview is illustrated in Table 2. Patients' online feedback was anonymous and confidential, and was not reported in any other form than its contribution to the re-writing of our patient brochure, to which they consented as part of the online participation. The web survey was advertised by hanging posters and flyers in the different oncology wards, by notifying self-help groups, and by posting content on the hospital's website and the website of 'Kom op tegen Kanker' (i.e., a cancer care and research charity in the local context). Patients, as well as healthcare professionals, provided additional oral or written feedback, as the patient information was re-written in subsequent versions.

Step 5: Planning for adoption, implementation and sustainability

Our primary intention for the intervention at this point was to conduct a pilot study instead of have the intervention immediately adopted in daily care.

To ensure treatment fidelity during the pilot study, we chose not to involve all clinical oncology nurses as possible programme providers but instead to have a limited group of trained intervention nurses conduct the intervention. Therefore, objectives for Step 5 were selecting the intervention nurses, planning their training programme, and coordinating and integrating the intervention with the usual care that would be delivered by the clinical nurses and doctors.

Next, a consultation and information plan was set up to present the project and to address possible concerns of clinical nurses, doctors, and paramedics who would be involved in the care for patients participating in the study.

Step 6: Planning for evaluation

The final step of the intervention development comprised the preparation of the evaluation of the intervention. A protocol for a mixed-method pilot study was written in order to capture the intervention effects and, at the same time, grasp the recipients' responses to the intervention and to explore explanations of the quantitative findings [39].

Table 2 Overview of survey used to reorient currently available patient information with proposed information for new intervention

	Topic	Question	Answer
Question 1	Symptom experience	What would you want to delete, adjust, add to the current patient information on (this side effect)? What would you want to tell fellow patients about (this side effect)?	Freely able to answer
Question 2*a	Self-care advice	To what extent is this advice helpful for (this side effect)?	4-point Likert scale
Question 2*b	Self-care advice	Why or why not is/was this advice helpful to you? What would you want to share with fellow patients about this advice?	Freely able to answer
Question 3	Self-care advice	Which other advices or strategies have helped you to deal with (this side-effect)? Which other advices would you share with fellow patients?	Freely able to answer
Question 4	Social support	How can your social network play a part in dealing with (this side effect)?	Freely able to answer
Question 5	Other	Which other suggestions do you have for patient information on (this side effect)?	Freely able to answer

*Repeated as many times as there was advice on the particular side effect

Results

In the results section, we present the outcomes and decisions made at each step of the intervention development process. Evidence and panel opinions supporting these decisions are available in Additional file 1.

Step 1: Needs assessment

The results of the needs assessment are presented in Fig. 1. The evidence underpinning the needs assessment is available in Additional file 2. The complete results of our qualitative study into how adult patients receiving chemotherapy deal with treatment-related symptoms at home is reported elsewhere [13]. Both panels agreed that

coaching patients to self-manage symptoms adequately was the appropriate goal for the intervention.

Step 2: Matrices of proximal programme objectives

Based on the needs assessment, the panels agreed on four patient performance objectives (POs) for the self-management intervention:

1. PO1: The patient performs preventive self-care behaviour, addressing the possible side effects related to his/her chemotherapy treatment.
2. PO2: The patient monitors the severity and duration of his/her symptoms.

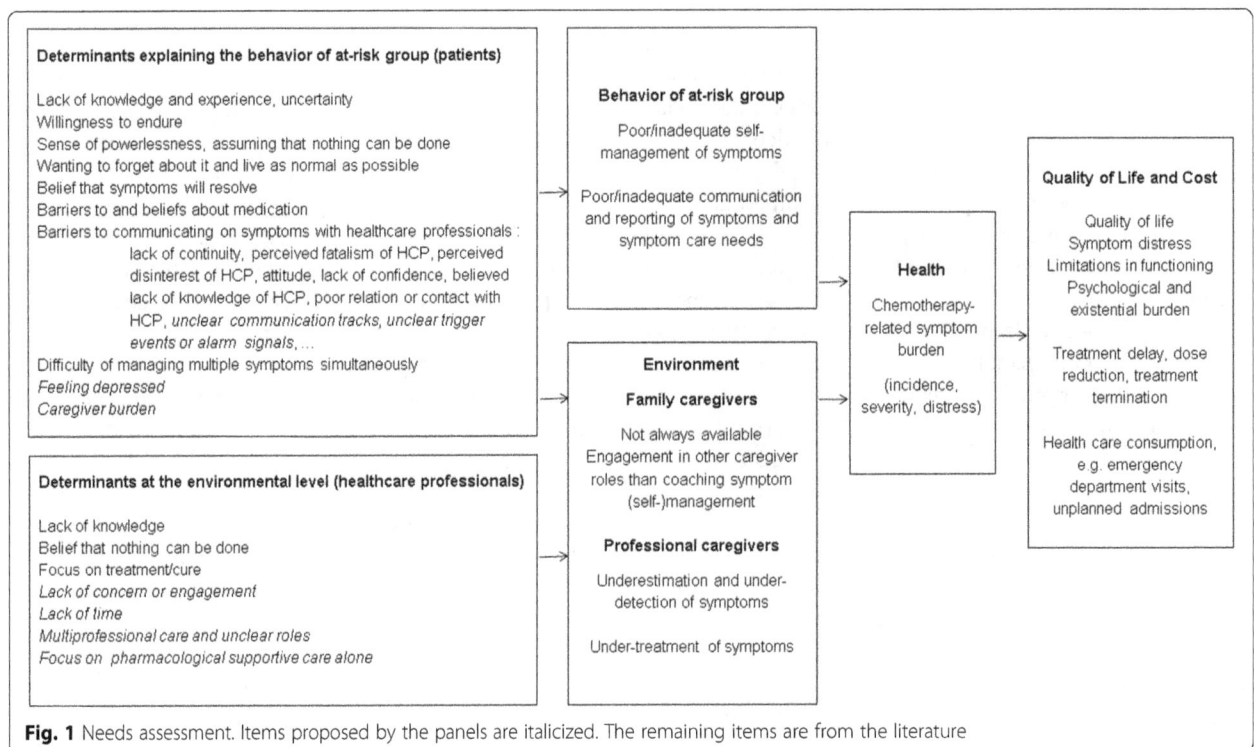

Fig. 1 Needs assessment. Items proposed by the panels are italicized. The remaining items are from the literature

3. PO3: The patient adequately reports in a timely manner and discusses his/her symptoms with healthcare professionals.
4. PO4: The patient performs self-care behaviour to manage symptoms.

Professionals and patients selected *self-efficacy, outcome expectations, knowledge* and *social support* as vital determinants for these POs. Interestingly, patients and caregivers suggested that tackling outcome expectations, self-efficacy, and social support would be especially able to increase the potential effectiveness of the intervention, as they believed the need for knowledge was already largely addressed in standard care. The professional panel shared this opinion on priorities.

Performance objectives and determinants were crossed in matrices to arrive at clear proximal programme objectives. An example for PO1 is provided in Table 3. To target the environmental factors and mainly the nursing role, the patient POs were translated into nursing POs.

Step 3: Selecting methods and strategies
Both panels agreed that tailoring was an important strategy to increase the intervention's potential efficacy. Naturally, this involved tailoring the intervention content to the particular treatment being started (and the possible side-effects associated with that treatment). It also meant taking into consideration the patients' personal symptom experience and symptom-management style [13]. More importantly, however, both panels agreed on the need to tailor the intervention dose. A standard intervention dose of two sessions was considered sufficient and feasible for patients who, with the help of the intervention, expressed sufficient knowledge, motivation and social support to perform the behavioural objectives. More sessions seemed warranted for those patients who

were more at risk (e.g., living alone or poor social support, poor understanding of information). Figure 2 presents an overview of the intervention.

Based on the panel meetings and the relevant determinants, motivational interviewing was believed to be the crucial foundation for the coaching intervention. Motivational interviewing (MI) finds its origin in the Transtheoretical Model, which presumes people are in different stages of readiness to make behavioural changes. It is a goal-directed counselling style for eliciting behavioural change, holding to the principle that motivation is elicited from the patient and not imposed from outside [40–42]. As a counselling style, MI itself encompasses other methods such as reinforcement and self-reevaluation that is applied in the intervention to elicit behavioural change.

Step 4: Producing programme components
For the intervention providers, a plan of action was developed that detailed the behaviour of nurses at every patient contact. Both motivational interviewing and tailoring were explicitly included and were outlined in the manual. Communication and motivational techniques were illustrated with examples of phrasings. The complete intervention manual is available upon request to interested readers.

One hundred-two patients between 27 and 78 years old, most of them (69%) women, participated in the online survey. Twenty-one survey respondents provided further feedback on rewritten information by email or during a personal meeting. Also, 17 healthcare professionals (psychologists, sexologists, dieticians, a physiotherapist, a revalidation therapist, and nurses and doctors) provided feedback on side effects related to their clinical expertise. The new booklet is called, "Dealing with side effects from chemotherapy at home".

Table 3 Examples from the matrix of proximal programme objectives for patients and nurses for PO1

PO1: The patient performs preventive self-care behaviour related to possible side effects of chemotherapy treatment.			
Determinant	Knowledge	Outcome expectations	Self-efficacy	Social support
Patient	Patient describes necessary self-care measures to prevent possible side effects from treatment. For example, finding balance between rest and exercise/activity to prevent fatigue	Patient expresses conviction that self-care measures will help to prevent side effects or to prevent side effect from getting severe.	Patient expresses confidence in their capability of performing the relevant self-care measures.	Patient involves his family caregivers to remind and support him in performing preventive self-care behaviour.
Nurse	Nurse instructs patient on relevant self-care measures to prevent possible side effects form his treatment.	Nurse explains effects and preventive mechanisms of preventive self-care behaviour. For example, importance of physical activity in maintaining physical condition and preventing fatigue from worsening	Nurse queries patients on perceived barriers for performing the self-care measures.	Nurse explores possible social support for reminding and supporting the patient with preventive self-care at home.

When?	Where?	What?	Why?	How?
Start of treatment		First nurse counselling session	- Preparing patients to deal (adequately) with side effects at home → elicit 4 behavioural strategies: - Preventing side effects - Monitoring side effects - Reporting and discussing side effects - Managing / relieving side effects - Getting to know the patient and estimating his/her symptom self-management profile	In-person Family caregiver present (if possible) New patient brochure Symptom diary Estimated duration: 30-60'
First days at home		Second nurse counselling contact	- Evaluating symptom burden and - Reviewing self-management strategies - Providing or planning professional symptom support - Reviewing and reinforcing adequate self-management strategies - Estimating his/her symptom self-management profile	Telephone Symptom diary (optionally) Estimated duration: 10-20'
At every later hospital appointment or patient contact		Evaluation of the need for further intervention	- Reviewing file reports on the patient self-management profile and actual symptom burden and/or consultation with clinical nurse - Planning and delivering of additional counselling sessions in hospital or at home	Assessment of patient file and/or consultation with clinical nurse Planning and delivery of further coaching intervention(s) if necessary
Throughout treatment		Patient brochure "Dealing with side effects from chemotherapy at home"	- Offering information and self-care advice on possible side effects from professionals and fellow patients - Describing professional support or resources - Formulating alarm signals for contacting health care professionals	
Throughout treatment		Acces to an on-call or online nursing service	- Offering continuous profesional support via an approachable nursing service to discuss symptom burden	Telephone, working days between 10 and 14 Email

Fig. 2 Intervention overview

Step 5: Planning for adoption, implementation and sustainability

We used the following criteria to recruit and select the intervention nurses that would deliver the intervention during the pilot study:

1. Having a bachelor's degree in nursing.
2. Having clinical oncology nursing experience. Having an extra degree in oncology nursing was considered valuable but not necessary.

Given the anticipated caseload of 2.3 new patients, or between 1 and 7 new patients per day, we sought 1.2 full-time equivalent positions so that one intervention nurse would always be available on every working day. We explicitly divided the mandate over six different nurses, since the allocation of one fixed nurse per patient was not the aim of the intervention and would potentially make the intervention more about the trust relationship between patient and nurse than about the intended active ingredients of the intervention. The six selected intervention nurses were all women, were between 37 and 50 years old, and had between 6 and 19 years of oncology nursing experience.

Nursing POs guided the content chosen for the training of the intervention nurses. A 2-day long training programme was organised to share knowledge and to provide training on the skills needed to meet the nursing POs. It included a thorough presentation of the intervention and the intervention manual, motivational interviewing, symptom management during chemotherapy, with a focus on self-care and (multidisciplinary) professional care, presentation of the new patient brochure, registration of patient care activities, and intervention fidelity.

Meetings were held to present the project to the ward nurses. The main purpose of these meetings was two-fold: first, to ensure that clinical nurses would have sufficient knowledge about the intervention; and second, to engender in them a positive attitude towards the intervention and its integration into standard care. Next, the project aims and its content were discussed at meetings of the board of directors of all medical wards involved.

Step 6: Planning for evaluation

The project team selected symptom distress as a primary outcome. We believed that it was sensitive to the components, and it matched the goals of the nursing intervention. Symptom severity and number of symptoms were selected as secondary health and quality-of-life outcomes. Next, the performance objectives and determinants suggested three intermediate outcomes for the study:

1. self-efficacy,
2. outcome expectations,

3. self-care or the adequacy of patient's self-management behaviour.

These were seen as especially important for gaining insight into the intervention's mechanism, or lack of an effect. Given the novelty of the intervention and given the recommendation of mixed methods research for the evaluation of complex interventions [43], the project team considered a qualitative evaluation of the patients' experience with the nursing intervention equally important as the quantitative pilot study to explore its potential effects. Finally, it was decided to monitor intervention fidelity by having the intervention nurses report on the completeness of and adherence to the intervention components at each patient contact. After every patient encounter, intervention nurses self-rated the contact on the extent they believed they had addressed the core elements of the intervention. Protocol of this mixed-methods evaluation and its results are reported elsewhere [44].

Discussion

We systematically developed a nursing intervention—called CHEMO-SUPPORT—aimed at reducing chemotherapy-related symptom burden that patients experience at home. This process resulted in an intervention including in-person coaching, telephone counselling, written patient information, and online/on-call access to nursing support. The intervention uses a tailored motivational approach instead of the educational approach for transferring standardized information and advice to the patient, unlike what is currently used in standard care.

Overall, earlier studies on nursing interventions targeting chemotherapy-related symptom burden have been unclear about intervention development methods [20]. Developing complex interventions using evidence and theory has been increasingly encouraged [30, 31], and by doing so, it is assumed that intervention developers improve the intervention's potential effects. Consistent with this hypothesis, the clinical utility of using a systematic development approach for our intervention should be judged on the results of the intervention, which will be reported later. However, reporting of the intervention development process alone has merit in clarifying the chosen objectives, methods, and strategies of the intervention. This will help readers and other programme developers not only to adequately interpret intervention results but also to replicate or build on research findings and further adapt the intervention content and delivery modalities [36].

Designing interventions using IM is a time-consuming process. Yet, we believe the mandate of having a clear focus, objectives, methods, and strategies, alongside stepwise planning of the intervention and inclusion of evidence and professional and patient expertise, is crucial in shaping the intervention toward its final content. For example, the complete make-over of our standard patient information was not anticipated at the start of this study but resulted from the patient panel's clear statement that reorientation of information material was necessary for better supporting patients in meeting their POs. As we moved through the six steps of IM, our decisions shaping the intervention were evidence- and theory-informed to the greatest extent possible. Meetings with the panels at each step of IM helped to complement the evidence with clinical and patient experience and to make clinically relevant and patient-centred decisions, all of which helped us to move forward in the development process.

It is important to note the limitations of our process of systematic intervention development and, as a consequence, of our intervention. First, social support as a determinant for adequate symptom self-management has received relatively little attention in the development of the intervention. While social support is clearly addressed in the counselling manual, the intervention could probably still benefit from better matching methods to change and mobilise social support [34, 40]. From what is known about the role of social support during treatment with chemotherapy, family caregivers' role, as well as patients' expectations, is very variable [45–48]. Caregivers sometimes act as co-managers of side effects, or sometimes as coaches. However, caregivers experience the patient's disease, treatment, and symptoms differently than the patient. So some patients feel that this difference prevents spouses and family members from developing a partnership to deal with all the burden. Also, some patients don't feel the need to have someone support their symptom management, while others simply have no one available. More in-depth research is needed to come to a better understanding of how to engage family caregivers in the symptom management process.

Secondly, our intervention development was mainly directed at tackling patient-related determinants of poor symptom self-management. Concerning the environmental-level determinants (see Fig. 1), lack of time and concern were addressed by hiring highly motivated auxiliary nurses who believed in the value of the intervention. Thus, the decision to plan an intervention study allowed us to delay dealing with some of the environmental determinants, specifically time and attitude. These issues will surface again as we discuss the adoption and sustainability of the intervention in daily practice. However, both quantitative and qualitative evidence on CHEMO-SUPPORT will facilitate the planning of further actions towards future programme providers and policymakers.

Finally, we did not pilot test the intervention or intervention components with intended programme receivers, as is recommended as part of step 4 of IM [34]. Given the active involvement of patients as well as professionals on the one hand, and our familiarity with the implementation of interventions in this clinical domain and in this clinical setting on the other hand, we were confident that the intervention could be delivered as planned. Also, we planned thorough qualitative evaluation of the intervention alongside our quasi-experimental study. However, pilot testing remains useful for getting a sense of the possible effects, determining how the intervention is perceived by naïve patients (i.e., those who have not participated in the intervention development process), and in determining problems with implementation [34]. Ultimately, our mixed-methods evaluation will guide the revision of the intervention before further implementation.

Conclusion

We used the IM Approach to design a self-management intervention aimed at reducing chemotherapy-related symptom burden at home. Given the impact of chemotherapy-related symptoms and the outpatient organisation of cancer treatment, self-management is a logical goal for nursing care. However, generally poor self-management suggests that well-designed nursing interventions are imperative. The combination of evidence, theory, and clinical and patient experience in the step-by-step IM Approach resulted in a clearly described self-management support intervention to be tailored according to the patient's self-management profile. The complete description of the intervention in this developmental study provides a foundation on which others can build on for future research and practice.

Additional files

Additional file 1: File presents evidence and opinions supporting decision-making throughouth the Intervention Mapping stages, from needs assessment to final CHEMO-SUPPORT intervention. (DOCX 98 kb)

Additional file 2: File shows evidence underpinning the needs assessment. (DOCX 66 kb)

Abbreviations
IM: Intervention mapping; MI: Motivational interviewing; PO: Performance objective

Acknowledgements
Funding for this study was provided by Kom op tegen Kanker, the campaign of the Flemish League against Cancer/Vlaamse Liga tegen Kanker VZW. We would like to thank all panel participants for their contribution in the development of CHEMO-SUPPORT.

Funding
Funding for this study was provided by Kom op tegen Kanker, the campaign of the Flemish League against Cancer/Vlaamse Liga tegen Kanker VZW.

Authors' contributions
AC, HW and KM carried out conception and design of the intervention development project, carried out the process of the Intervention Mapping Approach, and drafted the manuscript. TvA offered methodological guidance with regard to the Intervention Mapping Approach and carried out critical revision of the manuscript. BA and BDdC provided input on the design of the intervention development project and carried out critical revision of the manuscript. All authors read and approved the final manuscript.

Ethics approval and consent to participate
Patients, family caregivers and professionals were actively involved during this practice improvement process. Patient engagement, i.e. involvement of patients, their families or representatives, in working actively with health professionals to improve health and healthcare services is becoming more and more accepted at various levels across the healthcare system (direct care, organizational design / governance, and policy making). Since this participation did not imply the collection and reporting of study data, we did not apply the intervention development process to the Institutional Review Board. However, the principles of confidentiality, anonymity, non-binding and well-informed participation were carefully accomplished. Informed consent did apply for the qualitative study quasi-experimental that were part of steps 1 and 6. These studies took part with the approval Institutional Review Board and are reported elsewhere.

Competing interests
The authors declare that they have no competing interests.

Author details
Department of Oncology Nursing, University Hospitals Leuven, Herestraat 49, 3000 Leuven, Belgium. ²Department of Public Health and Primary Care, Academic Centre for Nursing and Midwifery, KU Leuven, Leuven, Belgium. ³Department of General Medical Oncology, University Hospitals Leuven, Leuven, Belgium. ⁴Department of Public Health and Primary Care, Academic Centre for General Practice, KU Leuven, Leuven, Belgium.

References
1. Deshields TL, Potter P, Olsen S, Liu J. The persistence of symptom burden: symptom experience and quality of life of cancer patients across one year. Support Care Cancer. 2014;22(4):1089–96.
2. Lowery AE, Krebs P, Coups EJ, et al. Impact of symptom burden in post-surgical non-small cell lung cancer survivors. Support Care Cancer. 2014; 22(1):173–80.
3. Ruland CM, Andersen T, Jeneson A, et al. Effects of an internet support system to assist cancer patients in reducing symptom distress: a randomized controlled trial. Cancer Nurs. 2013;36(1):6–17.
4. Hoffman AJ. Enhancing self-efficacy for optimized patient outcomes through the theory of symptom self-management. Cancer Nurs. 2013;36(1):E16–26.
5. Coolbrandt A, Van den Heede K, Clemens K, et al. The Leuven questionnaire for patient self-care during chemotherapy (L-PaSC): instrument development and psychometric evaluation. Eur J Oncol Nurs. 2013;17(3):275–83.
6. Dodd MJ. Assessing patient self-care for side effects of cancer chemotherapy–part I. Cancer Nurs. 1982;5(6):447–51.
7. Dodd MJ. Self-care for side effects in cancer chemotherapy: an assessment of nursing interventions–Part II. Cancer Nurs. 1983;6(1):63–7.
8. Given CW, Given BA, Sikorskii A, et al. Deconstruction of nurse-delivered patient self-management interventions for symptom management: factors related to delivery enactment and response. Ann Behav Med. 2010;40(1):99–113.
9. Coolbrandt A, Van den Heede K, Vanhove E, De Bom A, Milisen K, Wildiers H. Immediate versus delayed self-reporting of symptoms and side effects during chemotherapy: does timing matter? Eur J Oncol Nurs. 2011;15(2): 130–6.

10. Homsi J, Walsh D, Rivera N, et al. Symptom evaluation in palliative medicine: patient report vs systematic assessment. Support Care Cancer. 2006;14(5):444–53.

11. Pedersen B, Koktved DP, Nielsen LL. Living with side effects from cancer treatment–a challenge to target information. Scand J Caring Sci. 2012;27(3): 715–23.

12. Aranda S, Jefford M, Yates P, et al. Impact of a novel nurse-led prechemotherapy education intervention (ChemoEd) on patient distress, symptom burden, and treatment-related information and support needs: results from a randomised, controlled trial. Ann Oncol. 2012;23(1):222–31.

13. Coolbrandt A, Dierckx de Casterle B, Wildiers H, et al. Dealing with chemotherapy-related symptoms at home: a qualitative study in adult patients with cancer. Eur J Cancer Care (Engl). 2016;25(1):79–92.

14. Dodd MJ, Cho MH, Miaskowski C, et al. A randomized controlled trial of home-based exercise for cancer-related fatigue in women during and after chemotherapy with or without radiation therapy. Cancer Nurs. 2010;33(4): 245–57.

15. Given B, Given CW, McCorkle R, et al. Pain and fatigue management: results of a nursing randomized clinical trial. Oncol Nurs Forum. 2002;29(6):949–56.

16. Williams PD, Williams K, Lafaver-Roling S, Johnson R, Williams AR. An intervention to manage patient-reported symptoms during cancer treatment. Clin J Oncol Nurs. 2011;15(3):253–8.

17. Doorenbos A, Given B, Given C, Verbitsky N, Cimprich B, McCorkle R. Reducing symptom limitations: a cognitive behavioral intervention randomized trial. Psychooncology. 2005;14(7):574–84.

18. Molassiotis A, Brearley S, Saunders M, et al. Effectiveness of a home care nursing program in the symptom management of patients with colorectal and breast cancer receiving oral chemotherapy: a randomized, controlled trial. J Clin Oncol. 2009;27(36):6191–8.

19. Sherwood P, Given BA, Given CW, et al. A cognitive behavioral intervention for symptom management in patients with advanced cancer. Oncol Nurs Forum. 2005;32(6):1190–8.

20. Coolbrandt A, Wildiers H, Aertgeerts B, et al. Characteristics and effectiveness of complex nursing interventions aimed at reducing symptom burden in adult patients treated with chemotherapy: a systematic review of randomized controlled trials. Int J Nurs Stud. 2014;51(3):495–510.

21. Given C, Given B, Rahbar M, et al. Effect of a cognitive behavioral intervention on reducing symptom severity during chemotherapy. J Clin Oncol. 2004;22(3): 507–16.

22. Lev EL, Daley KM, Conner NE, Reith M, Fernandez C, Owen SV. An intervention to increase quality of life and self-care self-efficacy and decrease symptoms in breast cancer patients. Sch Inq Nurs Pract. 2001;15(3):277–94.

23. Jahn P, Renz P, Stukenkemper J, et al. Reduction of chemotherapy-induced anorexia, nausea, and emesis through a structured nursing intervention: a cluster-randomized multicenter trial. Support Care Cancer. 2009;17(12):1543–52.

24. Kearney N, Kidd L, Miller M, et al. Utilising handheld computers to monitor and support patients receiving chemotherapy: results of a UK-based feasibility study. Support Care Cancer. 2006;14(7):742–52.

25. Kearney N, McCann L, Norrie J, et al. Evaluation of a mobile phone-based, advanced symptom management system (ASyMS) in the management of chemotherapy-related toxicity. Support Care Cancer. 2009;17(4):437–44.

26. Maguire R, McCann L, Miller M, Kearney N. Nurse's perceptions and experiences of using of a mobile-phone-based advanced symptom management system (ASyMS) to monitor and manage chemotherapy-related toxicity. Eur J Oncol Nurs. 2008;12(4):380–6.

27. McCann L, Maguire R, Miller M, Kearney N. Patients' perceptions and experiences of using a mobile phone-based advanced symptom management system (ASyMS) to monitor and manage chemotherapy related toxicity. Eur J Cancer Care (Engl). 2009;18(2):156–64.

28. May C, Finch T, Mair F, et al. Understanding the implementation of complex interventions in health care: the normalization process model. BMC Health Serv Res. 2007;7:148.

29. Mohler R, Bartoszek G, Kopke S, Meyer G. Proposed criteria for reporting the development and evaluation of complex interventions in healthcare (CReDECI): guideline development. Int J Nurs Stud. 2011;49(1):40–6.

30. Craig P, Dieppe P, Macintyre S, Michie S, Nazareth I, Petticrew M. Developing and evaluating complex interventions: the new Medical Research Council guidance. BMJ. 2008;337:a1655.

31. Craig P, Dieppe P, Macintyre S, Michie S, Nazareth I, Petticrew M. Developing and evaluating complex interventions: the new Medical Research Council guidance. Int J Nurs Stud. 2012;50(5):587–92.

32. van Meijel B, Gamel C, van Swieten-Duijfjes B, Grypdonck MH. The development of evidence-based nursing interventions: methodological considerations. J Adv Nurs. 2004;48(1):84–92.

33. Bartholomew LK, Parcel GS, Kok G. Intervention mapping: a process for developing theory- and evidence-based health education programs. Health Educ Behav. 1998;25(5):545–63.

34. Bartholomew LP, Kok GS, Gottlieb G, NH Fernandez ME. Planning Health Promotion Programs: An Intervention Mapping Approach. 3rd ed. New Jersey: Wiley; 2011.

35. Kok G, Gottlieb NH, Peters GJ, et al. A taxonomy of behaviour change methods: an intervention mapping approach. Health Psychol Rev Sep. 2015;10(3):297–312.

36. Hoffmann TC, Glasziou PP, Boutron I, et al. Better reporting of interventions: template for intervention description and replication (TIDieR) checklist and guide. BMJ. 2014;348:g1687.

37. Glanz KR, BK, Viswanath K. Health behavior and health education: theory, research, and practice, 4th edition. New Jersey: Wiley; 2008.

38. Nutbeam DH,E, Wise M. Theory in a Nutshell: A Practical Guide to Health Promotion Theories. Australia: McGraw-Hill; 2010.

39. Lewin S, Glenton C, Oxman AD. Use of qualitative methods alongside randomised controlled trials of complex healthcare interventions: methodological study. BMJ. 2009;339:b3496.

40. Kok G, Gottlieb NH, Peters GY, et al. A taxonomy of behaviour change methods: an intervention mapping approach. Health Psychol Rev. 2015; 10(3):1–16.

41. Miller WR, Rollnick S. Ten things that motivational interviewing is not. Behav Cogn Psychother. 2009;37(2):129–40.

42. Rollnick S, Butler CC, Kinnersley P, Gregory J, Mash B. Motivational interviewing. BMJ. 2010;340:c1900.

43. Blackwood B. Methodological issues in evaluating complex healthcare interventions. J Adv Nurs. 2006;54(5):612–22.

44. Coolbrandt A, Wildiers H, Aertgeerts B, et al. A Nursing Intervention for Reducing Symptom Burden during Chemotherapy. Oncol Nurs Forum. 2018; 45(1):115–28.

45. Beaver K, Witham G. Information needs of the informal carers of women treated for breast cancer. Eur J Oncol Nurs. 2007;11(1):16–25.

46. Ellis J, Wagland R, Tishelman C, et al. Considerations in developing and delivering a nonpharmacological intervention for symptom management in lung cancer: the views of patients and informal caregivers. J Pain Symptom Manage. 2012;44(6):831–42.

47. Luckett T, Davidson PM, Green A, Boyle F, Stubbs J, Lovell M. Assessment and management of adult cancer pain: a systematic review and synthesis of recent qualitative studies aimed at developing insights for managing barriers and optimizing facilitators within a comprehensive framework of patient care. J Pain Symptom Manage. 2013;46(2):229–53.

48. Ream E, Pedersen VH, Oakley C, Richardson A, Taylor C, Verity R. Informal carers' experiences and needs when supporting patients through chemotherapy: a mixed method study. Eur J Cancer Care (Engl). 2013;22(6):797–806.

Permissions

All chapters in this book were first published in NURSING, by BioMed Central; hereby published with permission under the Creative Commons Attribution License or equivalent. Every chapter published in this book has been scrutinized by our experts. Their significance has been extensively debated. The topics covered herein carry significant findings which will fuel the growth of the discipline. They may even be implemented as practical applications or may be referred to as a beginning point for another development.

The contributors of this book come from diverse backgrounds, making this book a truly international effort. This book will bring forth new frontiers with its revolutionizing research information and detailed analysis of the nascent developments around the world.

We would like to thank all the contributing authors for lending their expertise to make the book truly unique. They have played a crucial role in the development of this book. Without their invaluable contributions this book wouldn't have been possible. They have made vital efforts to compile up to date information on the varied aspects of this subject to make this book a valuable addition to the collection of many professionals and students.

This book was conceptualized with the vision of imparting up-to-date information and advanced data in this field. To ensure the same, a matchless editorial board was set up. Every individual on the board went through rigorous rounds of assessment to prove their worth. After which they invested a large part of their time researching and compiling the most relevant data for our readers.

The editorial board has been involved in producing this book since its inception. They have spent rigorous hours researching and exploring the diverse topics which have resulted in the successful publishing of this book. They have passed on their knowledge of decades through this book. To expedite this challenging task, the publisher supported the team at every step. A small team of assistant editors was also appointed to further simplify the editing procedure and attain best results for the readers.

Apart from the editorial board, the designing team has also invested a significant amount of their time in understanding the subject and creating the most relevant covers. They scrutinized every image to scout for the most suitable representation of the subject and create an appropriate cover for the book.

The publishing team has been an ardent support to the editorial, designing and production team. Their endless efforts to recruit the best for this project, has resulted in the accomplishment of this book. They are a veteran in the field of academics and their pool of knowledge is as vast as their experience in printing. Their expertise and guidance has proved useful at every step. Their uncompromising quality standards have made this book an exceptional effort. Their encouragement from time to time has been an inspiration for everyone.

The publisher and the editorial board hope that this book will prove to be a valuable piece of knowledge for researchers, students, practitioners and scholars across the globe.

List of Contributors

Charles Ampong Adjei
Department of Community Health Nursing, School of Nursing, College of health Sciences, University of Ghana, Accra, Ghana

Collins Sarpong, Priscilla Adumoah Attafuah, Ninon P. Amertil and Yaw Abayie Akosah
Department of Nursing, Valley View University, Adenta, Accra, Ghana

Werku Etafa
Department of Nursing, College of Health Science, Wollega Unversity, Samara, Ethiopia

Zeleke Argaw and Endalew Gemechu
School of Nursing, College of Health Science, Addis Ababa University, Addis Ababa, Ethiopia

Belachew Melese
Department of Statistics, College of Natural and Computational Sciences, Arsi University, Asella, Ethiopia

Carol Bullin
College of Nursing, University of Saskatchewan, Room 4338 E-Wing, Health Sciences Building, 104 Clinic Place, Saskatoon, SK S7N 2Z4, Canada

Amit Arora and Narendar Manohar
School of Science and Health, Western Sydney University, 24.2.97 Campbelltown Campus, Locked Bag 1797, Penrith, NSW 2751, Australia

Amit Arora, Shilpi Ajwani and Sameer Bhole
Sydney Dental Hospital and Oral Health Services, Sydney Local Health District, Surry Hills, NSW, Australia

Amit Arora
Discipline of Paediatrics and Child Health, Sydney Medical School, Westmead, NSW, Australia

Amit Arora
Collaboration for Oral Health Outcomes Research, Translation, and Evaluation (COHORTE) Research Group, Ingham Institute for Applied Medical Research, Liverpool, NSW, Australia

Dina Bedros, Anh Phong David Hua, Steven Yu Hsiang You, Shilpi Ajwani and Sameer Bhole
Faculty of Dentistry, The University of Sydney, Surry Hills, NSW, Australia

Victoria Blight
Child and Family Health Nursing, Primary & Community Health, South Western Sydney Local Health District, Narellan, NSW, Australia

John Eastwood
Department of Community Paediatrics, Sydney Local Health District, Croydon Community Health Centre, Croydon, NSW, Australia
Sydney Medical School, The University of Sydney, Sydney, NSW, Australia
School of Women's and Children's Health, UNSW Australia, Kensington, NSW, Australia
School of Medicine, Griffith University, Gold Coast, QLD, Australia

Abebaw Jember, Mignote Hailu and Mohammed Hassen
Department of Medical Nursing, School of Nursing, College of Medicine and Health Sciences, University of Gondar, Gondar, Ethiopia

Anteneh Messele
Unit of Community Health Nursing, School of Nursing, College of Medicine and Health Sciences, University of Gondar, Gondar, Ethiopia

Tesfaye Demeke
Department of Pediatric and Child Health Nursing, School of Nursing, College of Medicine and Health Sciences, University of Gondar, Gondar, Ethiopia

Min Hyun Suk
Department of Nursing, CHA University, 30 Beolmal-lo, Bundang-gu, Seongnam-shi, Gyeongghi-do 13496, South Korea

Won-Oak Oh
College of Nursing, Korea University, 145 Anam-ro, Seongbuk-gu, Seoul 02841, South Korea

YeoJin Im
College of Nursing Science, Kyung Hee University, 26 Kyungheedae-ro, Dongdaemun-gu, Seoul 02447, South Korea

Brigid M. Gillespie
School of Nursing & Midwifery, Griffith University, Gold Coast, QLD, Australia Gold Coast Hospital and Health Service, Gold Coast, QLD, Australia

Brigid M. Gillespie and Emma B. Harbeck
National Centre of Research Excellence in Nursing, Griffith University, Gold Coast, QLD, Australia

Emma B. Harbeck
Menzies Health Institute Queensland, Griffith University, Gold Coast, QLD, Australia

Karin Falk-Brynhildsen, Ulrica Nilsson and Maria Jaensson
Faculty of Medicine and Health, School of Health Sciences, Örebro University, Örebro, Sweden

Sabine Homeyer, Wolfgang Hoffmann and Adina Dreier-Wolfgramm
Institute for Community Medicine, Department Epidemiology of Health Care and Community Health, University Medicine Greifswald, Ellernholzstr. 1-2,17487 Greifswald, Germany

Peter Hingst
Nursing Board, University Medicine Greifswald, Fleischmannstraße 8, 17475 Greifswald, Germany

Roman F. Oppermann
Department Nursing, Health and Administration, University of Applied Science Neubrandenburg, Brodaerstr. 2, 17033 Neubrandenburg, Germany

M. I. Loft, H. Iversen and L. L. Mathiesen
Department of Neurology, Rigshospitalet, Nordre Ringvej 57, 2600 Glostrup, Denmark

M. I. Loft, B. Martinsen and I. Poulsen
Institute of Public Health, Department of Nursing Science, Aarhus University, Aarhus, Denmark

B. A. Esbensen
Copenhagen Centre for Arthritis Research (COPECARE), Centre for Rheumatology and Spine Diseases VRR, Head and Orthopaedics Centre, Rigshospitalet, Glostrup, Denmark

B. A. Esbensen and H. Iversen
Falcuty of Health and Medical Sciences, Department of Clinical Medicine, University of Copenhagen, Copenhagen, Denmark

K. Kirk and L. Pedersen
Partner PAR3(consulting firm), Copenhagen, Denmark

I. Poulsen
Research Unit on Brain Injury Rehabilitation Copenhagen (RuBRIC), Clinic of Neurorehabilitaion, TBI unit Rigshospitalet, Glostrup, Denmark

Jaye Hampson, Cameron Green, Joanne Stewart, Lauren Armitstead, Gemma Degan, Andrea Aubrey and Ravindranath Tiruvoipati
Department of Intensive Care Medicine, Peninsula Health, Frankston Hospital, 2 Hastings road, Frankston, VIC 3199, Australia

Eldho Paul and Ravindranath Tiruvoipati
Department of Epidemiology and Preventive Medicine, School of Public health and Preventive Medicine, Faculty of Medicine, Nursing and Health Sciences, Monash University, Clayton, VIC, Australia

Eldho Paul
Clinical Haematology Department, The Alfred Hospital, Melbourne, Victoria 3181, Australia

Wendy Gifford and Barbara Davies
School of Nursing, Faculty of Health Sciences, University of Ottawa, 451 Smyth Road, Ottawa, ON K1H 8M5, Canada
Nursing Best Practice Research Center, 451 Smyth Road, Ottawa, ON K1H 8M5, Canada

Qing Zhang and Shaolin Chen
School of Nursing, Hunan University of Medicine, 492 Jinxinan Road, Huaihua, Hunan, China

Rihua Xie
Nanhai Hospital, Southern Medical University, 45 ZhenXing Road, Lishui Town, Nanhai District, Foshan 528244, Guangdong, China
OMNI Research Group, Department of Obstetrics, Gynecology and Newborn Care, Faculty of Medicine University of Ottawa, Ottawa, Canada

Shi-Wu Wen
Clinical Epidemiology Program, Ottawa Hospital Research Institute, Ottawa, Canada

Department of Epidemiology and Community Medicine, University of Ottawa, 501 Smyth Ottawa, ON K1H 8L6, Canada

Gillian Harvey
Adelaide Nursing School, The University of Adelaide, Adelaide, Australia
Alliance Manchester Business School, University of Manchester, Manchester, UK

Merete Furnes and Kari Sofie Kvaal
Faculty of Health and Social Services, Inland Norway University of Applied Sciences, Elverum, Norway

Sevald Høye
Faculty of Nursing and Health Sciences, Nord University, Bodø, Norway

Ingegerd Bergbom and Mona Ringdal
Institute of Health and Care Sciences at the Sahlgrenska Academy, University of Gothenburg, Gothenburg, Sweden

Ingegerd Berg bom
Faculty of Caring Science, Work Life and Social Welfare, Borås University, Borås, Sweden

Veronika Karlsson
Department of Health Sciences, University West, Trollhättan, Sweden

Mona Ringdal
Department of Anesthetic and Intensive Care, Kungälvs hospital, Kungälv, Sweden

Navideh Robaee
Student Research Committee of Nursing and Midwifery, International Branch of Shahid Beheshti University of Medical Sciences, Tehran, Iran

Foroozan Atashzadeh-Shoorideh
Department of Nursing Management, School of Nursing and Midwifery, Shahid Beheshti University of Medical Sciences, Vali-Asr Avenue, Cross of Vali-Asr and Hashemi Rafsanjani Highway, Opposite to Rajaee Heart Hospital, Tehran 1996835119, Iran

Tahereh Ashktorab
School of Nursing and Midwifery, Shahid Beheshti University of Medical Sciences, Tehran, Iran

Ahmadreza Baghestani
Department of Biostatistics, School of Allied Medical Sciences, Shahid Beheshti University of Medical Sciences, Tehran, Iran

Maasoumeh Barkhordari-Sharifabad
Department of Nursing, School of Medical Science, Yazd Branch, Islamic Azad University, Yazd, Iran

Kolsoum Deldar
Department of Medical Informatics, Faculty of Medicine, Mashhad University of Medical Sciences, Mashhad, Iran

Razieh Froutan
Department of Medical-Surgical Nursing, School of Nursing and Midwifery, Mashhad University of Medical Sciences, Mashhad, Iran

Abbas Ebadi
Behavioral Sciences Research Center, Faculty of Nursing, Baqiyatallah University of Medical Sciences, Tehran, Iran

Thokozani Bvumbwe
Faculty of Health Sciences, Mzuzu University, P/Bag 201, Luwinga, Mzuzu, Malawi

Ntombifikile Mtshali
School of Nursing, University of KwaZulu Natal, Durban 4041, Republic of South Africa

Katarina Sjögren Forss and Gunilla Borglin
Department of Care Science, Faculty of Health and Society, Malmö University, SE-205 06 Malmö, Sweden

Jane Nilsson
Malmö Town, Borough Administration West, SE-214 66 Malmö, Sweden

Sohila Seifi
Students Research Committee, Kermanshah University of Medical Sciences, Kermanshah, Iran

Alireza Khatony and Alireza Abdi
Nursing department, Nursing and Midwifery School, Kermanshah University of Medical Sciences, Kermanshah, Iran

Gholamreza Moradi
Department of anesthesiology, Medicine School, Kermanshah University of Medical Sciences, Kermanshah, Iran

Farid Najafi
Research Center for Environmental Determinants
of Health (RCEDH), School of Public Health,
Kermanshah University of Medical Sciences,
Kermanshah, Iran

Leanne S. Cowin and Robyn Moroney
School of Nursing & Midwifery, Western Sydney
University, Locked Bag 1797, Penrith Soutah DC,
NSW 2751, Australia

Faith Agbozo
Department of Family and Community Health,
School of Public Health, University of Health and
Allied Sciences, PMG, 31 Ho, Ghana

Faith Agbozo and Albrecht Jahn
Institute of Public Health, University of Heidelberg
Medical Faculty, Heidelberg, Germany

Esi Colecraft
Department of Nutrition and Food Science,
University of Ghana, Legon, Accra, Ghana

Timothy Guetterman
Department of Family Medicine, University of
Michigan Medical School, Ann Arbor, MI, USA

Annemarie Coolbrandt
Department of Oncology Nursing, University
Hospitals Leuven, Herestraat 49, 3000 Leuven,
Belgium.

**Annemarie Coolbrandt , Bernadette   Dierckx de
Casterlé, Theo van Achterberg and Koen Milisen**
Department of Public Health and Primary Care,
Academic Centre for Nursing and Midwifery, KU
Leuven, Leuven, Belgium

Hans Wildiers
Department of General Medical Oncology,
University Hospitals Leuven, Leuven, Belgium

Bert Aertgeerts
Department of Public Health and Primary Care,
Academic Centre for General Practice, KU Leuven,
Leuven, Belgium

Index